Ethnicity, Race, and Health in Multicultural Societies

Foundations for better epidemiology, public health and health care

Raj S Bhopal

CBE, DSc (hon), MD, MBChB, BSc (hons), MPH, FFPH, FRCP(E)
Bruce and John Usher Professor of Public Health, University of Edinburgh
and
Honorary consultant in public health, Lothian Health Board
and
Chairman, Steering group of the
National Resource Centre for Ethnic
Minority Health, Scotland

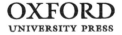

OXFORD
UNIVERSITY PRESS

OXFORD
UNIVERSITY PRESS

Great Clarendon Street, Oxford OX2 6DP

Oxford University Press is a department of the University of Oxford.
It furthers the University's objective of excellence in research, scholarship,
and education by publishing worldwide in

Oxford New York

Auckland Cape Town Dar es Salaam Hong Kong Karachi
Kuala Lumpur Madrid Melbourne Mexico City Nairobi
New Delhi Shanghai Taipei Toronto

With offices in

Argentina Austria Brazil Chile Czech Republic France Greece
Guatemala Hungary Italy Japan Poland Portugal Singapore
South Korea Switzerland Thailand Turkey Ukraine Vietnam

Oxford is a registered trade mark of Oxford University Press
in the UK and in certain other countries

Published in the United States
by Oxford University Press Inc., New York

British Library Cataloguing in Publication Data

Data available

Library of Congress Cataloging-in-Publication Data

Bhopal, Raj S.
Ethnicity, race, and health in multicultural societies : foundations for better epidemiology, public health, and
health care / Raj S. Bhopal.
    p. ; cm.
Includes bibliographical references and index.
ISBN-13: 978–0–19–856817–9   (alk. paper)
ISBN-10: 0–19–856817–7   (alk. paper)
1. Minorities–Health and hygiene. 2. Minorities–Medical care. I. Title. [DNLM: 1. Continental Population
Groups. 2. Ethnic Groups. 3. Epidemiologic Methods. 4. Health Services Accessibility. 5. Health Status.
6. Socioeconomic Factors. WA 300 B5756e 2007]
RA563.M56B56 2007
362.1089–dc22   2006038589

Typeset by SPI Publisher Services, Pondicherry, India
Printed in Great Britain
on acid-free paper by
Biddles Ltd., King's Lynn, Norfolk

ISBN 978–0–19–856817–9

1 3 5 7 9 10 8 6 4 2

Dedication

I dedicate this book to my parents-in-law, Subash and Anjani Mazumdar for raising my loving and beautiful wife Roma; to Roma for her unstinting support; and to my sons Sunil, Víjay, Anand and Rajan for making me such a proud father by their excellent contributions to our multi-ethnic world.

Contents

Foreword

Many years ago, in conversation over dinner with Raj Bhopal, I asked him why he had become academically interested in ethnicity. He replied cryptically: "I heard something...." The conversation was interrupted by the waiter placing our first course (squid cooked in its own ink) in front of us and so I never did learn how it all began.

The relationship between health, healthcare and ethnicity is uniquely complex, ever more so as the issues are explored.

By quoting Australian geneticist, Dr Steve Jones, in his opening chapter, Professor Bhopal focuses the reader's mind:

> The genetic differences between the snail populations of two Pyrenean valleys are much greater that those between Australian Aboriginals and ourselves. If you were a snail, it would make good biological sense to be a racist: but you have to accept that humans are tediously uniform animals.

Yet, until recently, the worth of an individual to wider society was defined largely by their heritage and the colour of their skin: race was a biological construct. 'Science' was used to justify racism and prop up the policies and regimes that relied upon it. Today, race is a social construct and the knowledge gained through biological science now acts to undermine racism.

In *Ethnicity, Race, and Health in Multicultural Societies*, Professor Bhopal explores the dynamic relationship between health and ethnicity (to which 'race' is but one contributor) with insight and skill. He presents a wealth of complex information such that it is palatable, and can be digested and retained with ease.

Nothing about ethnicity and its interplay with healthcare is simple: terminology, classification and how, when and why to collect ethnicity data all present challenges that are practical as much as they are philosophical. Confounders litter the path of researchers, publication bias hinders honesty and favours sensationalism. History casts a long shadow over medicine and ethnicity—grossly unethical syphilis research amongst African-Americans and medical collusion in eugenics at the time of the Third Reich serve as stark, and all too recent, reminders.

Professor Bhopal makes a persuasive case as to why valuing ethnicity is of real importance to health services; he provides readers with a solid grounding in history; and he equips them with a vision for the future and the tools with which to achieve it. He points out that valuing diversity in health services is not just about the services delivered to patients, but also about the positive experiences of healthcare staff. It is my belief that the medical profession and the wider health service still harbours and tolerates racism. This must change.

One of the founding principles of the National Health Service in the United Kingdom was that services should be equitable. This remains the case today, just as it was in 1948.

An equitable service is not one where the model of provision is inflexibly standardised across the country, where one primary care facility or hospital is a carbon copy of another. Just as the health needs of individual patients differ, so too do those of local communities. In an equitable service, variety is permissible, indeed, it is essential, to guarantee fair access to appropriate care.

In order to provide an equitable service, we first need to understand those critical differences. Only then, furnished with that understanding, will we stand any chance of delivering high quality services to fully meet the needs of all our citizens. Achieving this goal is undoubtedly challenging. It demands that we collectively have the intention, the vision and the ideas. It demands also that we exercise skill and determination in transforming those ideas into action.

Ethnicity, Race, and Health in Multicultural Societies will immediately become required reading for those who study ethnicity, health and healthcare. More than that, it will be of genuine interest and value to academics, clinicians, managers, policy makers and the public.

There can be no doubt that this textbook makes a significant academic contribution to the fields of public health and medical sociology. However, *Ethnicity, Race, and Health in Multicultural Societies* is the best sort of textbook: it is one that engages the reader and truly brings the material within it to life. And perhaps one day a biographer will discover in the mists of time what was said to inspire Raj Bhopal on the long and scholarly journey which led to this first class piece of work.

Chief Medical Officer   Sir Liam Donaldson
Department of Health
79 Whitehall
London SW1A 2NS

Preface

> Apart from a few small tribes in the South American rain forest every community on earth experiences influence from practically all others. Culture is an immensely dynamic entity. Cultural hybridisation and intermixture is the order of the day. There no longer exists any pure culture anywhere in the world.
>
> Azuonye (1996: 760)

Most of the industrialized world now comprises multi-ethnic societies i.e. of people from widely varying ancestry, cultures, languages and beliefs. With globalization of trade, increasing international travel and migration the whole world is destined to become multi-ethnic, probably within the next 20 to 30 years. This poses huge challenges for medical and social scientists, doctors, nurses, public health practitioners, health care managers and policy-makers. They have to meet social, ethical, legal and policy obligations to deliver evidence-based health care of equal quality and effectiveness to ethnic minority groups. To achieve this, they need a solid understanding of the underlying concepts of race and ethnicity and how these are applied to achieve robust and meaningful health statistics, workable health policies, effective health care systems, and better health for ethnic minority populations. They also need to have a high level of awareness of how things can go wrong; particularly taking into account the history of racism that permeates many societies to this day. This book lays the foundation for those wishing to acquire this knowledge.

Health care systems in multicultural societies aspire to provide a fair and high quality service to their multi-ethnic populations. For example, the health care system in Britain hinges on the National Health Service (NHS), a respected institution funded largely through taxation, and founded on the principle that it would provide quality comprehensive and equitable health care free at the time of use. Shortly after the foundation of the NHS in 1948, migration to Britain increased. People came to Britain from many countries but particularly the Indian Subcontinent and the West Indies, to work and settle. For most of its history, therefore, the NHS and its staff have had to meet the challenge of caring for recently settled British residents, some of whom were unfamiliar with local customs and how to access services, and for whom there were communication barriers.

Fifty-nine years later the NHS is still striving to develop and implement principles and policies to guide health care for ethnic minorities. Its initial challenges are only partially met, i.e., effective communication, quality of care, and equitable and effective use of services by ethnic minority groups. Issues such as interpreting and advocacy services, availability of educational materials in minority languages, the preferred format for consultation with ethnic minority groups, and agreement on service development priorities remain under discussion and matters for research, rather than ingrained and standard practice. There are gaps between need and provision that national policy initiatives are being designed to fill.

Progress on the development of policies and implementation of best practice has been slow but this is not simply a result of lack of effort or energy, research or even readiness to fund promising initiatives. Arguably, ethnic minority groups have had a share of each of the above. Certainly, the research effort, at least for descriptive studies, has been considerable, and it has been brought to wide attention through the main medical journals. The failure of previous efforts to bring about solid and lasting change in the NHS probably results from a lack of agreement on the answers to basic questions such as how much of a priority is ethnic inequalities in health and health care; which populations are to be targeted and why; how are they to be classified; how are valid data to be collected, interpreted and used to derive priorities, policies and action plans; how are services to be adapted, and how is effectiveness to be demonstrated?

For example, priorities have been deeply influenced by the comparative approach, whereby the problems of ethnic minorities which are more common than in the general population became high priorities, those problems which are less common than in the general population became low priorities. This approach is deeply flawed, for it focuses on differences and ignores similarities. This approach emphasizes the problem of tuberculosis as a problem of ethnic minorities, but not gastrointestinal disease. Betel nut chewing could become a higher priority than smoking, and surma use more so than alcohol. The comparative approach to setting priorities, combined with the ethnocentricity of key decision-makers, is considered as a core issue for this book. A planning approach based on actual, not relative, needs leads to different priorities, such as quality communication, and adaptation of services to ensure equality and equity.

This book starts with the premise that effective action needs to be based on sound understanding of the fundamental concepts of race, ethnicity and culture. It provides a conceptual framework, explores reasons for the incomplete success of past approaches and offers alternatives for the future. The book draws upon the author's work on the health and health care of ethnic minority groups in Britain, and close observations in other countries including the USA, but the principles drawn are generalized internationally.

This book explains the ideas underlying the race and ethnicity. For example ethnicity is not considered merely as an easy way to classify populations and generate data, but also in terms of the ideas and specific facets of humanity underlying the division of the global population into subgroups. The benefits of measurement of race and ethnicity, interpretation of data and application of information are considered alongside the dangers. While the underlying concepts are the same globally, the applications and examples differ very greatly by place and time and for this reason the book places emphasis on a historical and geographically based understanding, with examples spanning 200 years and many countries.

The purpose of this book is to help readers use the concepts of race and ethnicity for population-based research and practice, particularly in the setting of epidemiology, clinical services and public health. Readers are encouraged to consider these concepts in policy-making, health service planning and health promotion. The book emphasizes theory, ideas and principles and hopes to counter the study and use of ethnicity and race in an atheoretical, ahistorical and routine way.

The book will be of interest to science, social science, public health, epidemiology and medical students, and to practitioners and researchers interested in both fundamental ideas and applications. It is designed primarily for the postgraduate student. Undergraduates will find it helpful in deepening their understanding generally, or while studying some topics in a little depth. Health professionals (including busy doctors), who are caring for patients from a diversity of ethnic groups, will find this material an interesting adjunct to their study of clinical subjects. Finally, health service managers and policy-makers may find this book a source of insights that they need to confront the legal, policy and organizational challenges they face.

There are 10 chapters. Many courses are designed around 10–15 or so sessions. I envisage that the core of this book could be grasped in 10 days of committed study, preferably in the context of a taught course, but also independently.

The book is written in plain language but a basic understanding of epidemiology, public health, sociology and biology is needed, as is some familiarity with illness and disease. However, all terminology is explained and defined in a glossary. The learning objectives are expressed in terms of the reader acquiring understanding. I believe that achieving understanding is the highest form of learning—from that may flow a lasting and useable knowledge base, change of attitude and the achievement of skills.

There are exercises embedded in the text to help readers deepen their understanding. Readers are not expected to have the answers but to reflect on the questions as a prelude to effective engagement with the material.

Each chapter starts with a list of contents and educational objectives and ends in a summary, so that the reader can gain an overview of the subject in one hour.

The motivation to write this book came from two directions, one in academia, and the other in public health practice. The value of ethnicity and race research in health settings has been questioned by scholars and practitioners. Guidelines have been prepared on how to raise the quality of such research. Their adoption, however, has been patchy or non-existent. The quality of research, therefore, leaves much to be desired. This book aims to provide a single reference source that integrates the principles underlying the guidelines.

In my duties in the health service I have participated in many discussions on how the service needs to adapt to meet the needs of ethnic minority populations. Even where the goodwill is apparent, policy-makers and practitioners find it hard to act. This is understandable because the foundational understanding is too often absent e.g. the meanings of words such as ethnicity and the setting of priorities. Policy-makers and practitioners are eager to absorb the principles but these are too often contradictory. The need is to provide a sound foundation of knowledge which can be used to resolve contradictions and difficulties.

This book has a simple, intuitive but much-resisted message: priority-setting for minority populations follows exactly the same principles as for majority populations, and usually leads to similar conclusions on health care needs. The differences usually relate to the processes by which the priorities are to be achieved rather than priorities themselves.

If accepted, this simple message forces a completely new approach to the development of policy and the adaptation of practice. It also helps us to understand why so much research, thought and energy expended on health care for ethnic minority groups has led to so little. The message provides a new and firm foundation for research, priority-setting and service development in the future.

The conceptual frameworks of ethnicity and race required by practitioners are slightly different to those required by researchers. The nature of questions, the relative value of the various methods of race/ethnicity classification, and the approach to data analysis, presentation and interpretation differ. This book demonstrates these differences and makes the implications explicit.

This book differs in many ways from alternatives, for example:

- The concepts of ethnicity and race are discussed in detail, and are integrated with principles, applications and methods.
- Principles are emphasized and illustrated with examples drawn from both research and public health practice, including health care policy and planning. The idea is that the reader will acquire the depth of knowledge to use the concepts and not merely be aware of them.
- The book takes an international stance, although rooted in the UK experience.
- There are many exercises which require reflection.

This book shows how the study of health by the race and ethnicity can benefit the whole population, not just minorities, particularly by setting a new and demanding vision based upon the best health status, whatever the ethnic group. It rejects the time-honoured but narrow perspective of setting the majority population as a standard for minorities to aspire to. It asks us to grasp the vast opportunities for knowledge that are in our hands in multicultural, multi-ethnic societies.

Acknowledgements

A book writer performs the task with the help of far too many people to name, and even to remember. My thanks go to the people who helped me but are not specifically listed. Among these are the thousands of people whose papers, books, lectures and conversations have taught and inspired me. I hope you recognize your influence. I have recorded the contributions of co-authors separately.

The idea of writing this kind of book was Liam Donaldson's. He optimistically suggested in the early 1990s that I should be able to draft the book in a couple of weeks! Work started in earnest in 2004 when Helen Liepman of OUP guided my proposal through OUP's demanding peer review and committee stages. I thank her and her successor Georgia Pinteau and other staff at OUP for their unstinting help. I thank the OUPs referees for helpful feedback.

I was privileged in having four excellent readers of drafts. My research assistant Taslin Rahemtulla exemplified my target audience, so her carefully prepared constructive criticism together with the delivery of missing information was invaluable. Sonja Hunt's pointed and honest feedback was of immeasurable value—all writers need critics who are on their side. Aziz Sheikh is one of the busiest (and most productive) people I know so it was an honour when he volunteered precious time to read my drafts. I did not want to ask Gina Netto to read drafts for me even although I thought she was perfect for the task—but she volunteered, and even read some of the manuscript in the early hours. Surprisingly, she did not find it to be a cure for insomnia!

Needless to say, while the people who are acknowledged here may rightly share in any praise that may be due they take no responsibility for my errors, misjudgements or biases.

Normally book writers report that they occupied all the flat surfaces of their homes, forcing their families into a corner. I have behaved this way in the past but this book was prepared in the quiet of my study and my office at the University of Edinburgh. In the modern research-active university medical school books of this kind are seen as a luxury—best left to the years before or after retiral. As I did not do this I record my gratitude to my University, department and colleagues who supported me, uttering not one word of complaint even when there may have been neglect of other duties.

I am grateful for the dedicated and expert assistance of secretaries that worked with me on this book, principally Tori Hastie, Robyn Arsenault and Anne Houghton.

Delivery of a book such as this one has some resemblance to giving birth. It is a job that needs passion, knowledge, drive, partnership, sacrifices, pain, and labour but it ultimately gives a sense of fulfilment. My wife Roma gave birth to my four wonderful children

(Sunil, Vijay, Anand, and Rajan). I could not understand the drives that made her do this (but I supported her and have been the beneficiary). She has no drive for writing but she has supported me unquestioningly. I cannot find the words to thank her, but maybe dinner, flowers and champagne will convey the message, though a Caribbean cruise would be fairer recompense.

Sources and permissions

This book is nourished by the fruits of my own and many other scholars' work.

I have drawn greatly upon my published work, whether as sole author or co-author. Readers who have followed this work will spot this immediately. These older materials have been reviewed, torn apart and revised repeatedly for the purposes of the book. I hope readers will agree that this new context and reworking has added value. Sometimes I have used pre-publication drafts that have been free of the savage cuts usually required by academic journals. The terminology follows my published glossary on ethnicity (JECH), and in my textbook *Concepts of Epidemiology* (2002).

In particular, I acknowledge permission from Joan Mackintosh, Nigel Unwin and Naseer Ahmad, my co-authors of the *Step By Step Guide To Health Needs Assessment* (1998); and from Paramjit Gill, Joe Kai and Sarah Wild, co-authors of the chapter 'Health care needs assessment. Black and minority ethnic groups' (2005). These documents have not only helped me to write Chapter 5 but also many other parts of the book. I have used, with minor modifications, Mark Johnson's framework of thought to structure Chapter 4, but the writing is virtually all new.

Ideas first worked out about 15 years ago with my student Peter Senior, are dominant in Chapter 1. Chapter 2 reflects a fair bit of my thinking to be published in the forthcoming book of a symposium held in Minnesota in 2005 and incorporates some work with Taslin Rahemtulla on census classifications across the world. Chapter 7 reworks chapters and papers on priority setting published by me. Chapter 8 synthesizes a tidal wave of work done in Scotland, led by the Scottish Executive, and I am indebted to numerous people who have allowed me to see, at close quarters, the art of policy-making and implementation. In particular I thank my colleagues Rafik Gardee and Hector McKenzie. This chapter, more than others, is based on an array of existing documents that I have shortened, synthesized and revised to the purposes of the book. The original documents are referenced.

Chapter 9 uses structures and idea developed by me in my 'Black Box' *BMJ* paper, in a sketch of research methods ('Back to Basics'—reprinted in a volume edited by Ahmad) and my book chapter on centrality of context and purpose (in the volume edited by Macbeth and Shetty).

Specific debts are acknowledged in each chapter and the full bibliographic or web site details are given. I have used symbols to denote materials, cited, quoted, extracted or reworked.

This work seldom gives the references relating to the content of the particular sentence or section. There are three reasons for this. First, this is primarily a book about the principles of the subject, not a monograph for advanced scholars and researchers, and it develops the established tradition of the textbook, following the path of my book *Concepts of Epidemiology*. Second, writing with references forces a different style and alters the flow. Third, the chosen style allows me to work faster and accomplish a task that might otherwise have proven outwith my grasp—at least until retirement! Having said this, it would surprise me if the references list did not provide material that supports virtually the entire text. I have chosen a wide range of references not only from the UK and the USA, but also from many other parts of the world. The references span work done over 2000 years—from Hippocrates to 2006. I have chosen work that exemplifies the development of the field. In doing this, I hope I have added value to the Google and Medline searches that readers will no doubt want to do.

I have deliberately and liberally used quotations that interested, inspired or appalled me so readers can hear the voice of others, and not just mine.

I thank most sincerely both those granting me permission to draw upon my own materials and also those who have written the documents that have enriched my knowledge and enhanced this book.

I have cited my sources, being conscious that plagiarism is a hot topic in the academic and popular worlds of publishing. I would not wish to be accused of that. So, if readers find materials and debts that have not been properly acknowledged or referenced please let me know so I can repair matters as soon as possible. I would also greatly appreciate a note of any errors of fact or judgment. The easiest way to contact me is by e-mail: Raj.bhopal@ed.ac.uk.

Chapter 1

Introduction: The concepts of ethnicity and race in health

... medical research is arguably the last respectable bastion of racial ideology in science and one that makes a significant contribution to the contemporary scientific and social norms underlying discrimination

Ellison (1998: 2)

In South Africa, more so than in any other country, we have the widest divergence extant in the occurrence of a variety of diseases in our constituent populations.... If epidemiological information on vital statistics and prevalences of diseases is to become available only for the total population, then, apart from severely stultifying research on disease occurrence and its combating, it will diffuse the identity and magnitude of the very targets who are in most need of help.

Walker (1997: 329)

Chapter contents

- ◆ Chapter objectives
- ◆ Contemporary ways of conceptualizing race and ethnicity
- ◆ Overlaps and distinctions in concepts of race and ethnicity
- ◆ Historical evolution of the race and ethnicity concepts
- ◆ Prediction as to the likely evolution of the two concepts
- ◆ Related concepts—nationality, country of birth, immigration status, culture, ancestry, identity, racism, ethnocentrism
- ◆ Exercises to increase self-awareness of ethnicity and race
- ◆ Defining health, disease, health care, health promotion, health education, public health, clinical care and epidemiology
- ◆ Tracing the evolution of race and ethnicity in the health context
- ◆ Strengths and weaknesses of the race and ethnicity concepts in the health context
- ◆ Conclusions
- ◆ Summary of chapter

Objectives

On completion of this chapter you should be able to:

- Understand both the historical and contemporary basis of the concepts of race and ethnicity
- Understand the overlaps and distinctions between the two concepts
- Define these two concepts in relation to other related concepts such as nationality or country of birth
- Analyse your own background and identity using the concepts of race and ethnicity
- Appreciate the potential problems in using these concepts in health and health care
- Appreciate the potential benefits of these concepts in the health context

1.1 **Introduction**

Despite all their splendid variety, individual humans and human societies are actually most remarkable for similarity, itself a reflection of the unity of our species, as reflected in the quotation from Steve Jones.

> The genetic differences between the snail populations of two Pyrenean valleys are much greater than those between Australian aboriginals and ourselves. If you were a snail it would make good biological sense to be a racist: but you have to accept that humans are tediously uniform animals.
>
> Dr Steve Jones, *The Independent*, 1991 Reith lectures

This similarity goes beyond obvious and physical features such as body shape and posture and applies to emotions, culture and behaviour. Social scientists have defined hundreds of attributes that all human societies studied so far possess. As Pinker (2002) discusses in 1991 Donald Brown published a list of human universals, attributes possessed by all human societies as observed by ethnographers, comprising several hundred items. Among these universals are the following: insulting, leaders, music, play, poetry, the husband older than the wife on average, taxonomy, trade and empathy. The list is being added to. Some of these similarities are extremely surprising, and many of them are relevant to the subject of this book. You may wish to reflect on other potential universals, with particular emphasis on those that might lead humans to place emphasis on differentiating themselves, both as individuals and as groups. Before reading on, reflect on Exercise 1.1.

Exercise 1.1 Human universals and social subgrouping

- If every aspect of human life was a universal would there be any
  - (a) ethnic
  - (b) racial subgrouping?
- Reflect on some characteristics of human societies that you think are universals, that might underpin a human tendency to subgroup populations
- Reflect on some characteristics that are not universals that might promote subgrouping

---

If every aspect of human life was a universal there would be little or no way of differentiating human groups and societies, although individual differences would remain. Differences between individuals would not only be in physique e.g. height, but also in psychology e.g. temperament. Such differences would, however, by the law of averages be distributed evenly between societies, making them indistinguishable.

Several of the human universals, however, indicate both a capacity and emphasis on differentiating people, both individually and as groups, from others. For example, the universals include: classification, ethnocentrism, collective identity, recognition of individuals by face, formation of social structures, judging others, making comparisons, and awareness of self-image, including a concern for what others think. Colour terms, including white and black, are also universals. Golby and colleagues in 2001 did brain function studies and reported that recognition memory was superior for same-race versus other-race faces.

Alongside these universals there are many specific differences between human societies e.g. dress codes, marriage customs, and behaviours in relation to drugs such as alcohol and tobacco. Humans are skilled at distinguishing both obvious (different dress codes) and subtle (nuances in the accent) differences between themselves and others, both as individuals and as members of social groups.

These differences have permitted the subgrouping, or stratification, of human populations. One of the most fundamental questions is whether humans comprise one or more species, and this was a contentious one in Europe, but not necessarily at other times or in other parts of the earth, in the eighteenth and nineteenth centuries. Reflect on Exercise 1.2 before reading on.

Exercise 1.2 Human species

- What is a species?
- Do humans comprise one or more species?
- If one, what are the prospects of evolving into more than one?
- If more than one, what are the prospects of evolving into one?

In biology, a species is a class of animal or plant having certain permanent characteristics which clearly distinguish it from other groups. One of the most important of these characteristics is the capacity to produce fertile offspring from sexual unions in natural circumstances. All human groups meet this characteristic and belong to one species, i.e. *Homo sapiens*. This has now been agreed, and has been reinforced by modern genetics, although the debate is reopened periodically. Having said this, science has not satisfactorily explained why and how different human populations developed different physical characteristics over the last 50–100 thousand years. It is not surprising, perhaps, that in the early days of global exploration there was fierce debate about this fundamental issue—after all, outwardly people in different continents looked very different.

There have been many other human species that have now died out. There is a great deal of evidence that some tens of thousands of years ago three or even more human species coexisted: *Homo sapiens*, *Homo floresiensis* and *Homo neanderthalis*, but the latter two species are now extinct. Since physical or social separation, preventing interbreeding within a species, is a driver for the formation of new species, it seems unlikely that humans will, at least on earth, form separate species.

Similar to humans but very surprisingly, all dogs belong to one species, that of wolves, *Canis lupus*. Within this species, there are clearly differences of varying importance, both physical and temperamental. Nonetheless, humans have found it useful to differentiate different kinds of dogs, and they come with a number of labels such as Alsatian, Labrador, spaniel etc. Using the apparent differences between dogs, biologists and other scientists, breeders, farmers and the general public have tried to define subgroups, or more scientifically, subspecies, of dogs.

Humans have also tried to differentiate different kinds of their own species, but this practice has not been universally useful and the quotation from Richard Cooper exemplifies a powerful view shared by most scientists.

> Use of the category of race in epidemiologic research presupposes scientific validity for a system that divides man into subspecies. Although the significance of race may be clear-cut in many practical situations, an adequate theoretical construct based on biologic principles does not exist.
> Cooper (1984: 715)

There are, clearly, variants of *Homo sapiens*. Human beings place emphasis on differences relating to many factors including sex, age, height, weight, attractiveness, apparent social status, clothing, language, skin colour, facial features and hair type. These are among the characteristics which can be, and have been, used to create social subgroups. These differences are captured in a number of concepts (complex and interrelated ideas), which are in turn simplified as classifications comprising labels that are agreed, usually by powerful people.

Traditionally, differences relating to factors that define culture are clustered under the concept of ethnicity, and those relating to physical features under the concept of race. This is an extreme simplification of two very complex and contentious concepts of great importance to human societies, and this simplification will be subjected to analysis and development.

The division of people in any way, but particularly on the basis of race and ethnicity, raises questions about human values, for the consequences of such divisions have been, and continue to be, great. Neither local nor international ethical codes have prevented the disastrous consequences of racism and racial prejudice. Population growth, travel and rising global communications will require a radical shift in values in relation to ethnicity and race and stronger application of humanitarian ethics in the twenty-first century than in the twentieth. A renewed understanding of the risks and benefits associated with promoting these concepts in the twenty-first century is an essential step.

1.2 **Epidemiology—the author's professional perspective**

This book is about improving health using race and ethnicity in multidisciplinary settings. It is not solely about the epidemiology of race and ethnicity. Nonetheless, I come to race and ethnicity as a medical, public health epidemiologist, and personal and professional perspectives have a major influence on a person's stance. The epidemiological perspective of this book both reflects my interests, and the importance of race and ethnicity within this discipline. Epidemiology is one of the major and growing scientific disciplines underpinning public health and clinical medicine, and guides priorities in health care policy and delivery. Chapters 3, 5, 7, 8 and 9 are particularly influenced by my epidemiological viewpoint, and by my approach to the subject as in my textbook *Concepts of Epidemiology* (2002) (the central strategy is introduced below, and principles and methods are given as required throughout the text). My expectation is that the principles derived from this epidemiological viewpoint are widely applicable, particularly in other quantitative health sciences.

Epidemiology is the study of the patterns of disease and the factors that influence the emergence, propagation and frequency of disease in populations, with particular reference to causal understanding and prevention. Its major strategy, particularly for investigating the causes of disease, is to compare populations with different exposures to potential causes. These are known as exposure variables, in the sense that a change in exposure might alter disease incidence. Usually, the qualifying word exposure is dropped and epidemiologists refer simply to variables. Comparison lies at the heart of scientific reasoning: hypotheses are both generated and tested using the differences found. Similarities give less leverage for understanding causes.

Epidemiological exposure variables are measures which aid the analysis of disease patterns within and between populations, e.g. gender, age, occupation, social class, health behaviours etc. Most variables used in epidemiology indicate underlying phenomena of interest which cannot be measured easily, if at all. For example, social (occupational) class is a proxy indicator of various differences between populations including income, education and styles of consumption. Even apparently simple variables may reflect complex differences, for example, sex may act as a proxy for genetic, hormonal, psychological or social status in different studies. These variables may be used to define the distribution of disease and plan for service provision, or to generate hypotheses about the causes of disease. Such observations do not, in themselves, explain disease processes, and hypotheses generated need to be tested.

1.3 **Ethnicity and race as exposure variables**

Ethnicity and race are potentially valuable exposure variables and are, therefore, used to subdivide populations. Differences by ethnicity and race in both the characteristics of populations and their disease experience have been easy to describe and the scientific literature on ethnicity and health is large and growing. We will discuss the strengths and weaknesses of these variables throughout the book, but particularly in Chapter 9.

Based on these general principles, and the questions in Exercise 1.3, reflect further on the potential value of ethnicity and race in epidemiology before reading on.

Exercise 1.3 The epidemiological exposure variable

- What qualities should the exposure variables of race and ethnicity have to make them worth using in epidemiology?
- How do the purposes and uses of epidemiology help to assess the potential value of the race and ethnicity variables?

According to Senior and Bhopal (1994) a good epidemiological variable should:

- be an important factor in health and disease in individuals and populations
- be measurable accurately
- differentiate populations in their experience of disease or health
- differentiate populations in some underlying characteristic relevant to health e.g. income, childhood circumstance, hormonal status, genetic inheritance, or behaviour relevant to health.
- generate testable hypotheses on the causes of ill-health or disease, and/or
- help in developing health policy, and/or
- help plan and deliver health care and/or
- help prevent and control disease.

These attributes are closely related to the purposes of epidemiology. Ethnicity and race are contested and controversial variables in epidemiology and public health, and yet they are of central and growing interest. The quotations that opened this chapter are from two scholars immersed in the health and health care of South Africa a place where race and population categorization was deeply abused in the era of apartheid—yet they cannot agree whether to abandon or continue with race-based categorization. It is crucial for us to understand the strengths and weaknesses of these variables. Try Exercise 1.4 before reading on.

Exercise 1.4 Ethnicity and race as epidemiological variables

- Do ethnicity and race impact on health?
- Is ethnicity and race easily and accurately measured?
- Are ethnicity and race good at showing population differences in disease experience?
- What underlying differences between people do ethnicity and race reflect?
- How can these differences be used to advance understanding of disease causation, or health policy or health care planning?

There are many dangers of oil as fuel, particularly burning, but we cannot do without it. The fuel of epidemiology, and some other quantitative social and medical sciences, is

Table 1.1 Mortality for stroke given as standardized mortality ratios (95% confidence interval) in Bangladeshi-born men and women living in England and Wales compared to the standard population (England and Wales)

	Standard population	Bangladeshi men	Standard population	Bangladeshi women
SMR for stroke 1981 (ICD 9 430–438)[1]	100	267 (229–319)	100	139 (87–210)
SMR for stroke 1991 (ICD 9 430–438)[2]	100	281 (232–337)	100	151 (95–229)
SMR for stroke 2001 (ICD 10 I60–69)[3]	100	249 (213–292)	100	207 (164–258)

[1] From Balarajan *et al.*
[2] From Gill *et al.*
[3] From Wild *et al.* (unpublished data) (with permission).

the analysis of differences in the pattern of ill health and disease in populations. Ethnicity and race are rich fuels, providing a myriad of differences that are challenging to explain. Directly or indirectly, race and ethnicity have a major impact on populations' health patterns. This book has a selection of examples, including the findings of huge variations in stroke rates, as shown in Table 1.1.

Blood pressure is the single most important known risk factor for stroke. Bangladeshi men, however, have comparatively low blood pressure yet their stroke mortality is very high. This unexpected paradox forces the reappraisal of the causes of stroke, not just in this population but more generally, as discussed by Bhopal and colleagues (2005).

Public health policy is often founded upon such data, particularly where differences are inequitable in the sense of unjust. The central question that analysis by ethnicity or race leads to is this: why is a disease more or less common in one racial or ethnic group of people than in another? For example, why in comparison to the British population as a whole is diabetes so common in people who originate in India but live in Britain, and yet why is colo-rectal cancer relatively uncommon? Answers to these questions would help us to understand better the causes of disease, and would bring benefit to all populations. Epidemiologists are quickly intrigued by ethnicity and health research, and particularly the questions of why disease differences occur. Although differences are easy to describe, the mysteries behind the myriad of ethnic differences are not easily solved. The causes of differences in general will be discussed in Chapter 6, and the research challenges in Chapter 9. Chapters 5 and 8 will focus on appropriate responses to findings of such research.

Unfortunately, among many other difficulties that we will discuss, ethnicity and race are very difficult to assess accurately. Furthermore, there is no consensus on appropriate terms for use in the scientific study of health by ethnicity and race, and published guidelines on how to use these concepts are yet to be widely adopted. In view of the importance of terminology and classification, this matter will be discussed in Chapter 2.

In Table 1.2 race and ethnicity are reviewed in the context of other similar variables in epidemiology, showing why they are of interest, and in brief how one would like to measure them in an ideal world and how one does so in practice.

Table 1.2 Interest in and measurement of some important social variables in epidemiology, including race and ethnicity

Variable	Underlying epidemiological interest	Ideal assessment/measurement	Practical assessment/measurement
Age	Most diseases are strongly influenced by age, presumably through a combination of biological factors and environmental exposures	There is no reliable biological test for age, so the age is a chronological one, and not a biological one. The ideal is for age to be extracted from accurate administrative records e.g. birth certificate	Self-report at interview or self-completed questionnaire. Humans are good at assessing age. In clinical situations where it cannot be ascertained, e.g. the patient is unconscious or there is a language barrier, observer-assessed age is likely to be reasonably accurate.
Sex	The incidence of many diseases varies markedly by sex, presumably resulting from genetic, hormonal, lifestyle and environmental factors	There is a reliable biological test for sex but it is rarely used	Self-reported at interview or self-completed questionnaire; or extracted from administrative records e.g. birth certificate or passport. Humans are good at assessing sex. In clinical situations where it cannot be ascertained, e.g. the patient is unconscious or there is a language barrier, observer-assessed sex is likely to be extremely accurate
Education	Generally, the well-educated have better health than the uneducated	Testing of academic ability in the context of epidemiological studies would be the correct assessment of education, but it is not done	Self-reported data are usually used, usually at the level of—none, primary school, secondary school, further education and university education. Examination of records of educational achievement is unusual
Social class	Individuals belonging to higher social and economic standing in society have, with a few exceptions, better health than those of lower standing	Ideally, social class would be measured by a combination of assessment of social standing and economic worth, including wealth and income	Usually measured by occupation, or location of residence, or educational status, or ownership of a number of durable goods
Race	Individuals belonging to different groups on the basis of physical, biologically determined features can be demonstrated to have different disease patterns	The biological basis of the varying physical features would be measured and used to form human groups	Historical defined racial groupings underlie current classifications and these have been based on assessors' observations, with some modern day consultation with populations so defined.
Ethnicity	Individuals belonging to different groups on the basis of both physical and cultural characteristics have different disease patterns	Both biological and cultural characteristics would be measured and used, singly or in combination, to form human groups	Pragmatic classifications based upon a combination of external assessors' ideas and consultation with the populations to be defined

Table 1.3 Ethnicity as an epidemiological variable

Criteria for a good epidemiological variable	Criteria in relation to ethnicity
Impact on health in individuals and populations	Ethnicity is a powerful influence on health
Accurately measurable	In most populations ethnicity is very difficult to assess
Differentiate populations in their experience of disease or health	Huge differences by ethnicity are seen for many diseases, health problems and for factors which cause health problems
Differentiate populations in some underlying characteristic relevant to health e.g. income, childhood circumstance, hormonal status, genetic inheritance, or behaviour relevant to health.	Differences in disease patterns in different ethnic groups reflect a rich mix of environmental factors and may also reflect population changes in genetic factors, particularly in populations where migration has been high.
Generate testable aetiological hypotheses,and/or help in developing health policy, and/or help plan and deliver health care and/or help prevent and control disease	It is hard to test hypotheses because there are so many underlying differences between populations of different ethnicity Ethnic differences in disease patterns profoundly affect health policy. Ethnic structure of a population is critical to good decision-making. By understanding the ethnic distribution of diseases and risk, preventative and control programmes can be targeted at appropriate ethnic groups.

Table 1.3 summarizes the characteristics of a good exposure variable and analyses ethnicity in relation to these. An analysis for race, or indeed any other variable, would need to follow similar principles.

An emphasis on disease differences, so appropriate to the analysis required in the sciences, is also deeply influential in the health policy and management arena where it is sometimes, but by no means always, inappropriate (as will be discussed in Chapter 5). Since interest in, and the influence of, research on ethnicity and race is increasing it is important that the conceptual basis of the work is sound. As we will discuss throughout this book the concepts are currently mostly inadequately defined and used, and require further development. The starting point is an understanding of one's own and others' perceptions of race and ethnicity.

1.4 Ethnicity and race: self and others' perception of biological and cultural characteristics

1.4.1 Race

By inference, using the biological concept of race, your race is the group you belong to, or you are perceived to belong to, in the light of a limited range of physical factors. This type of race concept is deeply ingrained in human societies, and can be traced back in the roots of history, including in the writings of the great physician Hippocrates some 2,000 years ago, as translated by Chadwick and Mann. Hippocrates contrasted the feebleness of the Asiatic races to the hardiness of the Europeans. His concept of race was of human groups shaped by ancestry in different geographical conditions, especially climate. Race has played a major role in the way societies work and interact and the concept has been abused in the past to justify inequalities e.g. in slavery, colonialism, apartheid, separate education and restriction of medical care.

The still dominant, though deeply contested, idea of race is a biological one. Race in the biological sciences means one of the divisions of mankind as differentiated by physical characteristics. The concept of race was studied intensively by many scientists and scholars, particularly in the disciplines of anthropology and biology, in the nineteenth century with the development of classifications to provide a framework for understanding evolution and examining variation. The aim then was to extend to humans a taxonomic classification below the level of species.

The strategy for developing this classification was based upon observation and formal measurement of physical features. Many physical features were studied, but emphasis was placed upon some obvious ones including skin colour, hair type, eye colour, shape of the head and face, shape of specific features such as nose and lips etc. Indeed, the search for difference was intensive with few aspects of anthropometry (the measurement of the body's form) left unstudied.

Such classifications were not done in a social or political vacuum. Societies were already divided and distinguished on the basis of physical features. For example, this trend was apparent within northern European populations e.g. descriptions of 'criminal features' based on physiognomy which were supposedly beast-like characteristics. There were forces in place to take political or economic advantage of differences that could demonstrate the superiority of northern European populations which, in an era of colonization, was taken by some as a self-evident truth. While physical differences between human populations are quite obvious there was a deeper question underlying this work: were these human populations also different in relation to innate human capacities of overriding importance, including intelligence? If so, this would provide a scientific rationale for the maintenance of contested behaviours e.g. slave owning, control of immigration and colonization. A hierarchy of human races would be used to justify such policies, as reflected in the words of Ashley Montagu:

> It is a fact worth remarking that throughout the nineteenth century hardly more than a handful of scientific voices were raised against the notion of a hierarchy of races. Anthropology, biology, psychology, medicine, and sociology became instruments for the 'proof' of the inferiority of various races as compared with the white race. What H. G. Wells called 'professional barbarity and braggart race-imperialism' played a major role in the rationalization justifying the disenfranchisement and segregation of 'inferior races,' and thus prepared the way for the maintenance of racial thinking and exploitation of 'native' peoples, and the unspeakable atrocities of the nineteenth and twentieth centuries.
>
> Montagu (1997: 80)

Describing human variation by racial group ought, in theory, to help clarify the genetic and environmental basis of disease. Physical characteristics such as face shape and colour that were the primary features used to distinguish races, it turns out, result from a small number of genes and these physical characteristics have little to do with the deeper humans traits around intelligence, behaviours, attitudes, and decision-making processes. In practice, geographical variation in gene frequency is great, and however races are defined, large numbers of populations straddle boundaries. No race possesses a discrete package of genetic characteristics. Genetic diseases are not confined to specific racial groups, although the risk varies by region of ancestral origin. There is a great deal of genetic variation within races (indeed about ten times more than between them). Modern genetics has undermined the traditional scientific race concept by showing that there are no clearly genetically definable subgroups (subspecies) in the human species. At best, differentiation is at the continental level, reflecting ancestry.

In these circumstances, it is not too surprising that the massive effort over 150 years to classify races scientifically has largely failed, though we still use crude classifications which are based on continental groupings and which trace their heritage to Linnaeus, the great biologist who devised a biological classification of all living things. His grouping of humans had four categories. giving us the division of populations as follows: *Homo Afer* (later synonyms, black, African origin, negro, Negroid), *Homo Europaeus* (later synonyms, White, European origin, Caucasian, Caucasoid), *Homo Asiaticus* (later synonyms include Mongoloid, Asian) and *Homo Americanus* (later synonyms include American Indian, North American Indian, Native American). This work was developed by Blumenbach who added a fifth category, and most scholars trace current race classifications to his work. Variants of these classifications have a grouping for Australian aborigines.

Most complex classifications have been forgotten, even although some are very recent, for example the work of Carleton Coon, published in 1953. For example, the previous division of European White populations as Nordic, Alpine, or Mediterranean has become a relic of history. Though none of the numerous racial classifications have stood the test of time, there are echoes of them in current classifications. Since the mapping of the human genome, the controversy about the biological validity of such classifications has been reignited, and the bibliography points to some recent influential papers. As we will see in the next chapter when we examine terminology and classifications, race remains important in modern thinking, though increasingly it reflects geographical, social and class divisions, rather than biological ones.

Before reading on try Exercise 1.5.

Exercise 1.5 Race as a social category

♦ Reflect on whether there is truth to the view that races and ethnic groups are socially constructed, artificial ways of categorizing human beings.

Irrespective of the science, the idea of race as a marker of fundamental biological difference between human subgroups was destroyed by international outrage at the abuses of the concept of race, particularly by the Nazis (see Chapter 6). With the defeat of the Nazis at the end of the Second World War, and the ensuing international debate on the dangers of the race concept, under the leadership of UNESCO it was widely promoted that humans are one species, races are not biologically distinct, there is little variation in genetic composition between geographically separated groups, and the physical characteristics distinguishing races result from a small number of genes which do not relate closely to either behaviours or disease. Nonetheless, many individuals and governments (especially those using the race concept as part of institutions of government such as South Africa and Rhodesia) resisted these ideas – and some resist them even to this day. Ashley Montagu has been the most vociferous twentieth-century opponent of the concept of race, and the following quotation from his landmark publication *Man's Most Dangerous Myth* testifies to the persistence of the concept.

> More than half a century has passed since this book was first published in 1942, and more than a generation has gone by since the fifth edition was published in 1974. In spite of those five new editions, each larger than the one before, the race problem, like a malady that will not go away, seems to have grown more troubling than ever. . . .
>
> I have never before put what is wrong with the idea of 'race' in the form of a formula. Let me do so here. What the formula shows, in simplified form, is what racists, and others who are not necessarily 'conscious' racists, believe to be the three genetically inseparable links which constitute 'race:' The first is the phenotype or physical appearance of the individual, the second is the intelligence of the individual, and the third is the ability of the group to which the individual belongs to achieve a high civilization. Together these three ideas constitute the concept of 'race.' This is the structure of the current conception of 'race' to which most people subscribe. *Nothing could be more unsound, for there is no genetic linkage whatever between these three variables.*
>
> Montagu (1997: 31)

Many scholars, at least in the social sciences, have concluded that race is a social, rather than biological, construction. If so, it follows that racial categories are also socially constructed i.e. created from popular social perceptions and without biological foundation. The fact that so often ethnic categorization has been judged and imposed by observers is of interest in this debate, as will be discussed in the next chapter. It is evident, however, than even this social concept of race is ultimately based on physical and hence biological factors, though these are being de-emphasized by most scholars and researchers. As we have already discussed in relation to Exercise 1.1, if every aspect of human life was a universal, including physical appearance, we would have no biological concept of race.

For reasons which are not clear researchers often find genetic explanations for differences in health by race more attractive than social ones. Conclusions about genetic or biological factors as causes may be wrongly drawn from research showing health differences without proper consideration of factors which may be equally or more likely to be associated with ill-health including poor housing, racism, low income, or poor nutrition. The continued use of race classifications has legitimized them as acceptable descriptive labels for both populations, and individuals. In medicine using such labels as 'Asian', 'black', 'Chinese', etc. is common and seen by some clinicians as important to diagnosis and treatment of disease. The custom of beginning the medical case history with a racial label – this patient is a 43-year-old white/black/Asian—has often been questioned on scientific, medical and ethical grounds but the practice continues. Such labels are also important in social discourse and self identification, as shown by qualitative research by Catherine Campbell and colleagues, which is referred to in Chapter 2.

The biological concept of race is of some use in attempting to explain population variations in a small number of diseases, or other biological traits. Examples of diseases which illustrate this are mainly found in particular population groups, e.g. sickle cell disease in people of African origin (although not all African populations have a high prevalence of this trait, and many other populations evolving in places where malaria occurs have it), or cystic fibrosis in those of European origin (same limitations as for sickle cell trait). Usually, however, apparently racial differences in disease reflect differences in environmental and economic circumstances and not biology. Obviously, studies ought to indicate accurately the relative importance of genetic and environmental factors, but this does not happen because of a combination of conceptual and technical limitations of current research.

In retrospect, the biological concept of races as subspecies was ill-defined, poorly understood and invalid. The science based on it needed sharper criticism. In Chapter 10 I present two models of race. Whatever the underlying concept, race should be used with caution for its history is one of misuse and injustice. Still society has not been able to discard the race concept, and increasingly we see the adoption of the concept of ethnicity mainly as a synonym for race. A clear understanding of the race concept is, therefore, essential to understand the related concept of ethnicity.

1.4.2 Ethnicity

In their 1936 book *We Europeans* Haddon and Huxley recommended that race be replaced by ethnic type, an idea now enjoying much support and some criticism. The word ethnicity comes from the Greek word *ethnos*, meaning a nation, people or tribe. Ethnicity is a multifaceted quality that refers to the group to which people belong, and/or are perceived to belong, as a result of certain shared characteristics, including geographical and ancestral origins, but with particular emphasis on cultural traditions and languages. The characteristics which define ethnicity are not fixed or easily measured, so ethnicity is imprecise and fluid. Ethnicity differs from race, nationality, religion and migrant status, sometimes in subtle ways (see below), but may include facets of these other concepts.

The concept of ethnicity is complex and implies, according to most accounts, one or more of the following:

- Shared origins or social background.
- Shared culture and traditions which are distinctive, maintained between generations, and lead to a sense of identity and group-ness.
- A common language or religious tradition.

It follows that investigators who wish to study ethnicity should collect data on such underlying factors, especially language, religion and family origins, but often they do not. This need for further data will be discussed in Chapter 9.

While group allegiance is dependent on culture it also encompasses physical features, particularly facial features, as in race. In many respects this is reflected in the shared origins component of ethnicity.

The cultural melting pot changes and blurs ethnic distinctions. In multi-ethnic societies ethnic groups may remain distinct, however, while becoming different from the original migrant group that they descended from.

For practical and theoretical reasons, the current preference is self-assessment of ethnicity. (The alternatives include skin colour, birthplace of self or ancestors, ancestry, names, language, geographical origins or a mix of such factors.) Self-assignment poses massive problems, not least that people change their assignment over time, as is their prerogative. In a study following the 1991 British census 12 per cent of 'Blacks' altered their ethnic group, 22 per cent of the 'other' category did so, but only 1 per cent of White and South Asian groups did so. The self assignment changes in the USA are greater still (see Chapter 2).

While race and ethnicity are conceptually different, they are overlapping concepts that are often used synonymously, a trend which is being fostered by the increasing use, particularly in the USA, of the compound word race/ethnicity. This trend is unfortunate, but reflects both the conceptual and practical problems of separating the two concepts, and also the strong traditions of race-based analysis in the USA. In contrast, in Europe where the Nazis' abuses of race are still fresh and perceived as both shameful and dangerous, this word is being abandoned in favour of ethnicity. Whatever terms authors use, the underlying concepts ought to be discussed. In practice, a clear definition of what is meant by the terms ethnicity and race is often lacking making it difficult to compare studies, particularly internationally. This is not wholly surprising as race and ethnicity are complex, multidimensional concepts changing with time and therefore subject to varying interpretations. The study of ethnicity, race and health has, however, been weakened by the diverse and inconsistent use of terms and concepts, as reflected in the quotation from Fatimah and Jackson.

> Far too often ethnicity retains the flavour and tenacity of the old biological race categories, producing the same dismal results in loss of information, diminished insight, and stagnancy. By distinguishing the valid biological dimensions of ethnicity, we place this sociological construct within its proper integrated biocultural context, and we empower researchers to use the term effectively to explore its broad consequences on human health and disease.
>
> Fatimah Jackson (1992: 125)

This theme is developed in more detail in Chapter 2.

1.5 Problems in using the race and ethnicity concepts in epidemiology and other quantitative health sciences

Senior and Bhopal (1994) identified four major categories of problems with the concept of ethnicity in epidemiology, which are equally applicable to race, and in other quantitative health disciplines. These were measurement difficulties, heterogeneity of populations, ethnocentricity and ambiguity about the purpose of using these variables. Other variables used in population sciences may be subject to some of the same problems. However, Senior and Bhopal proposed that ethnicity is unusual because it suffers from the problem of measurement error, together with heterogeneity of the measured populations, and the additional complexity of cross-cultural research. The difficulties of measurement will be discussed in Chapters 2 and 3, and the remaining issues will be introduced here and referred to throughout the text.

1.5.1 The problem of heterogeneous populations

The populations identified by current methods of defining race or ethnicity are often too diverse to provide useful information. For example in the UK these populations include White, Indian and Pakistani, which have massive within-group heterogeneity, diminishing the value of ethnic categorization as a means of delivering culturally appropriate health care, and in understanding the causes of ethnic variations in disease. Even within one Indian-origin Hindu community in Dar es Salaam, substantial variations in socioeconomic and lifestyle characteristics and risk factor and disease prevalences have been demonstrated (Ramaiya, 1991). The term 'Asian' has been very popular in both North America and the UK but it is extremely broad and masks important variations by country of origin, religion, language, diet and other factors relevant to health and disease. Exactly the same criticism applies to categories such as Chinese, Afro-Carribean and African. A study postulating a causal role for diet in the aetiology of coronary artery disease which compared the risks of Indians and non-Indians would give only limited insights since 'Indian' diets are extremely diverse. By contrast, the findings of a study on first generation Punjabi Muslims, compared with another ethnic group of like age and sex, though more limited in its scope would, arguably, be more valuable both scientifically and would have more international generalizability (given that the population was described in detail).

The importance of social class variations within ethnic groups also needs to be considered. Unless research techniques can cope with the extreme heterogeneity of ethnic minority populations misleading conclusions may be drawn. Studies on broad, heterogeneous groups such as Afro-Carribeans, Chinese, African-Americans and South Asians may, however, have value as exploratory or pilot studies; as a first step to deeper understanding.

1.5.2 Ambiguity about the research purpose

There has been a tension between the needs of aetiologic research which relies on detailed information and focuses on measures such as relative risks, i.e the ratio of the rate of disease or death in the study population and in the reference (or comparison) population, and health services research which relies on a broad view and simple data, focusing on absolute risks, i.e actual numbers and rates and not a ratio. These ideas will be discussed in some detail in Chapter 5 and 7.

Research data cannot easily be collected and presented to achieve simultaneously the needs of aetiological enquiry and health care planning. Most researchers on ethnicity and health have emphasized the potential to illuminate aetiology rather than develop health policies and services. Aetiological research emphasizes study of relative excess in different populations, describing disease patterns by relative risk and odds ratios. Simple counts of cases, rankings of disease frequency and disease rates are not central to the aetiological approach. Ethnic group can be a key variable for implementing health policy, e.g. the need to identify, for the purpose of BCG immunization, infants of Indian subcontinent origin (other examples are considered in Chapter 5 and 8). One possible reason for the lack of emphasis on the value of ethnicity and health studies for service development is ethnocentricity, which is discussed below.

1.5.3 The problem of ethnocentricity

Ethnocentricity is the inherent tendency to view one's own culture as the standard against which others are judged. This has implications for all aspects of research on ethnicity and health. It will impinge on the design, aims and methods of studies and the presentation and interpretation of results; making 'value-free' observation impossible. The impact of researchers' values on the presentation and interpretation of results is illustrated in Table 1.4, which contains data originally presented by Marmot and colleagues in 1984.

Standardized mortality ratios (SMRs) are the summary outcome of a statistical method for taking account of differences in the age and sex structure of populations and allowing a comparison of the mortality in the population of interest relative to a standard population. In Table 1.4 SMRs for the Indian subcontinent-born population relative to the population of England and Wales provided the crux of the tables (presenting disease

Table 1.4 Deaths and SMR's* in male immigrants from the Indian subcontinent (aged 20 and over; total deaths = 4,352)

By rank order of SMR				By rank order of number of deaths			
Cause	SMR	No. of deaths	% of total (4,352)	Cause	SMR	No. of deaths	% of total (4,352)
Homicide	341	21	0.5	Ischaemic heart disease	115	1533	35.2
Liver and intrahepatic bile duct neoplasm	338	19	0.4	Cerebrovascular disease	108	438	10.1
Tuberculosis	315	64	1.5	Bronchitis, emphysema and asthma	77	223	5.1
Diabetes millitus	188	55	1.3	Neoplasm of the trachea, bronchus and lung	53	218	5.0
Neoplasm of buccal cavity and pharynx	178	28	0.6	Other non-viral pneumonia	100	214	4.9
Total	—	187	4.3		—	2626	60.3

*Standardized mortality ratios, comparing with the male population of England and Wales, which was by definition 100. Reproduced from Senior P, Bhopal RS. Ethnicity as a variable in epidemiological research. *British Medical Journal.* 1994; 309: 327–330, with permission from the BMJ Publishing Group.

ranking by SMR) and text of the key report by Marmot and colleagues. The left-hand column ranks diseases by their relative frequency based on the SMR, the right-hand column shows diseases among the same men ranked by the number of deaths.

A very different impression of the importance of various diseases amongst Indian men emerges, shifting the emphasis away from the diseases which are common relative to the comparison population, to those which are common independently of any such comparison. The primary perspective of Marmot and colleagues was to compare and contrast the performance of other ethnic groups to that of the majority population. This is the standard approach in ethnicity and health research. Less emphasis has been given to diseases where the standard population had an excess in relation to the minority population and still less to conditions which show no difference. The perspective of Senior and Bhopal was to consider the main problems of the Indian origin ethnic groups, without concern for excesses or deficits, but to find the common health problems confronting these groups. Both perspectives are based on valid research values but they lead to different emphases and interpretations of the same data. Researchers' and data interpreters' values are relevant in the collection and interpretation of data (see Chapter 10).

1.6 **Race ethnicity and social harm**

Race and ethnicity are not harmless concepts and variables, and it is worth reflecting on the potential dangers, as suggested in Exercise 1.6.

Exercise 1.6 Race, social abuses and ethnicity

- List and reflect upon abuses of the concept of race historically and currently
- Reflect upon the role of science in such abuses
- Why do you think scientists and health professionals participated in such abuses?
- In what way might ethnicity give rise to similar abuses?

In the nineteenth century, in particular, differences among races as then defined were usually assumed to be innate and irreversible biological features, interpreted to show superiority of White races and used to justify policies which subordinated non-White groups. In other words, differences underpinned racism, a topic which is discussed in Chapter 6. Briefly, racism results from the belief that some races are superior to others, which is used to devise and justify actions which create inequality among racial groups. It is self-evident that it requires power to implement such policies. In the absence of power it is difficult to put prejudices into action. Emphasis on differences is also a prequisite for racism. Disraeli, a British Prime Minister is famously associated with the quotation inextricably linking difference, superiority and dominance in the 19th century (p 150).

Research focusing on problems more common in minority groups, combined with data presentation techniques designed to highlight differences in comparison to the majority population, so easily portrays the minorities as weaker. When research implies genetic factors rather than environmental ones as the cause of racial differences in health, racial minorities may be perceived as biologically weaker.

As I have summarized in a British Medical Journal article in 1997(b), ideas that are developed in chapter 9, science that implied such weakness helped justify policies in favour of slavery, social inequality, eugenics, immigration control, and racist practice of medicine. Race-specific 'diseases' such as drapetomania (irrational and pathological desire of slaves to run away) were invented. John Down's theory of 'mongolism' (Trisomy 21 or Down syndrome) was that such infants were births from an inferior, Mongoloid, race. He interpreted this as indicating the unity of human races, as indicated in the quotations below

> A very large number of congenital idiots are typical Mongols.... The face is flat and broad, and destitute of prominence. The cheeks are roundish, and extended laterally. The eyes are obliquely placed, and the internal canthi more than normally distant from one another....
>
> The boy's aspect is such, that is difficult to realize that he is the child of Europeans; but so frequently are these characters presented, that there can be no doubt that these ethnic features are the result of degeneration....
>
> These examples of the result of degeneracy among the mankind appear to me to furnish some argument in favour of the unity of the human species.
>
> Down (1867 (reprinted 1995): 55–6)

The Tuskegee Syphilis study in Alabama lead by the USA Public Health Service from 1932 to 1972 deceived and bribed 600 black subjects into cooperating with research which examined the progression of syphilis without treatment, even once penicillin (a cure) was available. In May 1997 President Clinton apologized on behalf of the USA to the survivors of this experiment.

> The people who ran the study at Tuskegee diminished the stature of man by abandoning the most basic ethical precepts. They forgot their pledge to heal and repair. They had the power to heal the survivors and all the others and they did not. Today, all we can do is apologize. But you have the power, for only you—Mr. Shaw, the others who are here, the family members who are with us in Tuskegee—only you have the power to forgive. Your presence here shows us that you have chosen a better path than your government did so long ago. You have not withheld the power to forgive. I hope today and tomorrow every American will remember your lesson and live by it.
>
> Clinton (1997)

Tuskegee was not a unique racist research project. Osborne and Feit concluded that much American health research on race and ethnicity contributes to the idea that some human groups are inferior (1992). As Gladys Reynolds (1993) wrote 'We the scientific community...bring everything we have been taught by our culture—our xenophobia, our homophobia, our racism, our sexism, our "classism" our tendency to "otherise".'

The division of people on the basis of race and ethnicity raises important questions about human values, for the consequences of such divisions have been great. Studies of ethnic and racial variations in disease pose a challenge to the maintenance of high ethical standards in health research, themes I discuss in Chapters 8–10. The concepts of race and ethnicity are commonly applied to the study of the health of immigrant and ethnic minority groups in the hope of advancing causal understanding of disease. Contemporary race, ethnicity and health research is, however, mostly 'black box' research (see Chapter 9) concentrating on so-called ethnic health issues, and generating a multiplicity of interesting hypotheses. The idea of a package of specific racial or ethnic diseases that deserve special attention and research has unfortunate echoes in history. 'Negro' susceptibility to particular diseases, such as leprosy, tetanus, pneumonia, scurvy, and sore eyes was of great interest, and the differences were explained by hypotheses on causation centred around innate biological differences. These hypotheses were nonsensical as discussed by Kiple and King (1981).

Racial prejudice is fuelled by research portraying ethnic minorities as different, and differences being interpreted as showing their inferiority. Infectious diseases, population growth and culture are common foci for publicity. Following the release of statistics on the ethnicity of single mothers the *Sunday Express*, a popular UK newspaper, ran the headline *'The ethnic time bomb'* (13 August 1996). Toni Morrison wrote in her book *Beloved 'A whip of fear broke through the heart chambers as soon as you saw a Negro's face in a paper '* (for this signalled singularly bad news). Researchers cannot be responsible for media reporting, but epidemiologists must be aware of the attractions of their work to the media and of the potential impact of their work on race relations.

Race and ethnicity are variables that show, dramatically and unequivocally, the importance of historical, political and social awareness among health researchers. Although the term is rarely used, ethnicism, the idea that some ethnic groups are superior to others, is as much a danger as racism.

Table 1.5 identifies a few of the potential benefits and problems of ethnicity and race as concepts in the health sciences.

The greatest psychological barrier is in separating out the modest effects of biology, usually seen as central to the race and ethnicity concepts, from the huge effects of environment. Differences due to the environment are sometimes perceived as transitory and therefore unimportant, indeed possibly even unrelated to race or ethnicity, while biological differences are quite wrongly seen as, effectively, permanent and fundamental to race and ethnicity. This perception of permanence may lead to undue prominence. From another perspective, factors that can be controlled and changed should be given more prominence. Reflect on Exercise 1.7.

Exercise 1.7 The impact of similar environments on ethnicity and race

- Imagine, for any broadly defined ethnic group e.g. Indian, American Indian, African Caribbean, that following birth everything in the environment, defined as every non-genetic influence, was held constant.
- Would the health/disease outcomes be the same for all ethnic groups?
- Outcomes you may wish to consider include diabetes, lung cancer, coronary heart disease and schizophrenia.

Table 1.5 Potential problems and benefits of ethnicity and race in health sciences

Issue	Potential problems	Potential benefits
Credibility	Gives a powerful backing to scientifically difficult concepts that have been abused previously	Utilizing concepts in health sciences will lead to their development and improvement
Division of society	Reducing social cohesion, by an emphasis on differences	Helps heal existing social divisions by acknowledging and working on differences, as well as demonstrating similarities
Racism	Provides information that can be abused by those who wish to demonstrate superiority of particular groups	Information can combat past injustices, and guide future actions to prevent such racism
Ethnocentricity	Sets a standard usually based on the majority population that may be inappropriate for a particular ethnic group	By demonstrating that in some respects ethnic minority populations have better health, more challenging standards can be set for the population, including the majority
Emphasis on problems	Stigmatizing and stereotyping minority populations	By showing the heterogeneity within any minority population, and that in some respects health is better, this research can counteract existing stigmas and stereotypes
Scientific advances	As in the past, science might be led into unsound territory, and unethical practices	If the potential of studying race and ethnicity can be realized, important advances in population health could be achieved
Development of health services	Either as a result of faulty information or interpretation health services may veer away from true needs	With the appropriate data services might adapt to meet needs better
Individual clinical care	Clinicians might be misled by generalities, stereotypes and misleading research and scholarship	Armed with an understanding of ethnicity and race clinical care might become more effective

Even in identical environments health is going to vary between groups, although much less so than under normal circumstances, where there are huge differences in the environment. The result will differ by disease. Obviously, genetic factors are relevant though mostly modest. Non-genetic factors can also be transmitted across generations. Diabetes is a disorder where the interaction between genetic and environmental factors is particularly strong. It is also influenced by the fetal environment. Given identical environments, substantial ethnic variations will remain though these will decline over generations. Lung cancer is largely an environmentally acquired disease so given identical environments, especially identical smoking patterns, we would anticipate very little ethnic variation. This is also so for coronary heart disease (CHD), where the genetic influence is relatively small and diffuse. The causes of schizophrenia are poorly understood and the answer to my questions is unclear. While schizophrenia may well have a strong biological, indeed genetic, component, there will be an essential interaction with the environment. Given equivalent environments, ethnic variations in schizophrenia are likely to reduce very greatly.

1.7 Race and ethnicity in relation to ancestry, nationality, country of birth and religion

Before reading on you may wish to reflect on Exercise 1.8.

Exercise 1.8 Ethnicity and race in relation to nationality, religion and similar variables

Where are the overlaps and the similarities between ethnicity and race and:

+ ancestry
+ parental country of birth
+ country of birth
+ migration status
+ nationality
+ citizenship
+ religion
+ language?

Race and ethnicity are both closely related to ancestry. Race relates to ancestry for both biological reasons and the fact that the social concept of race emphasizes lineage, because it impacts on both identity and cultural and political heritage. These are retained across many generations. The characteristics traditionally underlying racial groups, e.g. skin colour, are largely inherited through the ancestral line. Where ancestry is mixed the relation between race and ancestry becomes complex, and undermines the concepts of race and ethnicity, as proclaimed in the quotation.

> Mixed race threatens the idea of racial difference. It also threatens ethnic boundaries and this seems to matter when groups wish to espouse and protect their uniqueness (for various reasons). All that is claimed for race—that it is a means of dividing and ranking humankind; that it is 'natural' to keep to 'one's own'; that the consequences of mixing race are dire—is disproved by the very existence of mixed race. Race is not the only difference that mixed race challenges. Differences in custom and religion, geographical and class differences can all be shown to have been mixed without adverse effect.
>
> Olumide (2002: 180)

Many of the factors underlying ethnicity are also inherited, although not biologically e.g. religion, taboos on behaviours, dietary preferences etc. Such factors are changeable yet tend to linger through generations. Factors that maintain identification with a particular group include physical features, so biology also contributes to ethnic identity.

Country of birth is closely related to race and ethnicity only when international migration is uncommon. This is no longer the case in many countries, particularly the richer ones and those where there is political strife at the borders creating large numbers of migrating refugees. Country of parental, or grandparental, birth may provide important additional information to add to self-reported ethnicity or race but these data are not a substitute. It may be, for example, that a person who is born in India, and whose parents and grandparents were all born there, is not ethnically Indian, and perceives their ethnicity as, say, Chinese or English. This situation is one outcome of colonization and globalization.

Ethnicity should not be confused with nationality or with migrant status. For example, immigrants from the Indian subcontinent may be British nationals but members of a particular ethnic group, say Sikh Punjabis. Their children, born in the United Kingdom, are members of their parents' ethnic group, but may perceive themselves part of a larger ethnic group such as Indians, Asians or Blacks. They may also perceive themselves to have an additional ethnic identity relating to the host community e.g. British, Scottish or Irish. This is particularly likely when people have the right of residence in the country. This additional qualification may help people to signal their citizenship and allegiance. While ethnicity, race, country of birth, nationality and citizenship are conceptually distinct, some countries place obstacles to (or make easier) acquisition of nationality and citizenship based on race or ethnicity. This is an abuse of the concepts of race and ethnicity.

Religion is of no consequence or relevance to the biological concept of race. It is, however, often a vital aspect of ethnicity, providing a strong sense of cultural and social identity, and governing important aspects of lifestyle and even language. Language is similar to religion in being of little importance to biological concepts of race, but is often vital to ethnicity. Table 1.6 shows the association between some characteristics of humans and the concept of race and ethnicity.

1.8 Analyse your own background and identity using the concepts of race and ethnicity

A good way for readers to reflect on ethnicity and race, particularly to contrast them and the related concepts discussed in Section 1.7, is to mull over the self-descriptions of ethnicity given by the author and close colleagues in the step-by-step guide by Mackintosh and colleagues (1998), and do this for themselves. Labelling of racial or ethnic groups can sometimes utilize terms relating to religion and language, not least because there is a link between territory, ancestry, race, ethnicity, religion and language. (The following are lightly edited extracts from Mackintosh and colleagues, 1998.)

RSB on ethnicity

I am of Indian birth, raised in Scotland, and enjoy the benefits of two cultures. I think others see me as an Indian, Pakistani or an Asian. I am a member of the Sikh religion by birth. My first language is Punjabi, in the sense that this was the language I learned first, but I am much more fluent in English. When in England I perceive myself as a British Indian, when in Scotland as a Scottish Indian, when

Table 1.6 Relationship between some attributes of humans and ethnicity and race

Relating mainly to concept of race	Relating mainly to concept of ethnicity	Sometimes related to ethnicity or race
Skin colour	Ancestry	Nationality
Other physical features such as hair texture and facial features	Language	Citizenship
Ancestral origin	Religion Diet Family origin Sense of group identity	Name Migration history Country of birth

at my parental home as a Punjabi Sikh, and when in India as a Punjabi. My behaviour, such as food eating and alcohol consumption, is context-dependent. I may wear a turban or traditional Indian dress on symbolic occasions such as weddings. The census classification of Indian does not do justice to my self-image, but when forced to choose I am happy to pick the ethnic group category Indian.

RSB on race

I do not know what race people think I belong to. They probably think I am Indian, although that is not a racial category. I am Indian born, to Indian parents. I have brown skin and black eyes and hair (sadly greying fast!). If forced to fit into the long-established racial categories I'd choose Caucasian (but not White) which I know will cause surprise because that word has been so closely linked to European or White. On the whole I believe I do not fit easily into a racial category. For sure, my race is *not* Asian. Others may see me as Asian. If I lived in the USA I would be classified as a member of the Asian race. That seems very odd.

Joan Mackintosh on race and ethnicity

I am British-born and I am classified by the census definition as 'White'. I am of Scottish ancestry (as far back as I know and before that almost certainly a mix of various others, e.g. Celt, Norman and who knows what else) and consider myself to be British, though when in Scotland I am seen as English and when in England I am seen as being from the north east. My first language is English. I was brought up to respect the traditions of the Christian church both at home and at school. I was baptized in a Methodist chapel and was married in a Presbyterian church. I do not consider myself particularly religious. I attend church on ceremonial occasions and my children are members of church youth groups. If asked to describe myself, I would say 'British' and if asked to define my religion from within certain recognized groups, will either tick the box 'Christian' or if further definition is required 'Church of England' because it is easier than describing 'other'. I am certainly aware that a person's social class has an enormous bearing on the type of health care they will receive—particularly in terms of patient-practitioner interaction—which is why I believe class and ethnicity are inextricably linked. Prior to starting this work I had never really given much consideration to the issue of ethnicity and self-defined ethnicity in particular (which probably speaks volumes). I found this quite a difficult exercise to undertake.

Nigel Unwin on race and ethnicity

This is very difficult. My ethnicity—depends very much on the context. Within a British context I am north of England, lower middle to middle class background, brought up within the traditions of the church of England (although I wouldn't describe myself as a Christian). You'll notice from the above that I think at least for me and probably for many people, class and 'ethnicity' are inseparable in some contexts.

Within a broader context, such as Europe or elsewhere in the world, I like to see myself as 'British'. This is a pretty vague notion, but for me hints at the diversity of cultures (over many centuries up to the present) in Britain and the creative public face of Britain, linked together with threads of common underlying values such as a tolerance, or at best a celebration, of diversity alongside an instinct for social justice. I don't like describing myself as 'English' because to me this smacks of the opposite of what I've described as 'British': of establishment, stuffiness, conservatism and colonial history and I don't see my background as being from that. However, I know that in certain contexts, particularly for example in North America, or in some parts of Ireland, being labelled as 'English' is something I can't escape. Accent and body language, if nothing else, all attract this label and the connotations that go with it.

In some contexts I think of myself as 'north European'. This is also a very vague notion, but like the sense of 'British' is based on a sense of common threads of culture and values in north European societies.

I haven't really seen myself in terms of race. Interestingly this is one of the criticisms sometimes levelled at white people—that they see themselves as 'raceless', race being an attribute of others (non-white people). If pushed I would say I'm of European ancestry (but probably for all I know a mixture of Celtic, Anglo Saxon, Roman, Norman and maybe other 'tribes' or 'peoples') and clearly within the context of a racist society, where people are prejudged on the basis of skin colour and appearance, I am 'White'. Certainly when travelling in Africa or the Caribbean I'm aware of often being seen as being of a different race i.e. 'White' or 'European' and I'm often referred to in those terms.

Naseer Ahmad on race and ethnicity

I do not see myself as British, or Pakistani, as I am not fully accepted by both. I'm too different to be Pakistani and too different to be British i.e. I don't speak the language and don't look the part, in both cultures.

So, after a long time of growing up (being called 'paki' and 'coconut' and being beaten up for being Muslim, all leave scars) and the 'culture clash' which many people my age are facing leads some to go to extremes i.e. deny their origin and see themselves as white through and through, or the other extreme where they love their origin and hate Britain. I do not ascribe to either of these views as extremism is not in my nature.

In short, I describe myself as Muslim. That's it. I go further and describe myself as a Muslim living in Britain as opposed to a 'British Muslim', as I am not sure what British Muslim means and after speaking to those who describe themselves as British Muslim know that they also do not know what British Muslim means. The reason for this is that the idea of artificial borders separating people i.e. those created by man, and then labelling those different based on these borders is just wrong, and dangerous. Rwanda and Bosnia show the dangers of labelling. It can be argued that separating based on religion i.e. Muslim-Kafir, Jew-Gentile etc are the same thing but in the end, I feel there is a deep-rooted need with man (and woman) to belong to something, and belonging to a thing that traverses colour, country and background and categorizing based on the actual person i.e. their thoughts, feelings, is somehow more just and more right, especially when it is emphasized that the 'others' have rights which must be respected e.g. right to justice and practising their religion.

However, if I had to choose, and have to be pushed to do this, I am a 'Pakistani' as this is my origin, but it has to be realized that I do not see myself as Pakistani. I am British by passport and if anything Britain is my home (I don't feel that any other country is my home, even the 'Muslim' countries, as my family is in Britain) but I do not see myself as British, especially not English (for the same reasons that NU describes) however, British has the same connotation for me i.e. British colonial rule etc.

The only label I feel comfortable with is Muslim. This is after a long, long time of being uncomfortable with myself. But, if I had to describe myself as anything, in Britain I am a Pakistani, and in Pakistan I am British. For statistics purposes, I am Pakistani, but it must be realized that I am uncomfortable with being described as British or Pakistani as I am neither!!

Ethnicity and race are such complex ideas (as the vignettes of the four authors of the *Step-by-Step Guide to Health Needs Assessment* show) that they ought to raise questions about the reliability of making assumptions that a person may (or may not) possess a particular behaviour or health characteristic on the grounds that they are a member of a particular ethnic or racial group. The limited usefulness of recording a patient's ethnic origin, using a simple label such as Indian, White, or Chinese, without taking account of other factors, has to be fully acknowledged. The vignettes show the importance of religion. Religions straddle ethnic and racial groups. As for Muslims (see vignette by Naseer Ahmad), the Jewish people originate from many countries and cultures and have a range of religious practices but may identify themselves as Jewish. Thus, on a Census which had a category Jewish, some would choose it over Black, Indian, White etc. In addition to the complexity which is shown in the vignettes, within every ethnic group there are significant variations in social class, culture and customs.

Now, reader, it is your turn to describe your race, ethnicity, and the related characteristics shown in Exercise 1.9.

Exercise 1.9 Self-analysis

- Analyse your own perceived
  - (a)   racial and
  - (b)   ethnic group
- How would your close associates, and perhaps new acquaintances, see your race and ethnicity? Would their own race or ethnicity influence their perceptions?
- How do your race and ethnicity, in your mind, link to your nationality, country of birth and religion?

1.9 The potential benefits of the race and ethnicity concepts in the health context

Studying ethnic and racial variations in health can, at least potentially, help to understand disease aetiology, tackle inequalities, assess need, make better health plans and direct resource allocation. The use of ethnic groups and race as variables in the health literature is increasing in recognition of this potential. The focus of race and ethnicity tends to be on those populations with comparatively adverse health outcomes. Clearly, it is not only non-White ethnic groups which are in this position.

To improve health policy-making and health planning, give new insights into the causation of disease and help the clinician in the differential diagnosis of disease Senior and Bhopal recommended in 1994 that:

1. Ethnicity is perceived as different from race and is not used as a synonym for the latter biologically discredited term.
2. The complex and fluid nature of ethnicity is more widely understood.
3. The limitations of all current means for classifying ethnicity be widely acknowledged, and the approach to ethnic categorization be made explicit in all reports. Definitions of ethnicity may need to be devised to suit the needs of the particular research project.
4. Investigators recognize the potential influence of their values, including ethnocentricity, on scientific research and policy-making.
5. The importance of socio-economic differences in explaining health differences between ethnic groups is considered at the same time and with at least equal weight as cultural or genetic factors.
6. Research on methods for ethnic classification is given higher priority.
7. As ethnicity is a fluid, dynamic phenomenon and research findings may rapidly become out of date, results should not be generalized across time periods, generations and populations with different migration histories, except with great caution.
8. Data from studies of ethnicity and health should, as a high priority, be analysed and applied to produce information of value in health care policy and service development.
9. Demonstrations of interesting disease variations should be followed by detailed examination of the relationship between environment, lifestyle, culture and genes to assess the relative importance of these influences.

Bhopal added several other recommendations in 1997(b) including:

◆ Researchers, policy-makers and professionals in the field of race, ethnicity and health should understand the ignoble history of race science, and be aware of the perils of its return.
◆ In the absence of consensus on the nature of ethnicity and race, researchers need to state their understanding, describe the characteristics of both the study and comparison populations, and provide and justify the ethnic coding.
◆ Editors must play a greater role in developing with researchers and then implementing a policy on the conduct and reporting of race, ethnicity and health research.
◆ There should be wide recognition that race and ethnicity data, as for social class, have a key role in raising awareness of inequalities and stimulating policy and action.

Throughout this book we will be returning to these and other guidelines.

1.10 **Conclusions**

Humans are mentally equipped to differentiate between individuals and groups. Race and ethnicity are only two of many ways that humans differentiate and group themselves and these are deep and lasting concepts. Scientific disciplines have studied these concepts and attempted to utilize them to advance scientific understanding and help in the applications of science. The sheer complexity of the concepts has made this task difficult, and the misapplication of race and ethnicity has often done more harm than good. Nonetheless, race and ethnicity are both excellent means of differentiating the health and health care status of subpopulations, and this property alone has given them central status in quantitative health sciences, and indirectly public health and clinical care. The challenge now facing us is to ensure the benefits of working with race and ethnicity far exceed the harms, and that our experience does not end in the same ignominious fate that met nineteenth-century research.

Purpose and context are the prime determinants of the way that race and ethnicity concepts are applied, classifications are devised and employed, and data are analysed and presented. Henceforth, we will consider the limitations and strengths of the concepts of race and ethnicity in relation to purpose and context. Ethnic and racial labels, as in national censuses, are no more than a first step to defining a person's ethnicity, and the remaining steps depend upon the purposes of data collection. Whatever the purpose, understanding the terminology we are using, and its origins, is vital to collecting the data. This is the subject of the next chapter. Some readers might find the historical and international background to the subject given in Chapter 4 useful preparation for reading Chapter 2.

> In describing racial/ethnic groups, authors should use terminology that is not stigmatizing, does not reflect unscientific classification systems, and does not imply that race/ethnicity is an inherent, immutable attribute of an individual.
>
> Kaplan and Bennett (2003: 2713)

Summary

Humans comprise one species, and their similarities globally are remarkable. Nonetheless, humans also have, and place considerable emphasis on, their differences both between individuals and between human groups.

Race and ethnicity are complex, intertwining, powerful and lasting concepts that are used by individuals and societies to identify and evaluate social groups and individuals. Traditionally, race was a concept focused around subgrouping humans based upon biological factors such as skin colour, facial shape and hair type. Your race, based on this concept, is the group you belong to, or are perceived to belong to, in the light of such factors. Racial classifications based on biology have proven of modest scientific value and questionable validity, and have been open to abuse socially e.g. the Nazi final solution. This concept of race is changing to incorporate social factors, and a shared history, and hence it is converging with ethnicity.

Ethnicity is a concept that, in principle, uses cultural and social factors such as language, diet and religion to subgroup humans. Your ethnicity, based on this concept, is the group you belong to, or are perceived to belong to, in the light of such factors. Ethnic classifications, in practice, do not tend to be founded on such cultural factors and usually include concepts such as ancestry that are akin to race. Ethnicity is the concept in vogue, particularly in Europe, partly due to the abuse of the race concept politically in both the nineteenth and twentieth centuries. In practice, race and ethnicity are often used synonymously, with the compound word race/ethnicity becoming more common. Both concepts are clearly separate from nationality (the nation you have chosen to belong to usually as identified by citizenship and/or passport) and country of birth. Both race and ethnicity are relevant to racism, the product of the view that some racial or ethnic groups are superior to others. Race and ethnicity are important components of identity in circumstances where people of different racial and ethnic groups mix. Reflecting on both one's own and others' perceptions of one's ethnic and racial group provides a route to understanding the strengths and weaknesses of the concepts.

Race and ethnicity are important in health and health care, particularly in demonstrating inequalities. The analysis of such inequalities can lead to insights into the forces causing them and hence point to the actions required to counter them. Such insights can add to scientific knowledge or stimulate new research.

Population health research, statistical analysis and clinical work, ideally, requires easy means of assessing, measuring and classifying variables but ethnicity and race are very complex. While race and ethnicity may be of value in clinical care, they can also lead to stereotyping, stigma and racism. The potential value of ethnicity and race in modern multi-ethnic societies will be achieved only if understanding and application of these concepts is advanced such that their advantages exceed their weaknesses. The first step towards this goal is the analysis of the terminology underlying these concepts and the classifications arising from it (the topic of Chapter 2).

Chapter 2

Terminology and classifications for ethnic and racial groups

If the term 'race' is used in scientific journals, such as the AJHB, then its use must be very clearly justified on the basis of human social or political affairs. I urge you as the Editor-in-Chief of the AJHB to treat this issue with the same care as you would issues of fraud or plagiarism. There is too much at stake regarding the reputation of the journal and the Human Biology Association.

Bogin (1998: 278)

Chapter contents

- The challenges of studying racial and ethnic differences without creating stigma or inequity
- Devising population groups using the concepts of race and ethnicity—historical and contemporary examples
- Analysing the facets of race and ethnicity that population groupings are based on
- The development of population groupings into comprehensive classifications of race and ethnicity, past and present
- The challenge of changing terminology in the development and application of classifications of ethnicity and race
- Trends in terminology and classification—examples internationally
- Conclusions
- Summary of chapter

Objectives

On completion of this chapter you should be able to:

- Understand that the concepts of race and ethnicity can be used to create population groups
- Understand that population groups created are, usually, utilizing one or a few aspects of the many that underpin ethnicity and race
- Appreciate that the set of population groups comprises a classification of race or ethnicity or both
- See how such classifications permit the use of race and ethnicity as epidemiological, public health and clinical variables

- Understand that numerous classifications have been created but none have stood the test of time
- Compare and contrast classifications of race and ethnicity with others such as sex, age, social class and education
- Understand the difficulty of creating acceptable, precise and lasting terminology to support such classifications
- Appreciate the underlying ideas, strengths and weaknesses of some current classifications in Europe, North America, South America and Africa
- Balance the dangers of creating stigma and further inequity against the potential benefits of operationalizing the concepts of race and ethnicity through classifications

2.1 Introduction: turning the concept of ethnicity and race into classifications

Concepts are by definition complex ideas. Obviously, before they can be used they need to be defined in words that explain, simplify and clarify the underlying complexities and allow the concept to be communicated easily. In this process the original, or underlying, meaning of the concepts may be altered, albeit in subtle ways. In particular, the interpretation of the concept may vary between time periods, places, disciplines and individuals. For example, in the modern era, many social and most public health scientists interpret race as a social or political concept, but most lay people and biomedical scientists see it as a biological one. In the past, say 150 years ago, the biological basis of race and its use to create a hierarchy would rarely have been questioned, except by the brave, as indicated in the quotation by Ashley Montagu (see p 10 for the context of this quotation).

> ... hardly more than a handful of scientific voices were raised against the notion of a hierarchy of races. Anthropology, biology, psychology, medicine, and sociology became instruments for the 'proof' of the inferiority of various races as compared with the white race.
>
> Montagu (1997: 80)

The historical position on race as a biological concept is echoed in most contemporary dictionaries and encyclopaedias, although change is underway.

To use the concepts of race and ethnicity, whether in research or practice, we need to create population groupings. In health and health care we need a terminology that not only describes the individual but also gives access, by association, to helpful information relating to the population from which the individual comes. For example, in medicine an ethnic or racial label is only of value if it helps in diagnosis, management or prediction of prognosis of the illness under investigation. To describe a patient as White is unlikely to be helpful, but to specify that a person is White of Greek origins may be relevant, whether in terms of practical matters such as language, or dietary advice, or the likelihood of haemoglobin disorders.

This process of moving from concept to classification is pragmatic, although it should be developed upon both scientific and logical grounds in so far as this is possible, and with a clear understanding of the purposes of the classification. There is a great deal of subjectivity in this process, with difficult choices needing to be made. The classification process will usually utilize only one or a few of the many facets of such complex concepts as race and ethnicity. For example, should the classification emphasize ancestry, language, religion or skin colour? The choice of emphasis will determine the classification arising. It is obvious that such classifications are constructed—but in this regard, race and ethnicity are by no means unique. Indeed, I cannot name any classification of any variable which is not. Even classification as male or female (sex) is social construction, and in that regard is reflected in the word gender.

Each group in the classification needs to have a name (or label) that is, ideally, both meaningful and acceptable, both to those creating and using the classification and those who are so classified. In the past, very often those being classified had little say, as their race or ethnicity was assigned by the observer, usually the census enumerator or a professional gathering administrative data. Alternatively, the assessment would be done on other data e.g. country of both. Presently, and increasingly, self-classification holds primacy. Nonetheless, the results of the classifications need to be, on the face of it, both valid and valuable, both to those being categorized, and those examining and using the data. Achieving this ideal is extremely difficult. The value of the classification achieved, as opposed to the many alternatives, should be judged by whether it serves the purpose(s). As the purposes may be multiple, and changing, even this is not a simple matter. Some of these points are developed in Exercise 2.1, which you should do before reading on.

2.2 Reflection on the word Asian and similar labels

Exercise 2.1 Reflection on the word Asian as used in countries such as the UK and the USA
- What do you understand by the word Asian as a label for a population group?
- To which general and scientific purposes might the word Asian be put?
- How might people described as Asians react?
- Why might they be annoyed or content with this label?
- How might the meaning of this label be differently interpreted in different countries?
- What are the disadvantages of such labelling in a scientific context such as epidemiology?
- What can researchers do to overcome such disadvantages?

The concepts of race and ethnicity are widely utilized in society for many purposes including politics, everyday and intellectual discourse, education, research, service delivery and entertainment. Each domain of activity may lead to a variety of labels to describe racial or ethnic subgroups. It is general knowledge that the word Asian means a person from the Asian continent, the largest continent on the earth that extends from

Turkey to Siberia. We would expect a schoolchild to know that. It is rare, however, for this word to be used in this way. Rather, the term has been commandeered as an ethnic label, with a much more limited meaning. In the UK the label is usually applied to people of Indian subcontinental origins, who mostly came from India and Pakistan, with smaller numbers from Bangladesh and Sri Lanka. (Asian has a very different meaning in North America—see below.) As a Punjabi-born Indian raised in Scotland I found the widespread use in the UK of the label Asian, particularly in the media, to describe people like me to be uninformed, simplistic and irritating.

The term Asian appeals to the media, possibly because it encapsulates a large and heterogeneous population within one easily understood word, which may sit well with the perceptions of the majority White European community. Some people of Indian, Pakistani and Bangladeshi origins find this label quite acceptable, and describe themselves as Asian. This is particularly, but not exclusively, so amongst younger people. The label must have meaning and value to the population so described, and this may be political, in the sense that it signals a unity in an otherwise highly diverse population. Context is clearly important in relation to self-identification. Some ethnic minorities who would not perceive themselves in this way in everyday life might be agreeable to the label 'Black' as a political statement of solidarity but not necessarily reflecting self-image or identity. Some qualitative research sheds light on the importance of such labels to communities, as indicated in the quotation from Campbell.

> Yet recent interviews we conducted with people who described themselves as African-Caribbean, Pakistani and White English suggested that beyond the world of academia, the discourse of ordinary people is replete with essentialist descriptions of their own and other ethnic groups. In this paper we examine such stereotypical representations. We will argue that they are very real in their effects—in so far as they play a key role in influencing the likelihood that people will participate in local community networks in the multi-ethnic communities which are increasingly a feature of multicultural Britain.
>
> Campbell and McLean (2002)

In 1984 I did my first research on ethnicity and health. I learned that the label Asian was embedded in the scientific literature too. It appeared that in the UK Asian was an ethnic category restricted by common usage to people whose ancestral origins lay in the Indian subcontinent but who were living in the United Kingdom. Clearly, this was the world of research reflecting a wider societal decision, almost certainly fostered by the White European origin majority population. The origins of this term are certainly not scientific. There were warnings even in the 1980s about the invalidity of such labels, including material published in the influential *British Medical Journal* by Shaunak *et al.* (1986).

By contrast, the term preferred by population science researchers for the same large population, South Asian, is rarely used in political and everyday discourse or by the people described by this phrase. The word Asian illustrates in a contemporary way how societies create racial and ethnic labels to suit social purposes, and how researchers might utilize such categories, thus apparently adding to their value. Which aspects of race and ethnicity does this Asian label refer to that might interest researchers? The precise components/facets underlying the label are seldom specified. We can infer, however, that in the UK setting it indefinitely includes ancestral origin on the Indian subcontinent (relating to race), and probably includes a characteristic brown skin and dark hair of varying hue (relating to race), a liking for a spicy cuisine, familiarity with a number of South Asian languages, and affiliation with Sikhism, Hinduism, or Islam (all relating to ethnicity). The amount of information is limited and most of it is probabilistic, and not certain. A simple label based on complex concepts of race and ethnicity serves the purpose of allowing self and other's identification, albeit in a partial, crude and somewhat unscientific way.

Just as in the UK the word Asian is commonly used to describe a circumscribed population, so it is in the USA, where Asian mainly refers to Chinese and Japanese and excludes, at least in practice, those from the Indian subcontinent. The inferences that would be reached from the label alone would be different there than in the UK. The phrase Indian Asian is common in the USA, thus differentiating from American (native) Indians. In the UK the phrase Asian and Chinese is heard and seen, which distorts geography, but meets the need for ethnic labels. There are obvious problems for doing useful research using such labels that will be lasting, amenable to future interpretation and be generalizable beyond the location of the study.

In my early publications in the late 1980s I took the step of defining my use of Asian in terms such as these 'For the purposes of this study, Asian refers to persons whose ancestry is from the Indian subcontinent.' I also tried italicizing the word Asian and putting it in quotations to alert the reader to the limited and specialized use of the word. In retrospect even these steps were insufficient. I followed general conventions used in the UK and, whenever appropriate, the terminology used by the original authors, and provided a statement on my use of terms. In recent work, I provided an explanatory paragraph usually as an appendix, which some editors demoted to a footnote or merged with methods. A typical paragraph is this one:

A note on terminology relating to ethnicity

There is no consensus on appropriate terms for the scientific study of health by ethnicity, and published guidelines are yet to be widely adopted. We have followed general conventions used in the UK and, whenever appropriate, the terminology used by the original authors. For example, in the UK the term ethnic minority group usually refers to minority populations of non-European origin and characterized by their non-white status. (We use it this way here.) The term South Asian refers to populations originating from the Indian subcontinent, effectively, India, Pakistan, Bangladesh and Sri Lanka. White is the term currently used to describe people with European ancestral origins. By ethnicity we mean the group a person belongs to as a result of a mix of cultural factors including language, diet, religion, and ancestry.

Popular terminology used to describe ethnic minority populations (Asians, Blacks, Chinese etc.) may suffice for everyday conversation or political exchange but is too crude for scientific studies on the frequency and causes of diseases. The continuing use in the

UK of the term 'Asian', to mean people from the Indian subcontinent but not Japanese, Mongolians and Siberians, is unacceptable unless there is widespread, explicit agreement on such usage and when terms are carefully defined. Otherwise the dialogue becomes parochial. Loose terminology encourages inventions such as the description of an ethnic group as 'Urdus' as has been done and published in respectable journals. It also leads to phrases such as 'Asians and Chinese' being used incorrectly, both from a geographical sense, and from the point of view of population sciences.

Similar arguments have been made in relation to other terms including White, Black and Hispanic as reflected in the following quotation.

> I argue that any standardized terminology is unavoidably flawed and conducive to the development of racist or, at best, trivial stereotypical analysis of the data thus produced. This 'Hispanic' label does not identify an ethnic group or a minority group, but a heterogeneous population whose characteristics and behaviour cannot be understood without necessarily falling into stereotyping. The label should be abandoned; social scientists and policy makers should instead, acknowledge the existence of six aggregates, qualitatively different in their socioeconomic stratification, needs and form of integration in the US economy: two minority groups (people of Mexican and Puerto Rican descent), and four immigrant populations (Cubans, Central American refugees, Central American immigrants, and South American immigrants).
>
> Gimenez (1989: 557)

The analysis of terminology in this chapter is designed to give readers a thorough grounding in principles and past practice, so they can join in the quest for better terminology and classifications.

2.3 Facets of ethnicity and race in classifications

It is easy to forget that categories are merely labels, and no more than a first step to understanding and defining a person's ethnicity or race. Labels such as White, Asian, Latino, Afro-Caribbean and Black need to be recognized as inaccurate and yet crude shorthand for potentially important information about a person's ethnicity. The ideal label would reflect important aspects of ethnicity or race. In the interests of simplicity labels usually reflect one aspect e.g. colour, the country or region of origin, or language, but the need for simplicity should be weighed against the dangers of stereotyping and inaccuracy. Authors should be describing the characteristics of the populations they are referring to. The label 'South Asian' should not, for instance, be used if the population referred to is a Bangladeshi one. Bangladeshis are very different from the many other South Asian populations. For example, Bangladeshi men have an extremely high prevalence of smoking, while some other South Asian groups of men (particularly Sikhs, but also Hindus) have a low prevalence, a vitally important fact lost by studies of smoking in 'South Asians' combined, and one that has led to misguided policies on smoking (see Table 3.1).

Most classifications put emphasis upon describing ethnic and racial minority populations, mainly because of the perception that they require special attention. This perception is usually, but not always, correct. A number of descriptions have been given to these groups, i.e. 'ethnic minorities', 'ethnic minority groups' or 'minority ethnic groups'. Sometimes, the phrase ethnic groups is used, wrongly implying that only minority populations have an ethnicity. Similar phrases are seen in association with the word racial.

The concepts of race and ethnicity are commonly put into operation in national censuses. Rather than developing their own classifications, modern-day researchers have mostly used such administrative categories for race and ethnicity, even when these are acknowledged by those developing them as having no scientific or anthropological validity (as is the case for the USA classification discussed below). I do not advocate a return to the eighteenth and nineteenth century approach when scientists developed apparently scientific classifications. This unsatisfactory state of affairs needs to be remedied by scientists becoming more deeply involved in the development of categories for the censuses and other major surveys, and not merely being end-users. Scientists should remember that their use of existing classifications of race or ethnicity can be interpreted as an endorsement of their validity. As a minimum, researchers should make clear their understanding of the concepts of race or ethnicity and the classification as they use them (e.g. one or a mix of ancestry, geographical origin, birthplace, language, religion, migration history, name, self-identity, observation etc). These tasks are difficult, and readers should grapple with this matter directly, by tackling Exercise 2.2 prior to considering the discussions of census classifications below. You may find the analysis of terms in contemporary ethnicity, race and health writings that is summarized in Table 2.1 of value in your work, and in the ensuing discussion.

Exercise 2.2 Creating and analysing a classification of ethnicity

- ◆ What principles would guide you in drafting an ethnic classification to meet the needs of population health research in your region?
- ◆ List labels that would describe the population groups.
- ◆ Compare your classification with those in the tables, and with that actually used in your nation (you may need to find it).
- ◆ In what respect are these classifications, including your own, based upon race, and, alternatively, upon ethnicity?
- ◆ What do you perceive to be the strengths and weaknesses of these classifications?

2.4 From concept, to category, to classification

Classifications vary between times and places, reflecting the social and political circumstances, the pragmatic nature of the processes of their development and the varying purposes for which they were designed. Many classifications of race and ethnicity, of varying complexity, have been created over the last 200 years or so. In regard to race, only those relating to broad continental groupings e.g. African, European etc., continue to hold influence. (In Chapter 9 I will consider current views on the genetic validity of

Table 2.1 An analysis of some of the terms currently in use in ethnicity and race research

Term	Dictionary-derived meaning	Usual meaning in ethnicity and health research	Relationship to race or ethnicity	Strengths	Weaknesses	Comment and recommendation
Afro-/African-Caribbean	No specific definition, but Caribbean relates to the territory comprising some West Indian islands	A person of African ancestral origins whose family settled in the Caribbean before emigrating and who self-identifies, or is identified, as African-/Afro-Caribbean	See African	The label differentiates Africans coming from two distinct places i.e. the continent of Africa and the West Indies	There is very considerable heterogeneity in the populations	Specification in more detail will be required e.g. the island of origin, and the migration history
African	A person belonging to, or characteristic of a native or inhabitant of, Africa	A person with African ancestral origins who self-identifies, or is identified, as African, but excluding those of other ancestry e.g. European and South Asian.	This population approximates to the racial group known as Negroid or similar terms (see Black)	This term is the currently preferred description for more specific categories, as in African-American, for example	In practice, Northern Africans from Algeria, Morocco and such countries are excluded from this category. (See also Black.)	Specification in more detail will be required e.g. the country of origin, and the migration history
Asian	A native of Asia i.e. anyone originating from the Asian continent.	In practice, this term is used in the UK to mean people with ancestry in the Indian subcontinent. In the USA, the term has broader meaning, but is mostly used to denote people of far Eastern origins e.g Chinese, Japanese and Philipinos.	The racial term Malayan, coined by Blumenbach, is forgotten as purposeless, but approximates to this label	It appeals to the general public and the media, possibly because of its capacity to simplify complexity	Asians comprise more than 40% of the world's population, with tremendous cultural and substantial biological diversity	More specific terms should be used whenever possible

Asian Indian	Belonging to or relating to India; native to India	In North America the term is being used synonymously with South Asian with the qualification Asian for differentiating from the original inhabitants of America or the West Indies	The term defines a broad ethnic group. There is no clear-cut equivalent in terms of racial classifications, though historically Northern Indians have been classified as Caucasian, and some Indian tribes as aboriginal.	This term is being used in North America to distinguish the population from Native Americans, previously known as American Indians	A term currently used synonymously with South Asian (see below), but with the important limitation that major South Asian populations such as Pakistani and Bangladeshi may not identify with it	Users need to state which South Asian populations are included and excluded
Bangladeshi	A person whose ancestry lies in the Indian subcontinent who self-identifies, or is identified, as Bangladeshi. (See also South Asian.)	As per dictionary meaning	Defines an ethnic group relating to a nation. There is no clear-cut equivalent in terms of racial classifications, though historically Northern Indians have been classified as Caucasian, and some Indian tribes as aboriginal.	Between 1947 and 1971 the land known as Bangladesh was East Pakistan and before that India. The term approximates to territory.	The recent political and geographical changes mean that identity with the country may be ill-defined	The term works reasonably well
Black	A person with African ancestral origins, who self-identifies, or is identified, as Black, African or Afro-Caribbean (see African and Afro-Caribbean)	People whose origins lie in sub-Saharan Africa e.g. excluding northern Africans, and settlers. In some circumstances the word Black signifies all non-White minority populations, and in this usage serves political purposes.	This use relates to race	The word is capitalized to signify its specific use in this way	The cultural, social, and genetic diversity captured by this term is vast	While this term was widely supported in the late twentieth century, there are signs that such support is diminishing

Table 2.1 (*Continued*)

Term	Dictionary-derived meaning	Usual meaning in ethnicity and health research	Relationship to race or ethnicity	Strengths	Weaknesses	Comment and recommendation
Caucasian	An Indo-European. Blumenbach's term (1800) for the White race of mankind which he derived from the Caucasus	Synonym for White	While often used in the context of ethnicity, it relates to race	Some relation to genetic composition. Defines populations by geographical origin in the distant past	Heterogeneous. Not geographically linked now. Not related to ethnicity	Means originating in the Caucasus region and refers to Indo-Europeans. Widely misunderstood. Widely used as synonym for 'White'. Abandon
Chinese	Of or pertaining to China. A native of China	A person with ancestral origins in China, who self-identifies, or is identified as Chinese	Usually used as an indicator of ethnic group. In terms of historical racial classifications, Chinese approximate to the group known as Mongolian or Mongoloid	Widespread appreciation of the grouping referred to	Massive heterogeneity	Combined with a description of the population under study, and possibly a qualification indicating population subgroup, this label seems to work
Ethnic minority group	Based upon the word ethnic, which has a number of meanings including pertaining to nations not Christian or Jewish	Usually, but not always, this phrase is used to refer to a non-White population. Alternatively, it may be used to describe a specific identifiable group e.g. gypsy travellers, and less commonly, Irish in the UK	Although relating to ethnicity, it is often used synonymously with race	Widespread use. Used with surprisingly little misunderstanding and easy to say	Some people consider the phrase inaccurate and prefer minority ethnic group, but the two phrases are used synonymously	Over time, this phrase is likely to be replaced with minority ethnic group

Term	Definition	Usage		Disadvantages	Comment
European	A native of Europe	It is usually used as a prefix to the term White e.g. White of European origin	Usually used in the context of ethnicity	Signifies geographical origin. Purports to describe a culture (though some would dispute its validity)	Describes heterogeneous populations. Ancestral origin may be difficult to ascertain	Comparable, in breadth, to terms such as Chinese, South Asian. Useful for international studies comparing large areas
Europid	Not defined but denotes origins in Europe	Rarely used, but it is a synonym for European origin	As above	Clear geographical status. New term; no past associations	Describes heterogeneous populations. Ancestral origin may be difficult to ascertain	Unfamiliar term. Comparable, in breadth, to terms such as Chinese, South Asian. Useful for international studies comparing large areas
General population	Not defined but epidemiological meaning is everyone in population being studied	Usually refers to a predominantly White population that is a comparison	Relevant to ethnicity and health studies	Makes no assumptions about racial/ethnic origin. Truly a whole population	Inaccurate unless it is a truly representative population	Excellent term for representative population samples
Hindu	An alien of northern India; of, pertaining to, or characteristic of the Hindus or the religion; Indian	An old, now seldom used term, for Indians. Rarely used, but in some countries such as Holland the term is used to describe the ethnicity of Surinamese of Indian subcontinent ancestry	Refers to ethnicity	None, other than the fact that some Surinamese identify with this term	The word describes a religion	Avoid

Table 2.1 (*Continued*)

Term	Dictionary-derived meaning	Usual meaning in ethnicity and health research	Relationship to race or ethnicity	Strengths	Weaknesses	Comment and recommendation
Hispanic	Pertaining to Spain or its people	A person of Latin American descent (with some degree of Spanish or Portuguese ancestral origins), who self-identifies, or is identified, as Hispanic irrespective of other racial or ethnic considerations	In the United States this term, often used interchangeably with Latino, is considered an indicator of ethnic origin	Widely accepted and used. Links heterogeneous populations	Massive heterogeneity	Needs a rigorous reappraisal, particularly with the intent of adding in detail
Indian	Belonging to or relating to India; native to India, with the qualification Asian in differentiating from the original inhabitants of America or the West Indies	A person whose ancestry lies in the Indian subcontinent who identifies, or is identified, as Indian (see South Asian)	Ethnicity	Widely accepted term that links heterogeneous populations	Major changes to India's geographical boundaries took place in 1947 when Pakistan was created. Massive heterogeneity	Qualify and describe the groups under study

Term					
Indigenous	Native or belonging naturally to a place. Pertaining to natives, aborigines	Various, but usually referring to the inhabitants prior to colonization	Unclear	Links to land and birthplace	Imprecise. Conflates concepts of place of birth, residence and ancestry	Some in the non-minority groups are not indigenous; some in the minority groups are. Abandon
Irish	The inhabitants of Ireland, or their descendants, especially those of Celtic countries	A person whose ancestry lies in Ireland who self-identifies as Irish but generally restricted to the White population (see, White).	Ethnicity	Meaning is self evident	As Ireland becomes a multi-ethnic society, the term will lose its specificity	The term works reasonably well
Other race or ethnic group	Self-evident	Groups not already included within the categories offered	Both	This term makes the classification inclusive in that either people excluded, or those who perceive themselves to be excluded, can offer a free text response	Another category seen in racial classifications is 'other', this permitting those not included to identify themselves, or be identified by the observer	While it is important to develop classifications that minimize the use of this phrase, it is likely to remain a vital component of any classification

Table 2.1 (Continued)

Term	Dictionary-derived meaning	Usual meaning in ethnicity and health research	Relationship to race or ethnicity	Strengths	Weaknesses	Comment and recommendation
Mixed race or ethnic group	The offspring of a couple from different races or ethnic groups	The term is relatively infrequently discussed, but its meaning is as per the dictionary one	Relevant to both	The increasing acceptance of sexual unions that cross ethnic and racial boundaries is adding both richness and complexity to most societies	The way to categorize mixed race people is unclear. Current approaches are inadequate, partly because the number of potential categories is huge	The increasing importance of the category mixed (ethnicity or race) is self-evident. One solution is to offer space for free-text responses for individuals to identify themselves. These responses, however, need to be coded, analysed, summarized, quantified and published. Without this, individually small but collectively large populations remain hidden when policy on ethnic diversity is made.

Native	One born in a place. One belonging to a non-European and imperfectly civilized or savage race	There are two usual meanings. First, the term may be used to define minority groups that originally populated the land e.g. native Americans, or to differentiate the (usually) White population from recent migrants e.g. native Dutch	The term relates to ethnicity and migration status rather than race	Links to land and birthplace	Historical connotations of being non-European. Conflates concepts of place of birth, residence and ancestry	Similar to, and used synonymously with, indigenous. Abandon except in historical treatises
Non-Asian/Non-Chinese etc.	Not defined but implies those not belonging to the group under study	The meaning is self evident	The term may fit either race or ethnicity	Logically correct	Extremely broad and imprecise	Avoid if possible
Occidental	A native or inhabitant of the Occident (West)	Rarely used, but usually a synonym for White or European	Either race or ethnicity	Geographically based	Heterogeneous. Unrelated to ethnicity	Means belonging to the West (Occident is where the sun sets). Abandon
Oriental	A term meaning a native or inhabitant of the Orient (East).	Most usually used to indicate far Eastern populations e.g. Chinese, Japanese	Either race or ethnicity	Geographically based	Heterogeneous, and unnecessary as better terms are available	This term is in occasional use in epidemiology, usually referring to Far Eastern populations. It is too general to be useful

Table 2.1 (*Continued*)

Term	Dictionary-derived meaning	Usual meaning in ethnicity and health research	Relationship to race or ethnicity	Strengths	Weaknesses	Comment and recommendation
Pakistani	A person whose ancestry lies in the Indian subcontinent who identifies, or is identified, as Pakistani (see South Asian).	This is usually used as a term of identity even for those born before the creation of Pakistan in 1947	It is a term of nationhood and ethnicity, and not race	Some Pakistanis may have birth or ancestral roots in the current territory of India but identify with Pakistan, a country created in 1947	Hitherto, the considerable heterogeneity within the Pakistani population has been largely overlooked, but it should not be	Users should be aware that this term is sometimes used as a form of abuse in the UK, usually in the abbreviated form 'Paki'. This said this is the correct term for populations who perceive themselves as Pakistani
Reference/ control/ comparison	The standard against which a population that is being studied can be compared. In science, a standard of comparison used to check inferences deduced from an experiment, by application of the 'method of difference'. To place together so as to note the similarities and differences of.	In practice, the terms are infrequently used, and usually denote a White, European origin population	Either depending on context	Neutral terms. Recognize purpose of the non-minority group in the research. Forces writer to describe population and clarify terminology of study or review	The nature of the reference/control population is not-self-evident. Could be misunderstood to mean closer matching than is actually carried out	Prefer these terms

South Asian	A person whose ancestry is in the countries of the Indian sub-continent, including India, Pakistan, Bangladesh and Sri Lanka	In practice, often used to describe populations from anywhere on the Indian sub-continent, and equally frequently confined to India, Pakistan and Bangladesh	Refers to ethnicity and nationhood	In terms of racial classifications, most people in this group probably fit best into Caucasian or Caucasoid but this is confusing and is not recommended	This is a good label, particularly when the population is truly from a mix of South Asian regions, when it should be qualified by a clear description	This label is usually assigned, for individuals rarely identify with it. (See also Indian, Indian Asian, Asian, Pakistani, Bangladeshi)
Western	Of or pertaining to the Western or European countries or races, as distinguished from the Eastern or Oriental	Rarely used, but when it is it is a synonym for White or European	Refers to geography, ethnicity and sometimes race	Refers to a culture and places	Not geographically specific. Describes heterogeneous populations	Abandon
White	Applied to those races of men (chiefly European or of European extraction) characterized by light complexion	The most commonly used term in ethnicity and health research	Ethnicity and race (as a synonym for Caucasian)	Used in census. Socially recognized and historically lasting concept. Antithesis of the term Black	Heterogeneous populations. Geographical links are historical i.e. Europe	Misnomer. In practice refers to European origin people of pale complexion. If used in the context of a reference/control population, use that terminology and describe this population

This table builds on the glossary of terms in Bhopal 2003 (see p 316)—with permission from *BMJ Publications*.

these race groupings.) Both historically and presently, censuses are the most important source of information relevant to ethnicity and health, and also the most influential in terms of shaping and implementing the concepts in the form of classifications. The use of censuses in health settings will be discussed in Chapter 3. However, particularly from a historical perspective the primary purposes of censuses include their use by governments for control of immigration and collection of taxes.

Table 2.2 provides summary information on the development of selected ethnic labels in censuses in seven different countries on five continents.

Try these three exercises before reading on.

Exercise 2.3 Tracing the evolution of the description of African-origin Americans in the USA

◆ Examine the column relating to African origin populations in Table 2.2. Why do you think the terminology varies between countries and changes over time within countries?

◆ Why do you think the basis of data collection changed from assessment by the enumerator to self-assessment?

Exercise 2.4 Facets of ethnic labels

◆ Examine each of the labels in the current census classifications of the UK, USA and New Zealand and your own country and note the underlying facets of either ethnicity or race that the label is emphasizing. (Do the same for other countries if you want to.)

Exercise 2.5 Sustaining terminology

◆ Look at the classifications in the UK, USA, New Zealand and your own country. What future limitations can you predict, knowing about the changing demography and social circumstances of these countries? (Do the same for other countries if you want to.)

◆ What ideas do you have for changing these classifications for the better?

Table 2 alone proves that numerous classifications with varying conceptual underpinnings are possible at any point internationally. There are also varying classifications within any country, although one tends to dominate, usually the one related to the census. Even government surveys might use different classifications. Mostly, there are relatively minor variants over time, with an evolutionary process. Nonetheless, sometimes major conceptual shifts occur, and some of these will be pointed out below. These usually respond to social and political changes, including shifting power relationships. In the first USA Census African origin people were mainly slaves, and they were counted as three-fifths of a person, while Native Americans who did not pay tax were not counted at all. Over time, and particularly from the 1960s onwards, we saw the emergence of the label

Table 2.2 Summary of census names for selected populations in seven countries on five continents

Country	Census year	Name for White populations	Name for Black populations	Name for mixed populations	Names for Asian populations	Names for indigenous populations	Other
USA	1850	White	Black	Mulatto	None	None	None
	1900	No options	No options	No options	No options	No options	No options
	2000	White	Black, African-American, Negro	None	Japanese, Chinese, Filipino, Korean, Vietnamese, Asian Indian, Guamanian or Chamorro, Samoan	American Indian or Alaskan Native (print tribe), Native Hawaiian, other Asian, other Pacific Islander	Some other race
South Africa	2001	White	Black African	None	Indian or Asian	None	Coloured other (specify)
England	2001	White (British, Irish, Any other White background)	Black, Black British, Black Carribean, Black African	Mixed (White and Black Caribbean) (White and Black African) (White and Asian) (Any other mixed background)	Asian or Asian British (Indian) (Pakistani) (Bangladeshi) (any other Asian background). Chinese	None	Any other ethnic group
Canada	1901	White	Black	(Mixed children were to be assigned to the appropriate non-White race)	Yellow	Red	None
	1951	English, Scottish, Ukrainian, Jewish, Norwegian	Negro	(Traced through the father except for mixed Indians living on reserves)		Native Indian North American Indian	

Table 2.2 (Continued)

Country	Census year	Name for White population	Name for Black population	Name for mixed population	Names for Asian populations	Names for indigenous population	Other
	2001	White	Black		Chinese, South Asian, Filipino, Latin American, Southeast Asian, Arab, West Asian, Japanese, Korean	None	Other (specifiy)
New Zealand	1916	European	Negro	Half-caste	Chinese, Hindu, Javanese, Polynesian	Maori	&c. as the case may be
	1951	European	Negro	Used fractions to denote percentage of racial mix	Syrian, Lebanese, Indian, Chinese	Maori	&c. as the case may be
	2001	European			Indian, Chinese	Maori, Samoan, Cook Island Maori, Tongan, Niuean	Other (please state)
Ceylon (now Sri Lanka)	1901	Not available					
	1946	English, Scotch, Irish				Low country Sinhalese, Kandyan, Sinhalese, Ceylon, Tamil, Ceylon Moor, Indian Moor, Malay	
Ghana	1901	Whites	Blacks	Mulattos			
	1948	No options					

Black as a matter of pride. Currently, African-American is the label that is favoured. Self-enumeration also responds to the increasing rights and power of individuals, in relation to those in authority, particularly on matters such as identity. Census classifications, rightly, respond to such important matters. Current racial and ethnic classifications tend to be more suitable for social and planning purposes than for scientific ones, and this is usually declared by those developing them. These issues are now discussed in relation to three countries on three continents with extra information on other countries in the appendix to this chapter.

The United States of America

The USA constitution required a census and this started in 1790. It collected data on race. In 1850 information on free and slave inhabitants was collected separately. The enumerator i.e. the person collecting the information, assigned race (white, black or mulatto). In 1870 additional groups were added—Chinese and Indian—that were not colour based, and foreign parentage was noted. In 1890 the word colour was dropped but the list was extended, with further graduations of racial mixture (quadroon, octoroon). Language was also assessed. The 1900 census asked of 'colour or race' but categories were removed. Of 28 questions in total, 8 attempted to describe aspects of ethnicity and migration status, reflecting the perceived importance of the issue. In 1950 the word race was used and colour dropped, with categories including negro. Completion of the form by the householder, as opposed to the enumerator, came in 1960. The householder was to report on the race (though this term was not specifically used) of the person using an extended list, including negro.

The 1970 census saw the return of colour and race with a request, for the first time, for the tribe of American Indians, and a question ascertaining whether the person was of Mexican, Puerto Rican, Cuban, Central or South American or other Spanish origin or descent (or none of these). This was the beginning of a question on Hispanic/Latino ethnicity. From 1977 the federal government sought to standardize data on race and ethnicity among all of its agencies through the Office of Management and Budget's (OMB) Statistical Policy Directive Number 15, *Race and Ethnic Standards for Federal Statistics and Administrative Reporting*. In these standards, four racial categories were established: American Indian or Alaskan Native, Asian or Pacific Islander, Black and White. In addition, an 'ethnicity' category was created identifying individuals as of 'Hispanic origin' or 'Not of Hispanic Origin'.

In 1980 the words 'colour or race' were again left out and the householder was asked to pick a race category on the basis of which one the person being classified 'most closely identifies' with. This was the first explicit link between race and self-identity. The centrality of ethnicity in its broadest sense was exemplified in this USA census.

The 1990 census explicitly used the word race. It encouraged specificity in Asian or Pacific Islanders and American Indian but not in the White, or Black/Negro categories. In preparation for the 2000 Census, the OMB revised these racial and ethnic categories, introducing new standards. In 2000, the Spanish/Hispanic/Latino question immediately preceded the race question. The race question introduced, for the first time and in the midst of great controversy, the opportunity to mark more than one category, hence indicating mixed race. The word African was introduced in the black/negro category.

Readers interested in how the USA's neighbour, Canada, has handled race and ethnicity will find a short account in the appendix to this chapter.

United Kingdom

In every census since 1841 a question has been asked about a person's place and/or country of birth; and most censuses in the UK have also included a question about nationality. However, neither are reliable guides to determining a person's ethnic origin. In the 1991 census a question on ethnic origin was asked for the first time although the authority for this was given in the Census Order of 1920. This authority was not acted upon for a number of reasons, including the view that country of birth was sufficient. Detailed plans to include a question on ethnicity in the 1981 census were cancelled because of opposition. The opposition was almost certainly because race relations were poor in the 1970s, partly because of the influence of the late politician Enoch Powell. His views are analysed below.

> According to Powell, the 'rivers of blood' will flow not because the immigrants are black; not because British society is racist; but because however 'tolerant' the British might be, they can only 'digest' so much alienness. This rather cannibalistic metaphor is instructive for (at least) two reasons. First, it fits in well with the assumptions of assimilation. If blacks could be 'digested' then they would disappear into the mainstream of British society. They would no longer be visible or different, and therefore no longer a problem. On the other hand there is also the inference—given the context in which such language crops up—that this alien food will not agree with a British stomach used to less 'exotic' fare. Consequently we can expect the violent ejection; the 'vomiting' up and out of 'all those ethnic lumps of Empire' which Mother England agreed to bring home and swallow. This idea, that the black cultures are not just different but so very foreign as to cause much discomfort in Mother England's digestive tract, is one point at which this racist ideology intersects with *common-sense* racism. Blacks are alien, aren't they? and because they are alien it is simply common sense that Britain can only assimilate a small number.
>
> Lawerence (1982: 81)

While the opposition to the 1981 question may have been motivated by concerns about immigration, it was needed because non-White ethnic groups were known to suffer discrimination and disadvantage. The 1991 Census question on ethnicity with its emphasis on non-White groups was justified by arguments emphasising the need for tackling inequity, inequality and racial discrimination. These arguments overcame opposition. The ethnic group question of 1991 was developed after consultations and debate with ethnic minority organizations. A broader set of ethnic categories was designed for use in the 2001 Census, including a specific 'mixed' ethnic group category. Each category can be broken down further into a much more detailed range of 16 ethnic groups.

The 1991 and 2001 censuses are compared in Table 2.3 and Table 2.4 provides the question for the 1991 version.

The 1991 Census question on ethnic group is a pragmatic, self-determined ethnic group question which was found to be acceptable despite conceptual limitations. For

Table 2.3 A comparison of the 1991 and the 2001 Census ethnic groupings in the UK's census (English version)

1991 Census—ethnic group	2001 Census—ethnic category	
0 White	White	
1 Black Caribbean	A	British
2 Black African	B	Irish
3 Black Other	C	Any other White background
4 Indian	Mixed	
5 Pakistani	D	White and Black Caribbean
6 Bangladeshi	E	White and Black African
7 Chinese	F	White and Asian
8 Any other ethnic group	G	Any other mixed background
9 Not known/not given	Asian	
	H	Indian
	I	Pakistani
	J	Bangladeshi
	K	Any other Asian background
	Black or Black British	
	M	Caribbean
	N	African
	P	Any other Black background
	Other ethnic groups	
	R	Chinese
	S	Any other ethnic group
	Z	Not stated

Table 2.4 The 1991 Census question on 'ethnic group'

Ethnic Group—please tick the appropriate box:

White	☐
Black—Caribbean	☐
Black—African	☐
Black—Other (please describe)	☐
Indian	☐
Pakistani	☐
Bangladeshi	☐
Chinese	☐
Any other ethnic group	☐

If the person is descended from more than one ethnic group or racial group, please tick the group to which the person considers he/she belongs, or tick the 'Any other ethnic group' box and describe the person's ancestry in the space provided.

example, the classification uses race and colour concepts (White/Black) together with national origins that are reflective of ethnic identity (Chinese, Indian, Pakistani etc.). The White group combines a number of groups which have distinct cultural, geographical and religious heritage, i.e. those of Irish, Greek or Turkish origin. The 2001 question is, with the exception of including mixed groups, a variant of the 1991 question. The 1991

Census ethnic question did not meet the requirements of users who argued that extra information was needed, such as languages spoken and religion, to properly describe the ethnicity of the groups. They also emphasized the need for an opportunity for people to describe mixed ethnic origins. In 2001, a religion question was included, although it was not legally compulsory. The inclusion of a language question in the 2011 census is likely.

Each of the four component countries of UK has made small variations in the nature of this question.

New Zealand

The 1906 census stated that a separate Maori census would be done. There was no other information on ethnicity, but country of birth and religion were recorded. From 1916 race and/or ethnicity has been recorded and have been prominent components of the census. In 1916 there was a European race, examples of others and reference to admixture (half-caste). In 1926 there was a Maori census, with the Maori language written in English script that also took note of admixture. There was little change until 1976 when ethnic origin replaced race (or in some forms there was either no term or descent). In 1981 we saw the first more structured, tick box, form of question, place much emphasis on mixed ethnic origin, with graduations of up to one-eighth e.g. 7/8 European. The 1986 census saw the progression of this approach to a range of questions, but the questions on mixture have been left out, although more than one ethnic group can be chosen. In 1991 there was a special emphasis on Maori ancestry and tribe. The 2001 questionnaire was in bilingual format—English and Maori. Maori background was specified as ancestry. In preparation for the 2011 census, there is considerable controversy about the continuing use of words such as European, with a clamour for a New Zealand identity.

2.5 Census categories are not necessarily a good match for identity

Census and other surveys' questions now usually allow respondents to choose their ethnic identity from a menu, but does the menu offer a good choice? Often this may not be so, and as Peter Aspinall says in discussing the 1991 Census, the options suggest there is a case for far more subtlety and more use of open responses.

> About one in four people from ethnic groups other than 'White' expressed a wish to describe their ethnic group.
>
> Given the important implications for determining the ethnic origin of the increasing numbers of people who choose not to fit into one of the standard predefined categories, write in answers should be reintroduced while there is still time for local implementation to do so.
>
> Aspinall (1995: 1006–9)

What sort of terms would people use? Data from a cross-sectional survey (the South Tyneside Heart Study) compared respondents' identification of their ethnicity using the Census question, a description in an open question, country of birth and country of family origin. Respondents (n = 334) first chose one of the categories from the UK 1991 Census question, then provided a description of their ethnicity. Respondents were also asked where they and their mother and father were born. The most striking observation was the rarity of the term 'Asian' and the absence of the term 'South Asian', both of which are commonly used in the UK to describe people originating from the Indian subcontinent. These labels do not capture ethnic self-identity. From the Census ethnic group categories, 130 (39 per cent) of respondents chose Indian. Only 81 (62 per cent) of those who were Indian on the Census question described themselves as Indian when given the open choice. Only 52/93 (56 per cent) of respondents born in India described themselves as Indian. Using Census categories for ethnic groups is insufficient to capture

Table 2.5 Respondents' descriptions of their ethnic origin by 1991 Census category

Self-description	Ethnicity according to the 1991 Census categories[‡]		
	Indian no. (%)	Pakistani no. (%)	Bangladeshi no. (%)
Indian	81 (62)	2 (5)	—
British/English/Anglo Indian	12 (9)	—	—
Indian Christian	1 (1)	—	—
Kashmiri Indian	1 (1)	—	—
Born in India but lived in Pakistan	1 (1)	—	—
Pakistani	—	29 (67)	1 (1)
Sikh	12 (9)	—	—
British Sikh	2 (2)	—	—
Indian Sikh	2 (2)	—	—
Bangladeshi	—	1 (2)	118 (94)
Bengali	—	—	5 (4)
British Bengali	—	—	—
Muslim	1 (1)	2 (5)	1 (1)
Kashmiri Muslim	2 (2)	—	—
British Muslim	—	1 (2)	—
British	6 (5)	5 (12)	1 (1)
British/ English Asian	4 (3)	3 (7)	—
Asian	4 (3)	—	—
Black or Asian	1 (1)	—	—
Total	130	43	126

I = India, P = Pakistan, B = Bangladesh, O = Other, UK = United Kingdom.
[‡] 15 missing values.
From Rankin and Bhopal (1996).

self-identification fully. Some sample results for Indians, Pakistanis and Bangladeshis are shown in Table 2.5.

The categories offered in the UK census are too few to reflect the true heterogeneity of ethnic groups. Similar issues also apply to other labels, e.g. 'Black', 'White'.

2.6 Towards a common international terminology

Table 2.1 provides a commentary on some terms in the glossary that serves as an example, but needs development in terms of geographical specificity, scope and precision. It will be clear that the terms and definitions are based on an amalgam of both the concepts of race and ethnicity. This glossary is used in this book, in full understanding that it is a work in progress. Clearly, using the principles evident in the glossary e.g. giving primacy to self-identity while acknowledging ancestry and the link to racial classifications, additional terms can be added. A deeper and longer glossary with truly international applications is, however, required. Then we would have a foundation for an internationally acceptable glossary. The task is enormous but if the subject of ethnicity and race studies is to mature it needs to be tackled. In the field of health there is a case for leadership from a partnership including the WHO, International Epidemiological Association, and an organization such as the World Association of Medical Editors. Research-funding organizations including The National Institutes of Health (USA), The Medical Research Council (UK) and equivalent organizations internationally also have a major role, working with national health care agencies.

2.7 Conclusions

Some two hundred years of effort in creating racial and ethnic classifications has led to numerous insights, particularly that the process is arbitrary, subjective, context-specific, purpose-driven, and imprecise. The process is atheoretical in that there is no coherent theoretical factor that underpins classifications. The view that the prime value of such classifications is in social, rather than biological, contexts and in service applications is clearly correct. Another insight is that these imperfect classifications provide a powerful tool for analysis of difference and similarity.

As societies are becoming more ethnically diverse such classifications are in increasing demand and use. The challenge is to create a suite of classifications that meet the purpose better and that have greater theoretical underpinnings than hitherto (see Chapter 10). Editors and writers are jointly responsible for ensuring scientific rigour and high quality writing, yet few journals or books have appropriate policies that are implemented vigorously. The *British Medical Journal* was one of the first journals to make progress on this. The guidelines were as follows:

Ethnicity, race, and culture: guidelines for research, audit, and publication

Authors should describe in their methods section the logic behind their 'ethnic' groupings. Terms used should be as descriptive as possible and reflect how the groups were demarcated. For example, 'black' as a group description is less accurate than 'self assigned as black Caribbean (Office of Population Censuses and Surveys category)' and 'Asian' less accurate than 'UK born individuals of Indian ancestry' or 'French born individuals of Vietnamese ancestry'.

If it is unknown which of ethnicity, race, or culture is the most important influence then an attempt should be made to measure all of them.

A range of information is best collected:

- Genetic differences (using relevant genetically determined polymorphism)
- Self assigned ethnicity (using nationally agreed guidelines enabling comparability with census data)
- Observer assigned ethnicity (using nationally agreed guidelines enabling comparability with census data)
- Observer assigned ethnicity (using OPCS or other national census categorisation or the researchers' own logically argued categories)
- Country or area of birth (the subject's own, or parents' and grandparents' if applicable)
- Years in country of residence
- Religion

McKenzie and Crowcroft (1996: 1094)

Research by George Ellison and colleagues has shown that these guidelines have not been followed by authors (2005). Similar efforts by the Journal of the American Medical Association have been partially successful in authors' reports of the ethnic labels, although they seldom explain the theoretical underpinnings of the use of the concepts of race and ethnicity.

Accurate use of concepts and words is an essential first step to good research, to improving the health of ethnic minorities and narrowing inequities. Helping achieve conceptual and terminological accuracy remains a major and challenging goal for authors and editors alike. The search for accurate terminology will remain controversial, however, for both scientific and social reasons, not least because of the tension between the differing needs of science, services and the public. There are other issues, e.g. whether international understanding and agreement on these concepts and terms is achievable, the comparative health of population subgroups within the populations defined by current categories, empirical demonstration that the benefits of data by ethnicity and race exceed the costs, and in particular that they help improve the health status of the study populations.

Accurate terminology in ethnicity and health research requires a consideration of concepts and terms beyond those referring to race and ethnicity. In comparative work, for example, terms such as reference, control or comparison population have advantages compared to those such as White or European. They raise fewer expectations and prior assumptions and require the writer to provide detail on the populations studied, including their heterogeneity and origins.

International collaboration for exchange of ideas and expertise, as well as technical information on definitions, is a necessary part of this endeavour. We will be returning to these issues, particularly in Chapter 9. In the next chapter, I consider the practical challenges of data collection by ethnic group. Some readers might prefer to read Chapter 4, which gives some historical and international background, first.

Summary

Concepts need to be defined and in this process we usually simplify and clarify them. In simplification the original meaning, and intent, of the concepts may be unwittingly altered. To utilize the concepts of race and ethnicity as variables in population health we create population groupings. This process is always pragmatic and, in the absence of firm scientific underpinnings, it is subjective and malleable, and designed to meet perceived needs. The grouping process will utilize only one or a few of the many facets of such complex concepts: the choice of which facets to emphasize will determine the grouping. The groups arising, collectively, comprise a classification. Each group needs to have a label. The label should be both meaningful and acceptable, both to those creating and using the classification and those who are so classified. Presently, most classifications are designed for self-report of race or ethnicity.

The value of the classification achieved, as opposed to the many alternatives, should be judged by whether it serves the stated purpose. In quantitative health sciences the purpose is to establish and explain differences in health status of populations, in public health it is to improve health through prevention and control of disease, and in clinical medicine it is to make diagnosis and treatment easier.

Classifications vary across times and places, reflecting both the pragmatic nature of the process of creation and the varying purpose for which they were designed. Many classifications of race have been proposed. Only those relating to broad continental groupings continue to hold influence. At any one place and time, though numerous classifications are possible, one tends to dominate, with minor variants. Usually, this is the classification used in the census.

Current racial and ethnic classifications, mostly based on the census questions, tend to be more suitable for social and planning purposes than for scientific ones. One of the biggest obstacles to scientific work is the heterogeneity of the populations described by current groupings.

The terminology supporting both concepts and classifications is problematic, and despite the difficulties of the task, progress towards an internationally agreed vocabulary is a prerequisite for progress. These challenges of classification, terminology and agreement on concepts are similar to those for other complex variables such as social class and educational status—race and ethnicity are not uniquely problematic. Despite their difficulties most classifications do work in the sense that they add to our capacity for analysis of similarities and differences in the health of populations.

Appendix

Canada

The Canadian census dates back to 1666. Data on ethnic or racial origins have been collected in all but one (1891) national censuses. In the 1901 census information was collected under four colour categories—white, red, black and yellow. Mixed coloured children were designated as non-white.

In 1981, 'Black' was not listed on the census questionnaire, though respondents could specify 'Black ethnic origin' in the write-in box. The mark-in response 'Black' was added to the 1986 Census questionnaire and included again in 1991. Some respondents objected to the presence of 'Black' as an ethnic group in the 1991 Census questionnaire. The removal of the 'Black' check-off entry in 1996 resulted in the decreased reporting of 'Black' and the increased reporting of African and Caribbean origins. This is one example of how political considerations are important in influencing classifications, and subsequently the interpretation and presentation of the statistics.

The idea of multiple ethnicities has been tackled since 1986. Since 1986, an instruction to specify as many ethnic groups as applicable has been included in the ethnic origin question.

With ethnicity, religion and language data, Canada has a rich data set on ethnicity to provide information that is required under the Multiculturalism Act, the Canadian Charter of Rights and Freedoms and other legislation. The amount of information has increased greatly, partly to meet the demand for information arising from federal government policy on multiculturalism, and this trend can be seen even between 1991 and 2001. Information on ethnicity in the 2001 census is in the section headed sociocultural information. The key question on ethnicity relates to the person's ancestors with exemplars based on countries. In addition there is a list of ethnic groups (Q19) that is justified by the need to promote equal opportunity. Several questions relate to original inhabitant/aboriginal status. In 2001, the 25 ethnic categories and subcategories used to classify individual ethnic origins included:

1. British Isles origins
2. Aboriginal origins
3. Caribbean origins
4. Latin, Central and South American origins
5. African origins
6. Arab origins
7. West Asian origins
8. South Asian origins.

The Canadian experience provides an excellent example of how complex ethnicity is, and how difficult it is to devise classifications in a scientifically objective, rational and consistent way.

Brazil

The Brazilian approach is unusual in modern times in being based predominantly on colour. The Census is held every ten years and it asks the question, 'what is your colour or race?' There are tick boxes for responses with no space for written responses. The response categories are white, black, brown, mixed, yellow and indigenous (referring to the indigenous Indian population). There is also a question 'what is your nationality?' with three tick boxes options: Natural Brazilian, Brazilian Citizenship, and Foreigner. There are three related questions: 'In which Brazilian state or foreign country were you born?' a question regarding uninterrupted stay in Brazil, and 'In which state or foreign country was your previous residence?'

India

The 2001 Census was the sixth since independence from Britain in 1947. No questions were asked regarding race or ethnicity but there are questions for mother tongue and other languages known and birthplace, specifying the state/country. There were two questions relating to caste and tribe.

Australia

Since 1961, the Census of Population and Housing has been held every five years. The census is collected from householders and is self-completed. Ethnicity has not been collected, although a question about ancestry was asked in 1986. A number of variables from 1996 may be used to derive ethnicity. Questions for 2001 asked for citizenship, country of birth, year of arrival, Australian or overseas birthplace of father and mother, language most often spoken at home, Australian indigenous origin, and ancestry. The question that is closest to ethnicity is 'what is the person's ancestry?' The example given include: Vietnamese, Hmong, Dutch, Kurdish, Australian South Sea Islander, Maori, Lebanese and there is scope to provide more than one ancestry if necessary. Australia analyses the variables ancestry, birthplace and parents' birthplace—Australia or overseas—as an indicator for first, and second-generation, Australians' ethnic background.

Fiji

A census has been held since 1881. Questions relating to ethnicity are place of birth and the ethnic group question. One response was accepted for ethnicity. The enumerator was instructed to 'record the group or race to which the person considers he or she belongs. If there is any doubt as to the person's racial origin, record the father' (Fiji Census 1996: 281). Enumerators used the classification code:

1. Fijians
2. Indians
3. Chinese and part-Chinese
4. European
5. Part-European
6. Rotuman
7. Other Pacific Islanders
8. All others
9. Not stated.

Mauritius

Mauritius has held a decennial census since 1846, and its last census was 2000. Information is collected on citizenship and linguistic group in the population censuses. According to the constitution, the Mauritian population includes a Hindu community, a Muslim community, a Sino-Mauritian community and the general population. The last time a question was asked on the ethnic composition of the community at a population census was in 1972. The question was: 'To which of the following communities does this person claim to belong? Hindu, Muslim, Sino-Mauritian (Sino is a descriptor for Chinese), General Population'.

South Africa

The census takes place every five years and it uses categories that arise from the apartheid era. Traditionally, the enumerator or the household member completing the questionnaire is asked to judge how each member of the household would describe themself i.e. there is no requirement to ask them.

Now, interviewers are instructed to accept the response that is given even if they don't agree. In 1996, there was no reference to the nature of the question but in 2001 the categorization was described as population group. In 1996 only four options were available with no 'other' category, which became available in 2001. A range of related questions—religion, country of birth and languages spoken in the home—allow a fairly detailed analysis of ethnicity.

Singapore

The definition used by Statistics Singapore was that 'ethnic group refers to a person's race as declared by that person. For those of mixed parentage, they are usually declared under the ethnic group of their fathers.' Ethnic group data came from the household register and was pre-printed on the census forms in 2000 for verification with the respondent. The Singapore government and statistical departments classify the population under four main ethnic groups: Chinese, Malay, Indian and Others, with many subcategories falling under each main category.

The Chinese category lists 22 subcategories, including Hokkien, Teochew, Cantonese, Hakka, Hainanese, Hockchia, Foochow, Henghua, Shanghainese plus 'other Chinese'. The Malay category refers to persons of Malay or Indonesian origin and contains 18 subcategories, listing Javanese, Boyanese, Bugi and 'other Malays'. The Indian category contains groups that have origins in India, Pakistan, Bangladesh and Sri Lanka. It lists 24 subcategories: Tamils, Malayali, Punjabi, Bengali, Singhalese plus 'other Indians'. 'Other' refers to all other groups not already listed including Eurasian, Caucasian, Arab and Japanese.

Chapter 3

Challenges of collecting and interpreting data using the concepts of ethnicity and race

The racial classification of health statistics in the United States is an anachronism.

The public health movement, which has spoken out vigorously against segregation in health services and in other aspects of American life, needs to examine carefully the issue of segregation in health statistics.

Terris (1973: 479)

The data that already exist show that disadvantage and discrimination are part of the everyday lives of ethnic minority people. This message has been clear for many years. In the formulation of legislation, therefore, there is no need to wait for more information. Indeed, it might be argued that there is no point in producing more data until such legislation exists or at least until there is an expression of political will.

Data have not been instrumental in reducing racial disadvantage.

Booth (1984: 20)

One of the reasons why policies and services have failed Black and Minority ethnic groups in the past is the lack of information available about them. Much information that is currently collected is not broken down by ethnic group. In addition, because people from Black and Minority ethnic communities make up a small proportion of the population, their representation in many surveys is so low as to make it difficult to use the results with confidence. The resulting lack of detailed, local and robust data that covers the whole country means that it is often difficult to adequately diagnose problems experienced by Black and Minority ethnic groups, better target policies or services at addressing their needs, and monitor and evaluate the impact on them.

(SEU 2000: p. 66; para 9.16)

Contents

- Chapter objectives
- Why collecting ethnicity or race within health data systems and health research is justifiable
- Relationships between concepts, classifications and methods of data collection on ethnicity and race
- Strengths and weakness of alternatives methods for collection of ethnic code data:

    (i) Self-assigned
    (ii) Assessed on the basis of self-reported data
    (iii) Other assigned
    (iv) Proxies such as the country of birth
    (v) Assessed on the basis of self-reported data

- Interpretation of ethnicity and race data

    (i) Questions to ask
    (ii) Essential and desirable supporting data to help interpretation of data

- Explanations for similarities and differences in health states by ethnic or racial group
- A conceptual framework for the analysis of ethnic or racial variations in health status
- Interpreting data in the face of incomplete examination of alternative explanations for variations
- Using data to formulate responses—exemplars, pitfalls, and challenges
- Conclusions
- Summary

Objectives

On completion of this chapter you should be able to:

- Understand why the concepts of ethnicity or race underlying your data collecting system are crucial to the method of data collection and data interpretation
- Accept that useful data collection by ethnicity or race requires that individuals provide, and data systems record, the relevant data items
- Understand that the interpretation of data rests upon the concepts underpinning the classification and validity of the data
- Be able to apply a framework of analysis to list the most important explanations for differences in health status
- Be able to offer appropriate policy, health planning or clinical care responses to observations on the patterns of health status by ethnic group

3.1 Introduction

As the quotations opening this chapter illustrate, it is not absolutely self-evident that data by ethnicity or race are necessary or helpful. Arguably, the only current ethical justification for collecting data by ethnicity within health information systems, and for holding such data on clinical records, is health and health care improvement for the ethnic groups being recorded, either directly through better service delivery or through research and clinical audit (see Chapter 10). This justification is, in my view, a sufficient reason for collecting such data, but see Box 3.1 for some more specific reasons. Box 3.2 gives some circumstances requiring such information.

Box 3.1 Health and health care improvement needs ethnicity data to

◆ establish the extent of health inequalities and inequity in health service provision
◆ monitor the impact of efforts to reduce these inequalities
◆ tackle racism
◆ make good decisions based on evidence
◆ grasp scientific opportunities

Box 3.2. Contexts and purposes

◆ Political
◆ Health policy
◆ Health care planning
◆ Clinical care
◆ Surveillance and monitoring
◆ Health services research
◆ Causal research

An explicit statement agreeing such an understanding ought to be in place before collecting data. Before reading on try Exercise 3.1, which encourages you to reflect on the reasons why ethnicity data is necessary for health and health care improvement and what would be lost if such data were not available.

Exercise 3.1 Data on smoking

◆ Examine the data in Table 3.1, making the assumption that the findings are correct.
◆ What potential benefits are there in having such data, particularly from the point of view of the communities under study and those providing health care and public health services?

Table 3.1 The Newcastle Heart Project. Current self-reported smoking prevalence in Indians, Pakistani, Bangladeshi and European populations (%)

	Indian	Pakistani	Bangladeshi	South Asian groups combined	European
Men	14	32	57	33	33
Women	1	5	2	3	31

Source of data: Bhopal *et al.* BMJ 1999; 319: 215–20. Similar to table published in Bhopal (2006). J Law Medicine and Ethics.

The data in the exercise come from a cross-sectional study in Newcastle in the 1990s, which was one of the earliest to put an emphasis on the differences within the South Asian population, as in the paper on heterogeneity of cardiovascular risk factors by Bhopal and colleagues in 1999. Here, a relatively simple classification of ethnic groups based on that of the 1991 census in the UK shows massive differences. The variations are far greater than are usually demonstrated by other commonly used epidemiological variables, e.g. sex, social class etc. Such differences cannot be quantified except by using the concepts of ethnicity, or a closely related variable such as religion. In this instance, dividing the Indian population by religion e.g. Hindu, Muslim, and Sikh would have produced even sharper variations because there are firm and effective taboos against smoking in the Sikh community. However, as most Pakistanis and Bangladeshis are Muslim, only analysing by religion would lead to a loss of the demonstrated difference between Pakistanis and Bangladeshis.

Such uniquely important differences cannot be ignored in public health programmes. Clearly, the health promotion message for women will need to be very different from that for men, and, indeed, that for European (White) UK women. The data also reinforce the point that minority ethnic groups may be extremely heterogeneous—as shown in Table 3.1 combining the three South Asian groups into one loses the ethnic variation in men-the combined prevalence was 32 per cent, i.e. more or less the same as for European (White) men. The data emphasize that using broadly defined ethnic groups may result in the loss of important data. The usual, and cruder classification, of these populations as South Asians would have missed important variation. The lessons from examining Table 3.1 are summarized in Box 3.3.

Box 3.3 Lessons from the Newcastle Heart Project data

- ◆ Such important differences cannot be ignored in public health programmes
- ◆ Such differences can only be quantified using the concepts of race or ethnicity
- ◆ Ethnic groups can be extremely heterogeneous—combining them into broad populations may lose important data
- ◆ For self-reported data we need to maximize cross-cultural validity

There are many reasons why we need to examine such data critically, including problems of cross-cultural validity of self-reported data. We will return to these matters later, particularly in Chapter 9.

3.2 **Data as an agent for health improvement—making choices**

A vision for using data is vital to its collection and interpretation.
  Before reading on, do Exercise 3.2.

Exercise 3.2 Look at the images in Figures 3.1 and 3.2 and answer the questions below

- Image one is the cover of the WHO book Migration and Health. What does it portray?
- Why is this an apt picture for a book on migration and health in Europe?
- What feelings does it evoke in you?
- Image two is the cover of the Faculty of Public Health's 1988 scientific meeting proceedings. What does it portray?
- Why is this an apt picture for modern-day societies?
- What feelings does it evoke in you?

Moving from the position as symbolized in Figure 3.1 to that in Figure 3.2 will not be easy, but in my opinion it cannot be achieved without data. As outlined in Chapter 6, ethnic inequalities in health, if not health care, are inevitable. Our objective in this book, set within the wider aim of improving the health of all populations, is to move from a

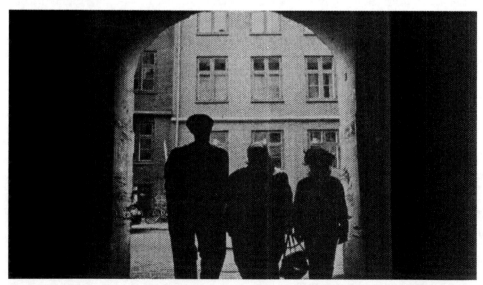

Fig. 3.1 Migrants in the archway. (Cover of WHO book Migration and Health (1983) edited by Colledge and Colleagues—see Books, p 318.)

Source: This image appears on the front cover of Colledge, M., Van Geuns, H. A., Svensson, Per Gunnar, *Migration and Health Towards an Understanding of the Health Care Needs of Ethnic Minorities*. The Hague, Netherlands. The original source is unknown.

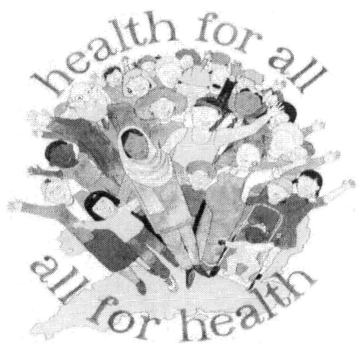

Fig. 3.2 Cartoon of a healthy society (front cover of the Proceedings of the 1988 meeting of the Faculty of Public Health).

society where minority populations are living on the margins of society (as symbolized in Figure 3.1) to a vibrant multicultural society with equitable health and health care (as symbolized in Figure 3.2). This is the topic of Chapters 6 and 8. In this chapter, we focus on the collection of data because information and research are the driving forces for change in the modern world.

Before reading on do Exercise 3.3.

Exercise 3.3 Information and research data

- What is the value of research data
- What purposes do they serve?
- What debates do they contribute to?

Health and health care data that can be analysed by ethnicity are essential to establish the extent of health inequalities in death, morbidity and well-being, to define inequity in health service provision, monitor the impact of interventions to reduce these inequalities and inequities, tackle racism in health care systems and in wider society that undermines health, make good decisions based on evidence, and grasp scientific opportunities for gaining insights into the causes of such inequalities and inequities (points summarized in Box 3.1). Unfortunately, collecting such data is not easy in practice, both because of lack of ethnic coding and lack of valid measurement instruments (the latter topic is discussed in Chapter 9).

3.3 Collecting data by ethnic monitoring: difficulties, choices and concepts

Examples of policies that underpin ethnic monitoring are discussed in Chapter 8. Here, we simply look at the difficulties of implementing the policies. In 1990 the Department of Health in England proposed that patients' ethnicity should be collected in general practice (known elsewhere as primary care or family practice) and forwarded in hospital referral letters. This seems a simple and efficient way of achieving comprehensive coverage of ethnicity in health databases, but it has yet to be achieved.

Recording of the ethnicity of patients admitted to hospitals in the NHS in England was made mandatory in April 1995. This has not been satisfactorily achieved. To some extent there is a resistance to collecting such data, including a view that their value has not been demonstrated. The data on smoking prevalence by sex and ethnic group, shown in Exercise 3.1 and discussed above, are a simple but powerful reminder that such data are vital for rational policies and plans.

As the quotations opening this chapter show, the need for data by ethnic group is contested, but usually because of the dangers of abuse, or almost as bad, non-use. Given an appropriate context (see Chapters 8 and 10) and agreement about the need for collecting ethnic group data in health databases and research studies, investigators must make choices on the concept that meets the purposes (i.e. race or ethnicity or both), and which aspects of race or ethnicity are to be emphasized and hence captured in the information systems. These choices must be governed by the purposes for which the data are being collected and the historical and social context. Without this essential first step the data are unlikely to meet the need. For example, if the purpose is to differentiate those born abroad, country of birth might be a reasonable indicator of ethnicity, and this is preferred in The Netherlands. Those born in Surinam, for example, comprise two major populations who differentiate themselves, and are differentiated by others, as Hindus and Creoles. Their health patterns are substantially different. Self-assessment of ethnicity might be more appropriate to differentiate them, as country of birth will not. It may be that in modern-day Netherlands, with its historical legacy of the colonization of Surinam, the purposes of the health system are best met by collecting information on the fact of birth in Surinam and on whether the person is Hindu or Creole. The former data could probably be obtained from administrative records, the latter by self-report. Once such basic decisions have been made, the method of data collection on race or ethnicity—whether self-report or some other indicator such as name—and the classification can then be chosen. The potential, interpretation and utilization of the data are dependent on these initial choices. The data system needs to be designed to record, retrieve and analyse data to meet the specified purposes (Box 3.2) and should include information on the underlying concepts and methods for the benefits of data users.

3.4 **Context, purpose and measures of ethnicity and race**

As Box 3.2 shows, there are many contexts and purposes for data collection on ethnicity and race. Before reading on try Exercise 3.4., which asks you to reflect on both ethnicity and race, in a number of contexts and for various purposes.

Exercise 3.4 Which concept, ethnicity or race, might prove the more useful in the following contexts:

- politics
- health policy
- health care planning
- clinical care
- surveillance and monitoring
- health services research, and
- understanding disease causation?

In answering this question, consider the purposes that the data might be used for.

My answers are summarized in Table 3.2 and in the text below.

For a fuller discussion, see my Chapter in Macbeth and Shetty (see book list p 317 and Bhopal, 2000), from where the following account is extracted and adapted.

3.4.1 **Political**

Historically, the most deeply rooted purpose of race-based data collection is political. Race-based data are used to identify individuals and groups so that policies can be applied differently (sometimes to the benefits of the minority groups, sometimes to their detriment) usually on political grounds. The history of the use of race in politics is mostly an unhappy one, so caution is necessary (see Chapter 6). The modern-day argument for the retention of the race concept is that it is necessary to guide corrective action to reverse the effect of past injustices. As the goal and purpose is social and political the racial classification ought to be a socially and politically generated one.

For political purposes the crude division of society as White and non-White, and other simple measures, may serve the purpose. The most common division in the USA is White/Black, and the groups assigned such labels are thought of as races, with the traditional biological construct increasingly giving way to the social one.

The concept of race as a physical and biological indicator of a population group, the physical features themselves having been in the past the foundation for racism, works, albeit imperfectly, as a basis for a classification to be used for such purposes. The problems with race, even here, should not be glossed over—physical features do not reliably identify population groups, they vary across generations and merge imperceptibly across geographical areas. The concept of race also becomes difficult to apply in people of mixed race. Nonetheless, the approach has some arguments in its favour and it is easier to

Table 3.2 Context, purpose and some potential measures of race and ethnicity

Context and comment	Purpose and potential measures of race and ethnicity	
	Purpose	Some potential measures
Political Markers sufficient. Race and colour-based division has been key	Discrimination, for or against, has been the perennial purpose Implement and monitor policy	Colour, and physical features Observer's assessment Ancestry Birthplace
Health policy Monitoring policy needs stable marker so race is better Both ethnicity and race needed for developing policy	Quarantine, segregation and port health Alleviation of inequalities in health and health care (fairness)	Nationality Country of origin Migration history Colour and physical features Colour as marker of discrimination Country of origin/ birthplace Self-perception of ethnicity or race Detail needed for causal understanding
Health care planning Race concept may suffice for access issues Ethnicity concept needed for assessment of need to adapt service	Restrict or target a service Add a new dimension to an existing service Evaluate a service Ensure quality	Migration status/nationality Observer's classification Colour Country of origin Name Language Religion Dietary preferences Self-assigned ethnicity Cultural health beliefs

Context / Issues	Purpose	Measures
Clinical care (nursing and medical) Race concept only rarely valuable Detailed data needed	Make diagnosis easier Communicate better Treat better	Colour Region/country of origin Travel history Language Health beliefs and behaviours Religion Dietary preferences Genetic indicators of disease risk and response to therapy
Surveillance and monitoring Race and ethnicity are low-cost markers. Race concept works; ethnicity is too variable to work well with some groups	Routine, low-cost data on previously agreed priorities to permit assessment of change and particularly whether problems exist	Migration status/nationality Observer's classification Colour Country of origin Name Self-report of race or ethnicity
Health Services Research and non-causal epidemiology Race and ethnicity as markers will often suffice for surveillance and other descriptive type HSR Details of underlying basis of ethnic differences needed when causal understanding needed	Raise attention to an issue Measure inequality in health or health care Develop a new service to meet needs Evaluate quality of care	Country of origin Migration status Observer's assessment Colour Name Language Religion Dietary preferences Self-assigned ethnicity or race Health beliefs and behaviour
Disease cause Race and ethnicity merely as markers are little value Detailed understanding of the interaction of biology and the environment requires direct measure of underlying facets of both ethnicity and race.	Test causal hypothesis Measure association between race/ethnicity and disease Distinguish relative contribution of environmental and genetic factors	Colour, and physical features Ancestry Birthplace Family tree/racial admixing Genetic indicators of disease risk and risk factors Valid and reliable measure of ethnicity and race (avoid misclassification bias) Measure of factors which relate both to ethnicity/race and to disease (confounders such as poverty, diet, exercise)

operationalize than the more complex idea of ethnicity. As is discussed in Chapters 6 and 8, the concept of race underpins much of law and policy, and is essential, if nothing else, to combat racism.

3.4.2 Health policy

Some health policies can apply the concepts of ethnicity or race as considered above for politics. For example in ethnic monitoring to assess whether minority group applicants for jobs in the health service are being considered, interviewed and employed, with the goal of equal opportunities in mind, race rather than ethnicity may be the better concept. This may be so both because physical features are the dominant factor that led to historical injustices that these policies seek to reverse, and because it is easier to collect information on. Labels of race and ethnicity in these circumstances are markers of groups of people, for some of whom the policy is relevant.

In policies designed to reduce inequalities in health status more data will be needed. Physical features such as colour are potential indicators of both historical and current discrimination on the basis of race, and will be highly relevant. The resultant health inequality, however, is a result of social factors including poverty, diet, employment, and cultural factors such as religion, smoking habits and dietary preferences etc. Such underlying factors, chosen carefully on the basis of the policy or research questions to be answered, need to be directly measured to make rational policy. Race and ethnicity are a means of both narrowing the search for populations and generating hypotheses for understanding why the disease or other health problem under investigation occurs.

3.4.3 Health care planning

Health care planners use race and ethnicity as a guide to assessing and meeting health needs. They require markers to identify groups they wish to consult with, or modify services for, in accord with health needs. In these cases ethnic or racial labels, colour labels, nationality and migration status are usually too crude. Country of parental or grandparental birth or the racial label do occasionally help, e.g. in the targeted delivery of BCG immunization at infancy, which in Britain is recommended routinely for children of Indian subcontinent origin as one step in the prevention and control of tuberculosis. Here the classification Indian, Pakistani, Bangladeshi or even South Asian as an overall term will do. Usually, however, more detail will be needed on racial/ethnic characteristics which impinge directly on the need for, or utilization of, a service. Sometimes needs will be the same across a number of racial or ethnic subgroups. If this is the case an umbrella term such as 'Asian', or 'Hispanic', may be applicable. Usually, there will be heterogeneity, in terms of language, religion, etc. making the provision of specifically targeted and appropriate services a huge challenge. The smoking data in Table 3.1 have demonstrated the importance of population heterogeneity in planning health promotion services Usually, the concept of ethnicity, rather than race, will be the more valuable, particularly because it can accommodate the complexity of factors that impinge on health care e.g. language, religion, and other aspects of culture.

3.4.4 Clinical care

Racial labels are sometimes used routinely to introduce the clinical history, as in 'This is a 45-year-old Indian/Caucasian/African/Chinese woman', etc. This practice is open to criticism, although there are counter-arguments in favour of its continuation. The practice is summarized in the American context in the following quotation.

> In regions of the United States such as ours, where the population is predominantly of European-American or African-American descent, the description of race is often distilled down to 'black' or 'white'. Thus, in our institution and in those with similar demographics, the fourth spoken word of many case presentations broadly describes the patient as black or white. Exactly when and how this form of introduction became common is unclear. In the United States, the format of the opening line seems to have been established in a priori in case reports in the early and mid-20th century.
>
> Caldwell and Popenhoe (1995: 614)

There are some circumstances where a racial label on its own may be helpful in diagnosis or case management. For instance, in the diagnosis of abdominal and joint pain in a person of African origin the diagnosis of sickle cell crisis ought to be considered more readily than in a European origin person (even though sickle cell disease does occur in European origin people, especially in the Mediterranean area). Even then, we must remember the huge heterogeneity in Africans. Sickle cell trait is not particularly common in Africans originating in the South, where malaria is uncommon. In these admittedly occasional circumstances the racial label might be valuable in triggering an association between the symptoms and the diagnosis. The clinician is simply using probabilities and potential problems such as stereotyping and misdiagnosis need full acknowledgement. Clinicians should be wary of routine use of race and ethnicity labels.

As a rounded understanding of the social and cultural circumstances of the patient is essential to good care, ethnicity is more likely to provide the level of complexity and flexibility required. For example, the physician treating diabetes in people originating from the countries of the Indian subcontinent will need to give advice on what to do during fasting. It is not uncommon among Hindus, particularly women, to fast for one day per week. By contrast, fasting during daylight hours is fastidiously observed by many Muslims in the month of Ramadan (even though the religion does exempt the sick, it is common for patients to fast nevertheless). Race is not helpful here. Ethnicity, based on identity, religion and origins is a reminder that the patient may need to be counselled on fasting. Religion is a more accurate means of assessment than the self-identified ethnic group since Indians, in particular, are heterogeneous in religion and culture. Even so, the physician could be seriously misled by an assumption that all Muslims fast in Ramadan or that the sick have exempted themselves from the religious requirement. A detailed cultural history from each individual is needed to ensure that errors are not made. For clinical work ethnicity is the key concept, but delving deeper than the ethnic label is almost always necessary. The purpose is to widen understanding of the culture and circumstances of the individual, which is very different from the research one.

3.4.5 Research

Chapter 9 discusses research challenges in detail. Different forms of research may apply different concepts of race and ethnicity. The racial and ethnic classifications are also likely to vary according to the type of research. Finally, the type of research will determine the depth of inquiry into the specific characteristics behind race/ethnicity, or in the words of La Veist (1996) 'those concepts believed to be measured by race'. Here, I consider causal research seeking to understand why something happens. For text relevant to the entries in Table 3.2 on surveillance, health services research and non-causal epidemiology see Chapter 9 and for further detail Bhopal (2000).

Ethnicity and race concepts may provide markers or indicators of a problem which merits causal investigation. They also provide a means of identifying relevant populations and interesting hypotheses, but they are not directly a source of causal knowledge. Since all disease arises from the interaction of the genome and the environment, here both the race and ethnicity concepts are potentially of interest. Historically, the role of biology has been invoked too readily as the prime explanation for racial differences. Unfortunately, contemporary research also gives prominence to genetic explanations and downplays environmental (and especially economic) ones. To take one example, the high rates of hypertension in African origin populations are often attributed to genetic factors with comparatively little effort to test other explanations, including stress, diet, poverty and racism. Cooper and colleagues (1997) have contested this kind of thinking and have examined hypertension in African populations across the world, and concluded that there is so much variation that genetic factors are outweighed by environmental ones.

Definitive work requires measuring directly the concepts reflected by the labels which define race and ethnicity. This task will often need to include genetic studies. For example, the rate of breast cancer in South Asian women is lower than in White women in England and Wales, as most recently shown by Wild and colleagues (2006). Since genetic factors are a demonstrated cause of breast cancer, it is important to ask whether the differences are attributable to genetic differences. It is imperative that the question is answered by direct measurements of the presence or absence of the relevant gene variants. The race and ethnicity of populations give no clue (at least to date) to their risk of possessing the genes linked to breast cancer, for the (few) genes which are responsible for the anatomic features which underlie the racial or ethnic classifications give no indirect clue as to the distribution of breast cancer causing genes. In future years when a large number of specific disease gene variants are identified and the population distributions are known this may change. Equally, the differences in breast cancer might arise from social factors which vary across the two groups e.g. diet, economic circumstances, contraception, the age at first pregnancy. Information on such social factors needs to be collected directly. Just as it must not be assumed that differences between ethnic groups are genetic, so it is with cultural hypotheses. The validity of these must also be tested and demonstrated.

Only when conceptual decisions of the kind discussed in 3.4.1–3.4.5 are made, and the purposes and contexts of the work have been defined, can practical issues in relation to data collection be tackled.

3.5 Collecting ethnicity and health data

Ethnicity is not easily assessed, as we would expect for any complex variable. Before reading on try Exercise 3.5.

Exercise 3.5 Assessing ethnicity

♦ Reflect on methods of assessing a person's ethnicity. Consider methods that would allow self-assessment and assessment by others.
♦ What method have you or would you use?
♦ What method would you prefer in the assessment of your own ethnicity?

Three broad approaches to collecting ethnicity and race data are used i.e. self-assessment, assessment by an observer on the basis of relevant data (whether self-reported or otherwise), and assignment by an observer on the basis of visual inspection. The last is becoming unacceptable now, though normal practice in the past and still seen today, particularly when staff feel embarrassed to ask the questions required. Table 3.3 summarizes the main approaches to assigning ethnicity and race, and these are discussed below. Table 3.4 lists the markers that would help assignment, sorting them by whether they are most relevant to race or ethnicity or both.

3.5.1 Self assessment of ethnic group

Over the last few decades the view has come to the fore, that ethnicity is primarily a matter of self-perception of identity, as influenced by factors such as ancestry, physical features, culture, religion, language and country of birth. Others' perception of our ethnic group is also factored into our self perception, as the vignettes in Chapter 1 illustrate. Voluntary, self-classification of ethnicity, albeit using a checklist, is rapidly becoming the most acceptable and most widely adopted method of collecting ethnicity data. As shown in the previous chapter, this principle has guided the classifications used in international

Table 3.3 Main methods of assigning ethnicity

Skin colour
Country of birth
Name analysis
Family origin, and
Self-assessed ethnic group

Table 3.4 Potential markers of race or ethnicity for self or observer assignment

Relating mainly to concepts of race	Relating to both concepts of race and ethnicity	Relating mainly to concepts of ethnicity
Skin colour, and other physical features, such as hair texture and facial features	Skin colour, and other physical features, such as hair texture and facial features	Name
Ancestral origin	Ancestral origin Family origin Migration history	Language Religion Dietary preferences and taboos Family origin Migration history

censuses, and was introduced in the UK in the 1991 census. The principle has been endorsed by the UK's Council for Racial Equality. The concept underpins the introduction of ethnic monitoring in the UK NHS.

As discussed in Chapter 1, ethnicity is a highly complex matter. The freely chosen responses generated by people describing their perceived ethnicity, such as those in the vignettes, are not suitable for statistical purposes, where easy aggregation is essential. The almost universally adopted compromise in epidemiological and statistical work is to invite self assessment of ethnicity using a limited set of categories. The development of these categories requires considerable work to ensure that they are acceptable, workable, and produce useful outputs. The ways that categories change over time and some of their strengths and limitations were discussed in Chapter 2.

From a scientific standpoint, self-assessed ethnicity is changeable over even very short time periods and is not subject to the control of the investigator, characteristics which are counter to the principles of measurement in science, including epidemiology. Having said this, it is remarkable that there is great stability in self-report of ethnic group amongst White, Indian, Pakistani, Bangladeshi, Chinese and many other populations. The greatest instability in self-report has been seen in Black/African, Hispanic, and Native American-origin populations. The quotation below is fairly typical of a number of studies examining this issue although the finding on Blacks is both encouraging and surprising.

> In our comparison of self-reported ethnicity with ethnicity recorded in the Northern California Kaiser administrative records, we found that the sensitivities and positive predictive values were excellent among blacks and whites; slightly lower, yet still high, among Asians; fair among Hispanics; and poor among American Indians. These patterns are consistent with previous studies of ethnic misclassification in administrative databases.
>
> Gomez *et al.* (2005: 76, 78)

The implication is that more research is required with these populations to find terms that are more consistent over time, and that probably means finding terms that fit better with self-perceptions.

While the question of how to categorize people of mixed origins is an extremely difficult one, self-report methods allow the respondents to resolve the matter, and the capacity to either describe their own ethnicity in free text, or to choose more than one category. Self-report assists, and may be the only solution, in what is undoubtedly a difficult matter.

3.5.2 Country of birth of self, parents and grandparents

Self-reported country of birth, coded on UK birth and death certificates, reported in the UK censuses, and held on population registries in continental Europe is commonly used as a proxy for ethnicity. It is, comparatively speaking, readily available because it is so often collected for administrative purposes. A question on country of birth is in most censuses, and in the UK it has been included in each census since 1841. It is a relatively objective but crude method of ethnic group classification for recent migrants.

The country of birth may not, however, relate to self- or other-perceived ethnic group at all. For example, a large number of elderly people living in European colonial countries were born in the colonies. In Scotland, for instance, at the 2001 census more than 50 per cent of those aged 65 years or more who were born in India classified their ethnic group as White.

People may be born abroad when their parents are travelling on vacation, on temporary work assignments, or working in the diplomatic service, to take a few examples. (Such a circumstance of birth gives rights of residence and nationality in some countries.) This method of assigning ethnicity does not take account of the diversity of the country of origin of the individual. India is, for example, culturally diverse, with innumerable distinct ethnic groups, a complex caste system, at least eight major religions and many official languages. Yet Indians are grouped as one by this method, a classification comparable in its heterogeneity to European.

The ethnic group of children of immigrants is not directly identifiable using this method. Country of birth as a proxy for ethnicity, therefore, becomes more inaccurate with time. One answer is to ask for the country of birth of parents, and/or grandparents and so on. The further back one goes the greater the difficulty of obtaining accurate data, and the greater the chances of parental/grandparental birthplace being in more than one country, creating difficulties in assigning a single ethnic group.

The St James survey in Trinidad and the Newcastle Heart Project used parental and grandparental national origin, and birthplace, respectively, to help assign more accurately the ethnicity of those being examined. Whilst it can help to more accurately assess individual origins and ethnicity by complementing other data sets, the method requires more information, adds rigidity to assignment, may override self-perception and yields a potentially large 'mixed' group (people with fewer than three grandparents from the same country, for example). Unlike self-reported ethnicity, there is no logical way of handling these mixed groups. In some places the father's country of birth takes precedence, in other places the mother's place of birth does. These decisions are arbitrary, and usually related to the politics of immigration.

Self-reported family origin has been used. This approach is also based upon ancestry and birthplace, usually of parents or grandparents. It is relatively straightforward and stable though individuals within particular groups cannot be considered homogeneous in respect of either ethnicity or health. Both self-perception and family origin are closely related. The difficulty with this approach occurs, as with many methods of assigning ethnicity, when an individual responds as having mixed family origins.

3.5.3 Assessment by an observer using relevant data

Methods of ethnic group classification that do not rely on direct contact with individuals are highly sought-after, particularly in societies and situations where people are uncomfortable about asking directly, or even giving out a self completion form.

3.5.3.1 Name search

An increasingly popular method is assignment of ethnicity using the name of an individual. Classification of ethnic status by inspecting names has been used to identify a range of populations including South Asian, Chinese, Hispanic and Irish. Experience of this method in the UK is fairly substantial where, in particular, it has been used to identify people with origins in the Indian subcontinent. South Asian names are distinctive, often relate to religion, region of India, occupation and caste. Marriage with other Indians is the norm even in Indians throughout the world. For South Asians the method is both sensitive and specific, i.e. it successfully identifies most South Asians from a list of names from a mix of ethnic groups (sensitive) and when a name is said to be non-South Asian that judgment is usually correct (specific). The method is by no means perfect. Some South Asian names are not distinctive (e.g. Gill), South Asians may deliberately Europeanize their names, South Asian Christians share names with White populations and marriage outside the South Asian community does occur and is increasing, meaning that South Asian women, in particular, may be difficult to identify by name, and women of other ethnic groups might be wrongly identified as South Asian.

Computerized name search algorithms are available e.g. to allocate Chinese and South Asian ethnic status. The performance of some computer packages has been studied in detail. The Nam Pehchan programme developed in Bradford performed well in that city and in other places in England. It was found to identify names of Pakistani ethnic origin better than those of Indian ethnic origin. The proportion of those judged by the computer program to be South Asian who actually turn out to be so (known as predictive power of a positive test) depends on the percentage of the population that is actually South Asian. The predictive power of this programme was found to be low in Scotland, because only 1 per cent of the population is South Asian. In places where the population is proportionately small it is essential that the ethnic group assignments of the programme are checked by expert observers. This is probably good practice everywhere.

The concept of name searching is, however, simple enough, and the methods could be adopted for other populations. The problem is that for some populations the name is not distinctive e.g. many people of African origin, and particularly those coming from the Caribbean, may have traditional European names, or names associated with religions they have adopted. Of course, this might help if one were searching for people with a particular religion. Muslims share a naming system that transcends countries of origin and ethnic groups. Such names are poor at identifying country of origin, or self-assessed ethnic group, but are excellent for identifying Muslims. The method's validity needs to be demonstrated in other ethnic groups, as experience is more limited.

It is not uncommon for researchers to do a name search on their lists of people with a disease or health problem (the numerator of the rate) but take information on the population at risk (denominator) from the census. This creates a mismatch between numerator and denominator. In a study in Canada examining mortality by ethnic group, Sheth and colleagues took the unusual step of validating name search against country of birth, as indicated in the quotation below.

> Our approach to this problem is unique in that we combined last names and country of birth criteria in classifying South Asian and Chinese ethnicity.
>
> This study is also unique in that we have selected self-reported ethnicity as the denominator for mortality rate calculation and validated its comparability to last name as a measure of ethnic status. We found that last names correspond to self-reported ethnicity among SA with high sensitivity and specificity. These results would suggest that last names and self-reported ethnicity are indeed comparable measure of ethnic status.
>
> Sheth *et al.* (1997: 293)

Even if such methods can be developed further, they fail fail to address the needs of all ethnic groups in an equitable manner and, therefore, are unlikely to meet the requirements of race relations legislation, e.g. the Race Relations Amendment Act 2000 in the UK, which requires public bodies to 'promote good relations between persons of different racial groups'. Self-evidently, name searching also ignores the increasingly common recommendation that ethnic group should be self-assigned.

3.5.4 Assessment on the basis of visual inspection

A classification based on physical traits (phenotype, or physiognomy) seems an obvious and logical way to assign race, if not ethnicity. The physical features most closely associated with race are the skin colour, facial contours, and colour and type of hair. These features are largely but not wholly, genetically determined, and are clearly related and relevant to the principle of race. Observers have classified people using such features, indeed this was the standard method until very recently.

This approach is generally judged as distasteful, subjective, imprecise and unreliable. Some of the criticisms, however, may derive from the political misuse of the concept of race in numerous societies throughout history (see Chapters 6 and 9). Clearly, many people would be difficult to differentiate and classify, even in broad groupings, on looks alone. This approach is currently out of favour, but it continues as shown in the following quotation.

> We found that although 85 per cent of hospital administrators surveyed reported always collecting patient data on 'race' in their hospitals, half obtained race by observing a patient's physical appearance and only 12 per cent allowed for multiple affiliations. This is consistent with findings from a New York City medical center showing that, despite decisions on the part of administrators to collect better ethnic data, admission clerks rarely requested ethnic information from patients.
>
> Gomez *et al.* (2005: 76, 78)

Perhaps observer-assigned methods should not be discarded, but seen as a component of a more sophisticated approach. In a recent study of myopia by Tung and colleagues in Australia, as part of a package of information to assign ethnicity, a photograph of the subjects was placed in the records (personal written communication). In practice, the photograph was not used, but the idea is a reasonable one. The greatest limitation, from a research point of view, of this approach is that it is crude; and is unlikely to differentiate at any more than the continental or subcontinental level, which is similar to modern-day genetic methods. It is most improbable that the method can differentiate between subgroups of Indians (e.g. Muslim Punjabi, and Hindu Punjabi), Chinese (e.g. Mandarin or Cantonese speakers), Africans from a variety of countries and tribes, and Europeans (e.g. Italian or French).

Observations can, nonetheless, help assign ethnicity. In addition to physical features, the observer can observe other clues e.g. the type of dress, the type of food eaten, or the language spoken. Some types of dress are highly distinctive e.g. the wearing of a kilt is closely associated with Scottish identity, the Hijab with Islam, the sari with being Indian etc. Even taking into account physical features and these additional cultural clues, an observer could not accurately distinguish, by observation alone, between Muslim and Hindu Punjabis, who are in several important respects culturally distinct though in others similar, or between people from Norway and Ireland. Given an opportunity to define their own ethnicity in health studies they would probably not place themselves in the same ethnic group. However, they are likely to be in the same racial group (though it is unclear which of the currently available racial groupings the South Asian groups above are in). Observation can be seen as a potential adjunct to self-report, but probably no more.

3.5.5 Combining self-reported data and observation

An observer might use a range of data to assign ethnicity including self-assigned ethnicity, reported country of birth and family origins i.e. self-report and observer assignment are not necessarily mutually exclusive. As ethnicity is a multifaceted concept it makes some sense to assign ethnicity using several variables. Hazuda and colleagues (1988) identified Mexican-American Hispanics using father's surname, mother's maiden name, birthplace, self-assessed ethnic identity and stated ethnicity of grandparents. The method was valid in reflecting both common origin and current identification, but such approaches require much data. Investigators would need to be sure that this adds value to simpler approaches before going down this path.

Even with detailed information of this kind the assignment might be wrong, as illustrated in the following quotation.

> The idea that certain 'scores' for a set of indictors will predict ethnicity has several associated problems. Even an exhaustive set of characteristics—for example country of birth, nationality, mother tongue or language spoken at home, parents country of birth, skin colour, national origin, racial group and religion—would, if measured in Yugoslavia in 1985, have failed to differentiate between Serbs and Croats who were personally atheist or agnostic but who would, 5 years later, have found themselves involved in a major interethnic conflict.
>
> Office for National Statistics (2005, p25, unpublished document, cited with permission)

3.6 **Practicalities of assigning ethnicity in health settings**

It is very difficult to put these ideas into practice. Assigning ethnicity in the context of censuses is demonstrably achievable, presumably because of the combination of a national integrated effort, earmarked funding, a long-standing research base and legislative force (Chapter 2). The bigger challenge is in following the same path in health care settings, particularly on a small scale, in places where the minority population is small (and where the need for data may be particularly acute). There are substantial gaps in the information available on the health status of, and the utilization of health services by, ethnic groups in most countries including the UK, and the main exception internationally is the substantial work on the Black/White population dichotomy in the USA. Monitoring the ethnic group of users of services is advocated to fill such gaps and to encourage a focus on the health needs of local minority populations. The main loci for such monitoring are primary and secondary care, administrative records, and through linkage. The policies underpinning ethnic monitoring are discussed in Chapter 8. The following account focuses on the UK scene, although the difficulties illustrated are widespread. Professionals have been calling for data for some decades, and the call was taken up by the English Health Department more than 15 years ago.

3.6.1 **Primary care**

In 1990, the Department of Health in England proposed that patients' ethnicity should be stated in GP referral letters. The rationale was that ethnic group data would be collected at patient's first point of contact with the National Health Service (NHS) and made available on referral. (Instead, recording of the ethnicity of hospitalized patients was introduced nationally from April 1995. This has not been wholly successful and the original proposal was probably better.)

Collecting ethnicity data in primary care settings makes sense because virtually everyone in many countries, including the UK, is registered with or regularly consults one general practitioner, or even if this is not the case most people have regular contact with the local primary care services. This gives an opportunity for capturing ethnicity data on a large proportion of the population.

Opportunities to promote health rather than treat diseases may be more realistic in primary care, and targeting such services would benefit from ethnicity data. Furthermore, when referrals are made to secondary care ethnic grouping can be sent with the referral letter. The problem is one of putting an apparently good idea into daily practice.

Sangowawa and Bhopal (2000) demonstrated the feasibility and acceptability of ethnic monitoring in primary care even in an area where a small proportion of the population was from ethnic minority groups i.e. north-east England. One general practitioner and one practice manager interviewed from each of eight general practices all supported ethnic monitoring in primary care, and thought that it may lead to improvement in

Table 3.5 Summary of responses to interview questions

Question	Number of responses (n = 16) (%)	
	Yes	No
Are you aware of ethnic monitoring in primary care?	5 (31)	11 (69)
Do you think that GPs may benefit from ethnic monitoring?	16 (100)	0 (0)
Do you think that patients may benefit from ethnic monitoring?	16 (100)	0 (0)
Do you feel that provision of health care services may improve with ethnic monitoring?	16 (100)	0 (0)
Do you support the implementation of ethnic monitoring in primary care across all Cleveland?	16 (100)	0 (0)

Extract from Sangowawa and Bhopal (2000).

provision of health care services and potential benefits for both patients and service providers (Table 3.5).

They thought it would be more beneficial to implement monitoring across the whole of their area rather than in selected practices. Other issues raised include the need for incentives to encourage compliance, for training staff, and education of the patient population.

A system for ethnic monitoring of patients attending two practices and inclusion of ethnic group data in GP referral letters was put in place. Effectively, the practice receptionists collected ethnicity data on attending patients, entering it on the computer system. In general practice A none of 2559 patients refused to indicate their ethnicity but more than one-third of patients were missed. In practice B, only 5 patients of 4096 patients refused to indicate their ethnicity and about one-fifth of patients were missed. Overall, of the 181 referral letters sent 160 (88.4 per cent) had a note on the patients' ethnic group. This demonstrated that ethnic group data can be collected and used to inform hospitals. The very high compliance achieved when a field was created in the referral letter template demonstrated the power of automation using computer technology. Scaling up this demonstration to a national level will bring its own challenges, but this is being attempted in Scotland at present. In the UK a small financial incentive has been provided for general practices that collect the ethnic code of newly registered patients.

3.6.2 **Secondary care**

It is widely accepted that, in a number of countries, a mixture of institutional racism and language and cultural barriers affect utilization and quality of hospital care of ethnic minority groups (see Chapter 8). Whether such beliefs are true or false is an important matter that needs to be evaluated using quantitative and qualitative research. A fundamental building block is ethnic monitoring of patients using the service. Ethnic monitoring was, as stated above, introduced in all hospitals in England in 1995. The codes were based upon census categories, though recognizing that they might be insufficient to meet the needs of the local population. The guidelines indicated that categories should be adapted for the particular service and the data system might include other relevant items such as religion, language, or dietary requirements.

Collecting valid data on ethnic group of people using hospital services has proven difficult even when ethnic monitoring is national policy, and generally the information remains incomplete and of variable quality making its interpretation difficult. This incompleteness may reflect variable commitment to collecting data; lack of awareness, or relevant training, about its importance; lack of custom-designed computer systems; and lack of use of data already being collected in research, clinical audit, service planning and delivery. Alternatively, there may have been an underestimation of the difficulties, sometimes interpersonal ones, of collecting ethnic group data in the context of busy hospitals dealing with large numbers of sick people needing urgent attention. The reasons include the possibility that staff do not like to ask questions about ethnicity because of the possibility that they might seem to be 'racist'. In Chapter 8, there is a table outlining some of the perceived obstacles and solutions, in the context of the implementation of the new Scottish ethnic monitoring programme. The new programme will replace one that has not worked.

Voluntary and optional completion of data does not work as shown by experience in Scotland. Between 1996 and 2004 a code for ethnic group was optional in the Scottish hospital admissions and discharges record. The guidance stated 'Although not mandatory, it is strongly recommended that these items be completed whenever the information is available.' Ethnicity was missing in around 94 per cent of records at the end of this period. Furthermore, it was not clear whether ethnicity was based on assessment of appearance by administrative staff or whether patients (or relatives) were asked to state the ethnic group. Ethnic group was recorded in only 18 per cent of Scottish cancer registrations.

An ethnic monitoring tool kit has been developed in Scotland and is currently being implemented. Ethnic monitoring is seen as vital and promoted by both the Race Relations Amendment Act 2000, and by the English health plan, and the Scottish Fair for All policy. It is also a central component of policies in other countries, including the USA.

Interpretation of data in ethnicity and health is often difficult, as illustrated in relation to mortality.

3.6.3 Mortality data

Death certificates seldom have ethnic grouping. Self-identified ethnicity is obviously problematic for mortality data, as it would need to be collected before death. One potential answer to this problem is data linkage, as discussed in the next section. In some places, including the UK, country of birth is recorded both on death certificates and census returns.

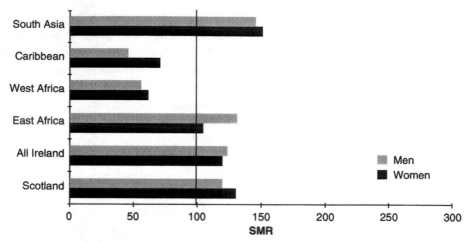

Fig. 3.3 Standardized mortality ratios for CHD by sex for selected countries of birth, 1989–92, in England and Wales
Source of data for figure: Wild and McKeigue (1997: 705–10). Reproduced from the British Heart Foundation, website http://www.heartstats.org/temp/PFigsp1.10bspweb06.ppt.

As country of birth is often recorded on the death certificates, information on mortality by country of birth is common, including the example in Figure 3.3, showing an analysis of coronary heart disease mortality by country of birth in England and Wales. Before reading on, try the following exercise.

Exercise 3.6 Analysis of heart disease mortality by country of birth in England and Wales

- What potential limitations can you see in accepting that the mortality variations shown in Figure 3.3 are true?
- Specifically, what errors might be present in the numbers of deaths, and the numbers of population at risk that are required to produce the disease rates that underlie the calculation of the standardized majority ratios (SMRs)?

Potential pitfalls in the analysis of mortality data will be discussed in more detail in Chapter 5 (Section 5.2.5). Country of birth provides a fair guide to ethnicity for recent migrants, particularly older people. However, even in relatively new immigrant groups, a large proportion of the population might be younger and born in the host country. The reason for this is that migrants tend to be in the age group (20–40 years) when raising a family is important. Currently, 40–50 per cent of people from UK non-White minority ethnic groups e.g., Indians, Pakistanis, and Chinese were born in the UK (with higher proportions among younger people) so country of birth information is becoming less useful. Most deaths, however, occur in the older age groups, so country of birth remains of some value even in these circumstances.

As discussed already, country of birth is potentially misleading for people who were born abroad but would classify themselves as of an ethnic group unrelated to the country of birth. For example, Scotland had a major role in the British Empire. While 98.9 per cent of White Scottish people were born in Scotland or England, this still means over 1 per cent (about 50,000 people) were born elsewhere. Some of them, especially the older ones contributing most deaths, were born in British colonies. Indeed, an analysis of the census data confirmed this, with most people born in India who were > 65 years of age in 2001 being self-classified as White. Many Scottish residents who perceive themselves as Indians, however, are born neither in Scotland nor India, but in a variety of other countries.

In the absence of valid ethnic group data, country of birth analysis has provided insights into health and disease inequalities. These analyses are also of value in their own right i.e. not merely as a proxy for ethnic group, but as a marker of migration status, and migration history, and in particular exposure to different countries at a particularly sensitive period in relation to health. For example, migration studies have shown that people born in northern Europe, e.g. Scotland, where there is a comparatively high risk of multiple sclerosis, but living in countries such as Australia where the risk is comparatively low, continue to have high risk if they migrated after childhood, but not if they migrated at a very young age.

The interpretation of country of birth analyses done using census denominators and death certificate data is complex, and has been discussed in some detail by Gill and colleagues (2006). In brief, the count of deaths (numerator) may be wrong because (a) some people may enter a country and die there but are not normally resident, e.g. they are tourists, business visitors, or have come for medical care (b) some people who are normally resident may prefer to leave the country to die elsewhere e.g. the country of birth (so-called salmon bias, as this fish tries to return to die at its place of birth). Even if such deaths are notified in the normally resident country, which is possible for administrative and other reasons, the cause of death may not be known. These effects are too seldom studied.

Cause of death may be incorrect. Diagnosing the cause of death without an autopsy is an imprecise part of the art of medicine. Whether there are variations by country of birth in the accuracy of the cause of death is not known, although on first principles one anticipates that there will be, for example, the medical history may be less accurate in those people born overseas who do not speak the local language well, making it more difficult for the doctor to identify the cause of death. The likelihood of gaining permission for an autopsy to ascertain more accurately the cause of death will vary by ethnic group.

The numerator (e.g. death) is turned into a disease rate using a population denominator i.e. number of people at risk. In some countries such as the Netherlands, this information is obtained from local government population registries. The death data and the population registries there can be linked exactly using a personal identifying number. This leads to an accurate assessment of the death rate by country of birth. In other countries, including the UK, this is not possible, and census data are used to estimate population size and structure. In most countries, the census is held once every 10 years, and the figures are most imprecise for mobile young adults and inner city populations (though the published figures may be adjusted for undercounts). There are, therefore, likely to be variations in the precision of denominators by country of birth group. The data from several censuses can be used to estimate the between-census population sizes by extrapolation.

Given appropriate interpretation the data are of potential value not least because they are available for a long period, as country of birth data have been, and remain, a central component of many censuses across the world. Try Exercise 3.7 before reading on.

Exercise 3.7 The value of data

◆ What value can you see in the data on coronary heart disease mortality by country of birth in Figure 3.3?
◆ Another way to answer this is to ask what would be lost without such data?
◆ What insights are gained by looking at these data?

International variations in CHD are well-documented, and although the rates are rising, generally mortality is comparatively low in the Indian subcontinent, Africa and the Caribbean. On the basis of such international studies we would expect ethnic variations in CHD within a multi-ethnic country. On first principles we would expect recently migrating minority ethnic groups living in industrialized countries to have, in comparison with the population as a whole, lower CHD. For example, we would expect relatively lower CHD in South Asian women, particularly Indians, who tend towards vegetarianism, and have low smoking prevalence.

Information on mortality by racial or ethnic group, in many countries including the UK, is not easily available. In these circumstances, country of birth offers an alternative. We see from Figure 3.3 that, as anticipated, variations are indeed present, but there is an important surprise—those born in the Indian subcontinent have a considerable excess of mortality, and not a deficit.

The lessons are that investigators need to be creative for information by race and ethnicity is not always easy to obtain; in this example country of birth is a reasonable proxy for ethnic group; general principles are inaccurate in predicting mortality patterns; and the differences shown have huge implications for public health, clinical practice and epidemiological research. Country of birth can continue to be of use in analysis of mortality data. Analysis of such data is recommended to add to our understanding of ethnicity and health for policy and service purposes, to contribute ideas for epidemiological and clinical research, and to compare and contrast findings with a large and growing international research literature. Box 3.4 summarizes these points. We need race and ethnicity but we need to do better than hitherto, and one potentially better approach is data linkage.

Box 3.4 Lessons from studies of immigrant mortality in CHD

- ◆ Coronary heart disease (CHD) is the dominant cause of death
- ◆ International variations in CHD are well-documented
- ◆ There are racial/ethnic variations in CHD
- ◆ On first principles, we would expect recently migrated minority ethnic groups to have lower CHD rates e.g. South Asian women, particularly Indians, tend towards vegetarianism, and have low smoking prevalence
- ◆ Information on mortality by racial or ethnic group is not yet published (but will be available in Scotland shortly)
- ◆ Several studies, including one by my Edinburgh colleague, Sarah Wild, have examined CHD by country of birth
- ◆ Investigators need to be creative as information by race and ethnicity is not always easy to obtain—here country of birth is a reasonable proxy for ethnic group
- ◆ First principles are inaccurate in predicting mortality patterns
- ◆ The patterns shown have huge implications for public health, clinical practice and epidemiological research
- ◆ We need race and ethnicity but we need to do better than hitherto

3.6.4 Linking data

There are some strengths in indirect methods of assigning ethnicity, e.g. name and country of birth. Notwithstanding the value of the data captured by such methods, they are not based on individual data including self-reported ethnic group. Record linkage provides a potential way to add self-assigned ethnicity to individual medical and death records. In some countries such as Norway, Sweden and the Netherlands locally based population registers have a unique identifying code that can be used to link data sets. As stated above, the Netherlands' data sets have country of birth but not ethnic group. In the absence of self-identified ethnic grouping, more complicated methods of data linkage are needed.

One major source of self-defined race or ethnicity data is the population census. Strictly speaking censuses tend to capture the ethnicity assigned by the person who fills in the census form, usually the head of household. There is an understandable concern about linking health data to census data, particularly as the uses of the latter are often tightly controlled by law. In a recent project in Scotland, such a linkage approach was considered acceptable only if the information on individuals remained strictly confidential except to those with previous authorized access. A strict protocol using computerized methods that prevents disclosure of personal information has been developed and tested. This study succeeded in its goals, achieving the pre-set standards for linkage (Bhopal *et al.* 2005).

Table 3.6 Directly standardized first acute myocardial infarction rates (incidence) using the matched population of 25 years and older from the Scottish census population 2001 as reference

Sex/ethnicity	Person years of observation	Adjusted rate/1000	95% confidence interval
Female			
Non South Asian	4557730	2.56	2.51–2.60
South Asian	24762	4.86	3.05–6.67

From Bhopal *et al.* (2005)—with permission from co-authors.

The methods created provided an innovative, cost-effective and ethical way to extract information by ethnic group from health databases. Cohort analyses can be done on data sets that link individuals to future outcomes on a one-to-one basis. On the assumption that the probability linkage is accurately linking individuals on the census to individual health outcomes, on a one-to-one basis, the output is a cohort analysis, with the census providing baseline data. The numerators are the morbidity and mortality counts based on the hospital discharge and deaths databases. As such we get an estimate of the incidence of disease based on new cases. Sample analysis is shown in Table 3.6.

What can we do, however, if there are no data and linkage is not feasible?

3.6.5 **Modelling data**

To prevent and control diseases it is necessary to know about the frequency and distribution of disease patterns and risk factors. However, there may be no such data, particularly in small areas. A potential way out of this dilemma is to extrapolate from data sources in other populations with a similar population structure. e.g. apply data from England to the ethnic groups in the Scottish population or from Oslo Norway to Bergen. The assumption behind this approach is that the distribution of diseases and risk factors is about the same in the ethnic groups in both populations except that demographic and social structures differ.

In England, data are available in relative abundance compared to Scotland and most other European countries e.g. from the 1999 Health Survey of England, country of birth mortality analyses, surveys such as the Newcastle Heart Project and many other sources.

The Scottish retrospective ethnic coding project, mentioned previously, aimed to use these data, together with population data on ethnic minorities in Scotland, to model the burden of some risk factors. The data source for this approach was the Health Survey for England 1999 with a boost sample for ethnic minority groups—see Erens *et al.* (2001). The project was able to demonstrate that it is possible to impute reasonable estimates for prevalence of health-related risks. Also, it was possible to estimate the distribution of continuous variables and present these as average (mean) in a distinct ethnic group and give confidence limits.

While conceptually this approach might work, it is unlikely, on its own, to satisfy the public, policy-makers, and researchers. It will certainly not meet legal and policy obligations.

3.6.6 Retrospective addition of ethnic codes

Routine health data generally provide incomplete information about ethnicity. The Scottish retrospective ethnic coding project was the result of a collaboration between several Scottish agencies between 2002–2005. Its objective was to see whether we could use existing databases to create analyses by ethnic group, particularly by adding ethnic codes retrospectively. It demonstrated that the data can be obtained at relatively low cost, and reasonable timescales, given cooperation between agencies and appropriate skills within the research team. Bhopal and colleagues' (2005) conclusions and recommendations from this project included these:

1. Name search methods offer some benefits but need considerable extra refinement if they are to be used in automatic mode i.e. without visual inspection by experts.

2. Country of birth is a reasonable proxy for ethnicity for recent ethnic minority migrant populations in the middle years of life and is of interest in itself.

3. Modelling has shown its value as a stopgap measure.

4. Linking ethnic codes on the census to mortality and morbidity databases is an approach that has great potential. The probability linkage method is likely to be exportable internationally wherever there is a census recording ethnic codes and an electronic health database with administrative details.

3.7 Interpreting data

The above discussion of approaches to collecting ethnicity data, and the examples of the strengths and weaknesses of the resultant outputs, should make it self-evident that data systems need to be designed to record, retrieve and analyse data to meet specified purposes, and should include information on the underlying concepts and methods for the benefits of data users. The users need to interpret the data and come to valid explanations for differences and similarities, or at least valid questions that guide interpretation.

Systems for data interpretation are fundamental to the science and art of epidemiology, and the real/apparent framework detailed in the textbook *Concepts of Epidemiology* (Bhopal 2002) will help interested readers. In brief, disease variations are often illusory, and arise from data errors and artefacts. A systematic approach to the analysis of variation in disease begins by differentiating artefactual change from real change. Differences can arise from data and system error; random error; bias in data collection; socio-economic and lifestyle difference; other cultural factors and genetic factors. Over-interpretation, particularly reaching unsubstantiated conclusions that differences arise from genetic factors, needs to be avoided. Real differences occur because there are differences in host susceptibility, in external agents' capacity to cause disease, and in the influence of the environment. In these circumstances, the epidemiological challenge is to pinpoint the causal factors.

Most quantitative research on ethnicity and health is epidemiological, or it uses closely related survey methods in social sciences. Epidemiological studies are prone to error, because they study human populations in natural settings and this is a complex matter especially when faced by time and cost constraints. The potential problems will be discussed in some detail in Chapter 9. In brief, three broad problems confront epidemiologists: selection of population, quality of information, and confounding. Confounding causes an error in the assessment of the association between a disease and a postulated causal factor. It results from comparing groups which differ in characteristics other than the postulated causal factor under study. In the following quotation, there is an example of failing to account for confounding. Essentially, an investigator jumped to the conclusion that the Irish population had a high rate of insanity. Once, however, social class differences were taken into account—so that like was being compared with like— their rate of insanity was lower than in the comparison population. We will discuss other examples in Chapter 9.

> Jarvis also proposed explanations for what he supposed, mistakenly, was an increased prevalence of insanity among the Irish in the lower social class. 'Besides these principles (low vital force), which apply to the poor as a general law there is good ground for supposing that the habits and condition and character of the Irish poor in this country operate more unfavourably upon their mental health, and hence produce a larger number of the insane in ratio of their numbers than is found among the native poor. Unquestionably,' he wrote, 'much of their insanity is due to their intemperance, to which the Irish seem to be peculiarly prone, and much to that exaltation which comes from increased prosperity.'
> A more complete analysis of the data would have disconfirmed Jarvis' prejudices: the slight increase in the unadjusted crude prevalence of insanity he observed in the Irish disappeared, was even reversed, upon adjustment for social class.
>
> Stoep (1998: 1397)

Principles which apply to all studies and help minimize these errors include: construct research questions and hypotheses carefully, so as to benefit all the populations equally; study representative populations; measure accurately and with equal care across groups; compare like with like; and check before assuming that inferences and generalizations apply across groups.

The importance of interpreting health data on ethnic minority groups with care cannot be overemphasized, especially when these apparently show a higher degree of disability or disease than the population as a whole. It is still a normal practice to compare health data in minority ethnic groups with those of the ethnic majority, usually the White/European origin population, as in Figure 3.3 and Table 3.1. A comparative approach has many strengths. This is potentially, however, an ethnocentric approach that can be misleading by concentrating on specific issues and diverting attention from the more common causes of morbidity and mortality. For example, while there may be some differences between ethnic groups in health patterns, generally the big picture will follow that of the whole population e.g. in most of Europe and North America cardiovascular, neoplastic and respiratory diseases are the major fatal diseases for all ethnic groups. In a recent analysis of mortality in England and Wales by Gill and colleagues, the top five causes of mortality by the chapter headings of the International Classification Of Diseases (ICD) in all minority ethnic groups were:

◆ Diseases of the circulatory system (ICD 390-459)

◆ Neoplasms (ICD 140-239)

◆ Injury and poisoning (ICD 800-999)

◆ Diseases of the respiratory system (ICD 460-519)

◆ Endocrine, nutritional and metabolic diseases, and immunity disorders (ICD 240-279).

It is important that actual (or absolute) and relative disease patterns are both examined because they give a very different picture. This issue is discussed in some detail in Chapter 7 on priority setting.

3.8 Making use of data

Collecting data has a cost. This is, obviously, partly financial, but sometimes it is less tangible e.g. public perceptions. To justify the cost it is imperative that the data are analysed and used well. In health care, public health and epidemiological contexts, there is an ethical obligation to use data to do good (see Chapters 8 and 10 for further discussion). Turning data into useful recommendations that can be used to alter policy, strategy or plans, in turn to improve services or health status, is no easy matter. Usually, the benefits are intangible, long-term and diffuse. In the above examples of variations in smoking and in coronary heart disease we saw how a lack of data could be seriously misleading, and how such information can change perspectives, priorities, and in turn service delivery. This will be a recurrent theme throughout this book, but will be tackled specifically in Chapters 5 and 8.

3.9 Conclusion

Collecting data by race or ethnicity is difficult, and requires both excellent information systems and excellent communications and understanding between data providers and data holders. The choice of classification should be driven by the purposes to which the data are to be put, though pragmatism will be essential. In practice, classifications will follow, at least in past, those used in the national census. There should be a widespread understanding of the concepts underlying the classification to permit valid interpretation and utilization of data. It is, in fact, unlikely that exact explanations for population differences will be achieved, and more likely that the findings will raise questions that focus attention on priorities. In the next chapter, as a foundation for moving from theory to practice, we trace an evolutionary pattern in the development of interest in ethnicity and health, using the UK as an example, before turning to the use of data in health needs assessment.

Summary

The only ethical justification for collecting data by ethnicity and health is health improvement either directly or through research. People setting up health databases and research studies need to make choices on which aspects of race and ethnicity are to be captured. These choices ought to be governed by the purposes for which the data are being collected. The method of data collection on race or ethnicity—whether self-report or some other indicator such as name—and the classification can then be chosen. The interpretation and utilisation of the data are dependent on these choices. Purpose and context will influence the concepts of ethnicity to be adopted, as well as the methods applied, and how data are interpreted and used.

There are three main approaches to collecting ethnicity and race data: self-assessment, assessment by another on the basis of relevant data, and assessment by another on the basis of observation. The last is not acceptable in contemporary societies, though normal practice in the past.

The data system needs to be designed to record, retrieve and analyse data to meet the specified purposes, and should include information on the underlying concepts and methods for the benefits of data users. The users need to interpret the data and come to valid explanations for differences and similarities, or at least valid questions that guide interpretation. A conceptual framework for such interpretation includes data and system error; random error; bias in data collection; socio-economic and lifestyle difference, other cultural factors and genetic factors. Over-interpretation, particularly reaching unsubstantiated conclusions that differences arise from genetic factors, needs to be avoided.

Chapter 4

Historical analysis of the development of health and health care services for ethnic minorities

It is these twin and entangled legacies, indelibly inscribed in our nation's history—of conquest, slavery, colonization, and immigration on the one hand and a commitment to liberty and equality on the other—that permeate our changing beliefs and understandings and constructions of the very notion of 'race/ethnicity'.

Krieger (2000: 1688)

Contents

- Chapter objectives
- Outline of the historical response to the challenges of minority ethnic group health in the UK, USA, South Africa under apartheid, the Netherlands and Australia
- The importance of political, social, research and health care context in the response of countries to the challenge of minority ethnic group health
- Analysis of the patterns of response and derivation of principles
- The role of research data and routine information systems in guiding a response—dangers and benefits
- The pressing need for ethical research and the implementation of any recommendations arising
- The rationale for continuing to develop the concepts of race and ethnicity and the classifications and related terminology
- Conclusions
- Summary of chapter

Objectives

On completion of this chapter you should be able to:

- Trace the development, using case studies internationally, of the social and institutional response to minority ethnic group health and health care challenges, and based on this, see and discuss a pattern of response and action

♦ Understand the crucial role that both research data and case studies play in instigating and directing social and institutional responses
♦ Understand that without ethnic group and race-based data a directed and rational response is not possible: hence the need to make progress on the complex task of conceptualizing ethnicity and health and devising terminology and classifications

4.1 **Introduction: migration and ethnicity**

Migration is the driving force that creates multi-ethnic societies. Migration and exploration are fundamental human behaviours, possibly relating to the evolution of humans as hunters and gatherers, moving from place to place both as a way of life, and as a way of meeting the need for food and other resources. This drive has permitted humans (who all originated in Africa) to inhabit the entire earth and adapt to local environments as diverse as the tropics, the mountains, the desert and the Arctic. There are many reasons for migration in the modern world including trade and commerce, the need for work and the demand for workers, colonization, education, aspirations for a better life, political refuge and curiosity. All are worthy and important motivations.

Migration and the health of ethnic minority populations are closely linked. The *Oxford Dictionary of Current English* defines an immigrant as 'one who immigrates; descendant of recent (especially coloured) immigrants' and to immigrate as 'come into a foreign country as a settler'. The emphasis here upon coloured immigrants is an important acknowledgement of a reality, illogical though it is. Race, the concept so closely related to 'colour', is important in relation to migration. The immigration experience of a White person migrating to the UK from northern Europe, even though unschooled in English, is likely to be more favourable than for an African or Indian person educated in English. Whether consciously or subconsciously, immigrant health is usually focused on non-White people. This is unfortunate for White disadvantaged migrant minorities. Immigrant and ethnic minority health cannot be disentangled easily, if at all, although the issues change over time and generations (so-called 'second generation, third generation' and so on).

Generally, even in the absence of data, ethnically diverse societies are conscious that the health status and health care needs of their populations vary by ethnic group. The direction of variation will not be known precisely, but there tends to be a perception that the minority is disadvantaged compared to the majority. Such perceptions of disadvantage may not exist in relation to immigration of businessmen, academics, senior professionals, colonizers and even descendants of ex-colonizers (it is amazing, for example, how warmly welcomed the British are in India). The response of the society will depend upon the prevailing values towards immigrants.

Historically, most if not all societies have been suspicious of immigrants as outsiders, and as potential harbingers of disease, and have been particularly fearful about contagious diseases. There are many historical examples but the slaughter of Jewish people to control infectious diseases is particularly gruesome. The contagion theory was once one of two dominant theories in explaining the occurrence of plague (the other being based on miasmata). Jews, a minority population in Europe that was discriminated against in many ways, were incriminated in a poorly defined causal pathway of contagion and thousands were executed in organized efforts in various places and times to control plague, particularly in the fourteenth century. Tesh (1988) gives a figure of 16,000 Jews killed in Strasbourg alone while the historian Roy Porter gives a figure of 2,000 Jews slaughtered in Strasbourg, and 12,000 in Mainz (Porter 1997). Suspicions, prejudices and stereotypes can be very dangerous to minority populations.

Societies do in fact have good reason to be suspicious of migration, of both humans and animals, because infectious diseases can be transmitted quickly over large areas, before immunity can develop. Influenza and measles are killing disorders in populations previously unexposed to them and therefore lacking in immunity. Over the last few hundred years isolated groups have been rapidly exposed to populations of strangers with devastating consequences for their health. The Tasmanian aborigines, for example, were made extinct largely by their interaction with European settlers and North American Indians were decimated by the new patterns of disease arising from both the interaction with Europeans, and later the new demoralizing social expectations and roles imposed upon them. In more modern times, the British colonized the Andaman Islands (East of India, West of Thailand) in 1857 when 5,000 people comprised the tribe Great Andamanese. In 1988, 28 were left. Measles and influenza took a major toll. The record shows that when populations mix the smaller, rural, isolated groups fare worse than urban populations—at least from infectious diseases.

Migration and population mixing have a profound effect on the disease patterns of society even for non-infectious conditions. As a generalization, over some generations, the migrant population takes on, or at least converges towards, the pattern of disease prevailing in the country to which migration takes place. The process of change is usually slow, but it can be very fast. Sometimes the incoming people can overshoot the rate of disease seen in the host population, and two of the best examples of this are the high prevalence of hypertension in West African origin populations moving outside Africa, particularly those living in the USA, and the high rate of heart disease in South Asians in numerous countries outside the Indian subcontinent. In both instances a low rate is converted to a very high one by migration. The explanations are highly complex and contested (see references for further reading e.g. book by Patel and Bhopal 2004).

Populations that are physically different, whether in terms of biology (e.g. facial features) or culture (e.g. wearing a burqua), are destined to be seen as immigrants and minorities. This is reflected in the persistence of illogical terminology such as second, third (etc.) generation immigrant—offspring of immigrants born in the receiving country are not immigrants. Immigrant health is, nonetheless, usually focused on immigrants and their descendants i.e. ethnic minorities, and in the case of Europe and North America this primarily means non-White people. This may disadvantage some White migrant populations who are themselves disadvantaged e.g. the highest all-cause mortality rates in England and Wales are in Scottish and Irish immigrants, as demonstrated by Wild and McKeigue (1997).

Most non-White immigrants, in general and in comparison to the White populations, tend to live on the margins of society, occupying the poorly paid jobs, the lower quality housing and a lower social status. This is particularly true in the early years of migration but it may persist over long periods. Arguably, many African-Americans are still shrugging off the disadvantages of the legacy of their immigration in the era of slavery and historical racism.

The key potential contribution of race and ethnicity in epidemiology and public health is to point to actions that can help these minority populations directly, and contribute to the well-being of the whole population indirectly. Some of these points are summarised in box 4.1. In so doing, a consciousness of the harm done by the concept of race in the past is necessary. As discussed in Chapter 1, race has been used in justifying slavery and colonialism, abetting eugenics, contributing to the unfortunate and damaging debate on the IQ of human subgroups, underpinning harmful medical research, and promoting genocide as in Nazi Germany, to list some of the harms. (Figure 4.1 lampoons the IQ and race debate.) This burden now lies heavily on the shoulders of those who advocate the active use of race or ethnicity to promote well-being of populations, and the creation of harmonious, dynamic, multi-ethnic societies. In the next section I consider how five countries have responded to the issues of race and ethnicity. I focus on the UK and the USA, the countries I know best, with some other illustrative and complementary observations on the other three countries.

Box 4.1 Population data

- ◆ Migration is dynamic, with surprisingly rapid changes in population composition
- ◆ Data by country of birth, ethnic group and religion only available for limited census years
- ◆ Census incomplete, numerically, and in terms of population categories
- ◆ Population projections make estimates of births, deaths, migration but do not give local information
- ◆ Immigrants and their families comprise a population of special interest in public health

Before reading on try Exercise 4.1.

Exercise 4.1 Potential responses of societies to ethnic variations in health status or health care

- ◆ What range of responses can you foresee – in general terms, and
- ◆ Can you outline the likely chronological order for these responses:

   (a)   in practice
   (b)   ideally?

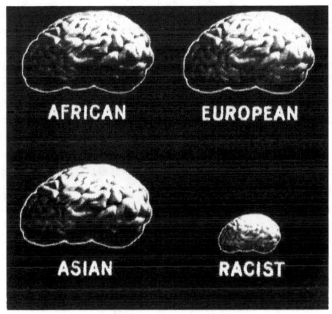

Fig. 4.1 A Cartoon published by the Council for Racial Equality, UK.
Source: CRE, origins unknown.

4.2 Characterizing society's response to the health aspects of migration

In an ideal world, where migrants were welcomed and perceived as new and necessary contributors to the receiving community, one might anticipate that there would be a rapid assessment of needs followed by the delivery of the services needed to prepare the newcomers for their roles. In a health setting newcomers might be introduced to the health threats facing them, i.e. pressures to drink alcohol, smoke cigarettes and eat a high fat, high energy diet, and helped to use the health services they needed. In due course, these newcomers might be invited to participate in health research and to participate in the health services as volunteers or as employed, trained staff. The reality tends to be different.

Mark Johnson (1984) has identified four broad phases in the development of interest in the health of ethnic minority groups in the UK, and these may be internationally generalizable. There was early interest in the unusual diseases ethnic minority groups had, particularly unusual infections. Johnson called this the port health or exotic disease phase. In many respects, this phase builds upon an interest in the colonial era in tropical and international health, not to mention the continuing importance of infections. It is not surprising that migration was, until recently, focused in seaports, particularly in the days when merchandise was often transported by sea, and shipping was the main means of international travel. Now, migration of people is mainly through air and land travel, and health units tend to be established in these locations.

The second phase, according to Johnson, was around biological differences, with a focus on genetically inheritable diseases, such as the haemoglobinopathies. There was also an interest in the relationship between genetics and cultures, as in cousin marriage. This interest was easily linked to mother and child health, including congenital abnormalities.

Third there came a focus on the population patterns of disease, including attention to mental health, with a strong emphasis on ethnic group comparisons. In trying to explain variations, it became necessary to examine the impact of immigrants' culture, and social and economic standing, on their health. Comparisons of the patterns of diseases were usually, if not invariably, with the majority White population. These variations drew the attention of researchers, professionals and policy-makers. Once noted, such variations were not easily ignored. (In Chapter 3 we examined some of the strengths and limitations of this approach, and will develop the theme in Chapters 5 and 9.) The response varied from blaming the minority population for their health problems, excluding them from services, setting up special initiatives, adapting services to meet needs, and a general policy of equality—equal service for equal need. The response depended largely on the social context and political and public views on race and ethnicity.

Johnson notes that following this there was an interest in the issue of adapting health care policy, research and services to meet the needs of ethnic minority groups, and arguably this fourth phase was surprisingly late. Even then the aim was to adapt policy and services to meet specific needs, rather than to try to ensure the NHS as a whole was primed to meet the challenges of multicultural health care. This latter more ambitious goal was set very late (in the late 1990s), and remains a current challenge.

In Johnson's view two issues were under-emphasized in this evolution: racism, and acknowledgement of the delivery of substantial amounts of health service by ethnic minority staff.

While Johnson's framework does not necessarily work as a rigid chronological account, it makes sense, assuming an ongoing interaction between the four phases. The framework predicts that the society's response follows a pattern: an awareness of problems and especially of a risk of infectious disease harming society as a whole; formal study of health status and health care by ethnic or racial group; articulation of policy and plans, sometimes backed by legislation; a move from policies of indifference towards, and even exclusion of, minorities, to the promotion of the welfare of minorities; specific actions to redress inequities; and, finally, an attempt to adapt general service to meet needs.

With this framework in mind, we will examine, briefly, the response of five countries to the issue of ethnicity and health. Before reading on you may wish to reflect on whether this framework fits your country, and then reflect on your knowledge of the evolution of the response to ethnicity and health in one or more of the following: Australia, the USA, South Africa, the UK and the Netherlands.

4.2.1 UK

As trading nations in command of the biggest empire in world history, the countries of the UK were hubs for international travel and migration—particularly emigration, but also immigration. Ports in the UK have been home to small multi-ethnic populations for centuries. The country was also deeply involved in tropical medicine, both from the perspective of safeguarding the health of British emigrants, particularly those holding important roles in empire or serving in the Armed Forces, and the local people being governed. Until 1962 there was, apparently, a free flow of people across the Empire and Commonwealth as there was no legal or institutional block to immigration (in practice, obtaining passports and visas was not always easy).

In the nineteenth and early twentieth centuries Britain was home to large numbers of immigrants, mainly from Europe, in particular Ireland. This changed after the Second World War when substantial numbers of non-White people from the Commonwealth or Empire, particularly from the Caribbean and the Indian subcontinent, settled in the UK. The reasons for this immigration are complex but include Britain's need for labour for post-war reconstruction. Also, there was a great deal of political and social turbulence following decolonization e.g. in the creation of Pakistan in north-west and north-east India. This either compelled or motivated tens of millions of people to migrate, and some went abroad. Relatives and friends followed.

The National Health Service was formed in 1948 with the aim of providing high quality, comprehensive health care for all people in Britain. Although, in truth, there is no such thing as a culturally or genetically homogeneous population or nation, the NHS at that time provided a model of care for, comparatively speaking, a fairly stable culture, rooted in northern European traditions and based on the English language and the Christian religion. In its early years the NHS was not expected to adapt itself to meet the needs of ethnic minority groups. Such populations were small-scale and expectations were, compared to the present day, low. Some conference reports and papers in the UK research literature discuss the challenges of meeting the health needs of ethnic minority groups in the 1960s. Many of the issues of concern observed then remain a challenge today, for instance the need for communication between professionals and patients which bridges language and cultural barriers. Interest in the health and health care of immigrants then accelerated, at least partly in response to the rise of the ethnic minority population following immigration from the 1950s through the 1970s.

Mark Johnson's analysis of the evolution of interest in the health of ethnic minority groups was based on his observations in the UK. Numerous documents demonstrate that there was interest, first, in the unusual diseases ethnic minority groups had (the exotic diseases phase), second, in the impact of their culture on their health, and, third, in comparing the patterns of their diseases with those of the majority White population. Interest in adapting health care policy, research and services to meet the needs of ethnic minority groups came late. Even then the aim was to adapt policy and services to meet specific needs, rather than to try to ensure the NHS as a whole was primed to meet the challenges of multicultural health care. This latter more ambitious goal was the prime purpose of the NHS Ethnic Health Unit which served in England for three years from 1994 to 1997, closing down with the task only begun. Following the Race Relations

Amendment Act 2000 the urgency of this task has been renewed in all the devolved nations of the UK, as discussed in Chapter 8.

Despite the multi-ethnic and multicultural nature of modern Britain, and notwith-standing the enormous efforts of both institutions and individuals, NHS health care provision and training are still largely based on the concept of a relatively homogeneous, 'British' population. Health service provision in Britain is largely based on an under-standing of what constitutes illness, disease and health care in terms of so-called 'Western medicine', and this is firmly based on the teachings of British medical schools.

Throughout the UK many projects on ethnic health and health care start and stop each year and their subject is usually basic e.g. communication (usually health promotion projects) services. Nationally, even basic services such as translation have not yet become integral, properly funded, effective and accountable parts of routine NHS care. While there have been attempts to adapt services to take into account Britain's multiracial, multicultural and multi-faith society, inequitable health care for ethnic minority com-munities continues as a consequence of linguistic difficulties and social and cultural differences between patients and staff. Often the ethnic minority groups are blamed for their failure to adapt, e.g. for not learning English faster or for their behaviours. Such barriers to equity of access and quality of care undermine the assumption that because the National Health Service is free to all then it is equally available to all.

In the UK, as in the USA, the issue of racism in health has been comprehensively discussed, particularly in relation to employment of staff (see Chapter 6). Laurence Ward reviewed the history of racism in the employment of staff in the NHS. Nurses were specially recruited for the NHS by waiving immigration restrictions in the 1960s but most overseas nurses went, or were channelled, into the lower status state enrolled nurse (SEN) rather than the higher status state registered nurse (SRN) grade. They were concentrated in the fields of psychiatry, geriatrics and mental handicap, which were unpopular and yet, at least arguably, needed an understanding of local cultures greater than would be the case for other higher status acute care specialties. British nursing schools trained very few local people from ethnic minority populations—the reasons for failure to recruit them are complex, and include the perception amongst some South Asian groups of nursing as an undesirable profession for women. This perception is partly to do with cultural views on modesty and handling of body fluids and excretions, particularly for people of the opposite sex. The recruitment and retention issue remains an acknowledged and priority challenge to this day.

Doctors were recruited from India and Pakistan from accredited colleges. In 1977, about one-third of all doctors were from overseas and most from the Indian subcon-tinent. Again, perhaps surprisingly from a sociocultural perspective, but not from an understanding of the competition for posts, many went into psychiatry and geriatrics. These might have been, comparatively speaking, inappropriate specialties for immigrant doctors but they were least popular for home-educated graduates. As problems with the quality of care were perceived, the overseas doctors were blamed, rather than the system of discrimination channelling overseas graduates into these specialties. The General Medical

Council's requirement for most overseas doctors to sit an examination (known as PLAB) to gain full registration was subsequently introduced.

Studies demonstrated that race and ethnicity, sometimes distinguished by indicators as crude as the name, not even the place of graduation, was a factor in obtaining entry to some medical schools and subsequent employment opportunities. The distribution of both merit awards (subsequently distinction and now in England clinical excellence awards), and specialist/consultant status, showed huge disparities by ethnic group, which are not easily explained. The charge of racism in health care in Britain is less vocal than in the USA but the issues are similar enough to learn from the experience there.

In the UK the focus in the area of ethnicity and health has been on immigrants and their descendants. Each group of immigrants, whether Irish, Jewish or Indian, has been associated with raising the risk to wider society of infectious diseases and environmental hazards. Since the 1970s the potential value of studying epidemiologically variations in disease patterns has increased attention on ethnic minority groups. This has been followed by a policy response to tackle health problems seen in excess in minority groups. Where minority groups have a lower prevalence of a problem, the issue is usually ignored—wider society thereby misses the chance to learn from the minority e.g. on the social forces that maintain a low prevalence of smoking in women from the middle east, South Asia, and China. A new and better approach to making comparisons is discussed in Chapters 6 and 9.

The 1990s and early twenty-first century has seen the rise of a social justice agenda accompanied by powerful legislation to promote equality in Britain's multi ethnic society. As predicted by Johnson some 20 years ago, the prime current interest in ethnicity and health is the challenge of delivering equitable services, and this topic is the focus of Chapter 8.

While it would be naive to portray the UK as a paragon of virtue, it has not, to my knowledge, in the last few centuries created laws and structures that embed racial inequality as, for example, has been the case in South Africa, Germany, or the USA, to mention a few countries. To counter the then pervasive socially generated racial discrimination that imposed barriers to employment, housing and social exchange ('No Coloured' signs in bars, for example) the Race Relations Acts of 1965 and 1976 were passed to outlaw such actions. The racist murder in London in 1993 of a British-born teenager, Stephen Lawrence, followed by an inadequate response by the police led to the MacPherson Inquiry that spurred the Race Relations (Amendment) Act 2000. This Act has required a major shift in the way all public bodies approach employment and service provision issues. Above all the Act places a duty on public bodies to actively promote racial equality. The Commission for Racial Equality is the lead body monitoring the implementation of the Act. One of the principal outputs from public bodies are Race Equality Schemes that comprise detailed plans of the actions to be taken, and then regular reports on progress. This legislation virtually mandates ethnic monitoring of both employment practices and service delivery. Furthermore, it requires a response to epidemiological demonstrations of health inequalities (see Chapter 8 for details).

In Scotland, in parallel to these legislative moves the Scottish Executive Health Department, in collaboration with academics and health service professionals, has created and is implementing a wide ranging policy called Fair for All. This policy requires NHS staff to meet the health and health care needs of ethnic minority communities and is being extended to other groups that are potentially at risk of discrimination. Amongst the many outcomes of this policy is the creation of the National Resource Centre for Ethnic Minority Health in the summer of 2002. The centre started its work by focusing on policy in health. The Scottish Health Service has responded enthusiastically, though goals are always difficult to achieve in the light of resource and expertise limitations, especially in the face of stiff competition from other areas of work. Nonetheless, the principles and processes established by the Fair for All policy are judged worthy of wider application e.g. in the fields of inequalities in services for the disabled, the elderly etc. (see Chapter 8 for details).

With legislation and policy backing that promotes equality epidemiological data can be both generated and applied to public health good, as will be discussed in Chapters 5, 6 and 9. Certainly, the risk of harm is reduced in this environment. These laws and policies have had an impact on local strategies, plans and services as will be discussed further in Chapter 8.

4.2.2 United State of America

The USA has a long and sustained tradition of race and health research, scholarship, and practice with a strong focus on African origin populations, especially in comparing them with the White population—the Black/White dichotomy is deeply ingrained (see Chapters 6 and 8 for examples).

Johnson's framework applies very well, but over a much longer timescale than in the UK. From the sixteenth to the eighteenth century when West Africans were imported as slaves the medical interest was on the exotic illnesses they had, and on biological differences, particularly those that made them effective slaves, e.g. endurance of long working hours, heat tolerance and their comparative immunity to tropical infectious diseases. Much of this work was, in retrospect, scientific racism as mentioned in Chapter 1, and discussed briefly below and in more detail in Chapters 9 and 10.

Medical practitioners were important contributors to racialized science i.e. a science that saw race as a primary means of analysis (see Chapter 10). As discussed by Kiple and King (1981), and referred to earlier, the idea of a package of specific 'ethnic' diseases was of much interest to medical science and practice. Africans' susceptibility to some diseases were sometimes explained by nonsensical hypotheses on causation that veered away from the probable and obvious ones of poverty, captivity, demotivation, lack of opportunity, overcrowding and lack of previous exposure to some infections etc. Impressive Latin labels such as drapetomania—defined as an irrational and pathological desire of slaves to run away—and dysaethesia Aethiopica (rascality) were used to label and explain such normal human behaviours.

These ideas, essentially based on an ideology of biological differences, were attractive as a way of maintaining differences in social positioning in which White people were superior and Black people inferior. They were not, of course, completely unchallenged. Krieger (1992) discusses the work of Dr. James McCune Smith who was the first Black USA-trained physician. In 1859 he challenged the assumption that Black inferiority was innate and pointed out, amongst other things, that rickets was similar in poor Black and White children. He also argued that the division of people into White and Black categories was artificial and that race was a social category. It is no coincidence, perhaps, that it took a Black person to state something so obvious.

Until the latter half of the twentieth century the research and health care work on race and health in the USA was, overall, detrimental to minority groups, with negative stereotyping the norm and open discrimination being common for limiting access to health care facilities. Black Americans have been legally free and equal citizens with voting rights only since 1968, shortly after the Civil Rights Act in 1964. This is a very short period in comparison to a history of 250 years of slavery and 100 years of segregation following the end of slavery. As a reminder of this it is worth remembering that Rosa Parkes, the woman who was jailed when she refused to give up her seat to a White person on a bus in Alabama, thus sparking the Civil Rights movement, died on the 24 October 2005.

Following the Civil Rights Act in 1964 the aim of narrowing the gap between the health of African-Americans and White Americans came to the fore. The USA's major classification for race and ethnicity, released as Directive 15 of the Office of Management and Budget, was created to help achieve this goal (see Chapter 2). Those who created it explicitly stated that is was designed for that purpose and did not have anthropological or scientific validity.

This goal of equality and equity has not, however, been achieved, and the gap has widened rather than narrowed in the twentieth century, as shown by La Veist and colleagues, probably reflecting increasing inequalities in wealth and incomes (1995). Black people are disproportionately represented in physical environments that are likely to produce ill-health. One of the staggering statistics that has been widely publicized is that males in Harlem, New York, have less chance of reaching 65 years of age than males in Bangladesh. Cirrhosis and homicide are the third and fourth causes of death in Harlem males.

Boys in Harlem who reached the age of 15 had a 37 percent chance of surviving to the age of 65; for girls, the likelihood was 65 percent.

Geronimus (1996: 1552)

The data we obtained in Harlem and Black Belt Alabama highlight the importance of accounting for social factors that are not represented in typical measures of socioeconomic status. Black Belt Alabama had the lowest excess mortality of the poor black groups, although it had the highest rate of poverty, whereas Harlem had the highest excess mortality but the lowest poverty rate. These findings remained valid after adjustment for cost-of-living differences between the rural South and the urban North.

Geronimus (1996: 1557)

Some citizens in the world's most powerful nation have worse health, as measured by life-expectancy, than citizens of one of the poorest countries. Yet, as a group, Native Americans are even worse off than African-Americans, with the worst health of any in America, even though they have their own Indian Health Service to help tackle the challenge. As with Aborigines in Australia (see below), Native Americans are a people who were displaced by colonists, often by the force of arms, with the catastrophic loss of population and from a historical perspective, loss of perceived and actual dignity, respect, status and resources. Fortunately, this is changing for some groups. For example, the Apache of Arizona and the Navaho have become well-organized and wealthy—but wealth is bringing its own problems e.g. the rise of diabetes and obesity in Pima Indians.

Such persisting inequalities pose political, social and ethical problems, and the analysis leads to many questions and potential explanations. Of the explanations those relating to racism are the most disturbing yet least amenable to open discussion and action. In Chapters 6 and 8 we will consider this matter in more detail, in relation to policy documents. Empirical evidence is complex to interpret but much public opinion and some scholarly analysis in the USA and the UK places racism at the hub of ethnic and racial inequalities in health and health care. Racism is most clear-cut, surprisingly, in health research and the most infamous example is the Tuskegee Syphilis Study which has done more to substantiate the charge of racism than anything else in North American medicine. As already mentioned in Chapter 1, this was a government-sponsored research study looking for differences in the response to syphilis which took place in Alabama during 1932–1972. The 600 subjects of the study were deceived and bribed into cooperating in an examination of the natural history of syphilis in poor 'negroes'. The study actively denied them effective treatments and hastened many deaths. Syphilis in Blacks had been a matter of long and considerable interest to the medical profession, and this work was done to test a viewpoint that the disease was less serious in Black people than in White people; a viewpoint that was wrong and predictably so, even then.

Gamble has painted a picture of a legacy of mistrust by African-Americans in health care and health research, showing that the Tuskegee Syphilis Study was not unique as a racist experiment. Gamble recounts Thomas Hamilton's experiments on a slave called Fed, testing remedies for heat stroke, and the work of Dr J Marion Sims on an operation for vesico-vaginal fistula. The slaves, of course, had no right to refuse as they were property. The legacy has meant, according to Gamble, that participation in research by Blacks is low, and it offers an explanation for distrust of health care workers in modern America.

The issue of racism in health care has been the underlying, if sometimes understated, focus of the extensive debate and research on the disparities in the intensity of activity in the health care received by Black compared to White Americans. 'We believe that inadequate health education, differences in patients' preferences for invasive management, delivery systems that are unfriendly to members of certain cultures, and overt racism may all play a part', said Whittle and Colleagues (Whittle *et al.* 1993, p 627). This matter will be discussed in Chapter 6.

A Panel on Racial and Ethnic Disparities in Medical Care has reviewed the evidence, making 24 policy and 11 research recommendations (Institute of Medicine 2003—see p 345). These recommendations are easily generalizable internationally. Among the observations were the following: the disparities in racial and ethnic disparities are persisting and may be widening; only recently has the focus turned to health care; there is evidence of both stereotyping and bias against racial minorities in the USA; there are inequities in relation to health insurance; data collection is vital to redress the balance, including data collection for clinical records; and the legal and policy basis for redressing racial and ethnic disparities is already in place, but underused. In particular, the Panel believed that narrowing these disparities is a civil right.

It appears that the USA is also at the crossroads where the attention is turning to the effective and equitable delivery of health care and health promotion. In Chapter 8 we discuss the policy response there. In terms of Johnson's framework, we see once again that the collection of epidemiological data has preceded the call for action to redress inequalities. We also see that action has been minimal, even discriminatory, until the social and political circumstances were favourable—i.e. after civil rights were granted.

4.2.3 Australia and the indigenous population—aborigines

Australia is a country of immigrants but, surprisingly, ethnicity and race have not loomed large in the health care response. The reasons for this may include the fact that the country promoted a White Australia policy through much of the twentieth century: the populace regarded the country as belonging to a homogeneous group of northern Europeans; and responsibility for health and health care is constitutionally by state, rather than central (Commonwealth) government.

In the last three decades of the twentieth century Australia became one of the world's most multi-ethnic nations, with migration from numerous countries but especially the south-east and eastern Asian countries. Despite this the academic and service response has been relatively muted, with only a few studies examining ethnic/racial/country of birth variations in health status and health care. As is so often the case following such migrations, there has been a political backlash with a rise to popularity of politicians advocating a pro-European stance in national life, culture and immigration.

There has been a focus, however, on the indigenous populations, especially the aborigines, who have exceptionally poor health. Currently, about 2 per cent of the Australian population is aborigine. This focus was boosted by a referendum giving responsibility for the welfare of these populations to central government. The poor social, political and economic circumstances of the Aboriginal people have been noted for a long time but sympathy has been in short supply. Instead political and institutional efforts were directed towards reducing the aboriginal presence and culture, either through assimilation, enforced settlement or resettlement, and at times even force and violence. At one time there was an acceptance that the Aboriginal peoples of Australia were dying out. This forecast was, fortunately, wrong except in Tasmania.

The late twentieth century saw an awakening to their appalling health status and limited health services and a resolve by central government to improve matters. Unfortunately, this has not proven easy to achieve. Whether seen in terms of general indicators of health (life expectancy, infant mortality), specific diseases (coronary heart disease, stroke, diabetes), social problems (alcoholism, tobacco use, illegal drugs, violence), or utilization of high quality preventative or curative services, the picture is grim. Inequalities appear to be widening. Life expectancy of aborigines is about 20 years less than the population as a whole. There is probably no equivalent disparity elsewhere in the world.

In terms of Johnson's framework, in relation to non-White immigrants and indigenous populations, we have seen a period of hostility and then indifference, followed by a curiosity around aboriginal culture and lifestyle, an examination of their health status, and finally a failed attempt to redress inequalities. While Australia is a multicultural nation that is slowly leaving its openly racist and Eurocentric era behind (despite some politicians' attempts to turn the clock back), social attitudes towards Aborigine populations remain largely negative or indifferent. The era of equality for them is in the distant future, but at least part of the solution is reflected in the following quotation.

> Social and cultural factors are mainly responsible for the higher levels of mortality and morbidity, including alcoholism, found in Aboriginal communities. The development of mutual respect and mutual participation in health and medical programmes offers the possibility for improving Aboriginal health.
>
> Hausfeld (1977: 1307)

4.2.4 South Africa (under apartheid)

South Africa exemplifies, par excellence, how race and ethnicity concepts can be applied over very long time periods to bolster a society's efforts to justify, institutionalize and sustain major inequalities in access to economic opportunities and services. South Africa has exemplified a struggle between populations—whether the indigenous ones living there when the settlers arrived, the African ones migrating there after that, or between the Dutch and British colonialists.

South Africa under apartheid exemplified the damaging effects of a policy institutionalizing, with the full force of the state, separate and unequal social development and services for different racial groups, defined in arbitrary and unscientific ways. South Africa's health researchers in the past expended much energy in studying racial differences in health and disease, using the statistics generated by the state-sponsored compulsory racial classification, itself designed to maintain the so-called purity of the White population.

The results of apartheid were, predictably, comparatively excellent services and economic development for the country's White population and comparatively inadequate services and relative poverty for the other groups, especially the Black African majority.

South Africa is the richest country on the African continent, with about five million people classified as White who were and still are in command of a large share of the resources, while the 30 million plus others were politically and economically marginalized. With the dismantling of apartheid the situation is changing, albeit slowly. While the public health sector does most of the training of staff, and most of the research and development for the population, the private health sector focuses its attention (and

50 per cent of the total spending on health care) on the 20 per cent of the population that has health insurance i.e. mainly the White population.

In some ways, Johnson's framework still applies, with the major difference being that for a long period of time the interest in race and ethnicity led to negative discrimination. In South Africa, we see an evolution from interest in infections, tropical diseases and exotica, to biological differences, to discriminatory practices under apartheid, and then to the study of epidemiological variations (partly generated by the apartheid policy) based on rigid, politically driven racial classifications. Once again, nonetheless, we see the appearance of an interest in equity and equality in health and health care. The Gluckman Commission Of Inquiry in the 1940s pointed to the need for a new direction but little happened, and the Freedom Charter of the African National Congress (1950s) offered a new vision for South Africa but at the time did not have the political power to deliver, until the arrival of democracy and the demolition of apartheid promised to deliver change. The current health and health care challenge is equality. As elsewhere, South Africa is finding that racial equality cannot be delivered without data and without racial classification. Ironically, the very racial classifications that suppressed ethnic minorities for so long are being put back into service to rectify the same problems. The quotations that opened Chapter 2 aptly summarize the tensions around data collection about ethnicity in South Africa.

4.2.5 Netherlands

The Netherlands became a multi-ethnic society with substantial numbers of non-White people in the late twentieth century, with the entry of people from its previous colonies, particularly Indonesia and Surinam, but also from the Antilles, Turkey and Morocco. As in other European countries, decolonization, the need for labour, and humanitarian asylum policies underpinned this immigration. The country has been famous for its egalitarian and liberal politics. Examples of this include legalizing gay marriage in 2001 (the first in the world), and liberal rules on euthanasia and the private use of drugs such as cannabis.

The Netherlands' policy response in relation to the welfare of ethnic minority populations has, however, been unstable in the light of political change. Initially, the response was minimal. The earliest major immigration of non-White people was from Indonesia, an ex-colony. These Indonesian immigrants seem to have settled and assimilated very well, both in terms of economic development and use of services. In the 1990s there was increasing awareness that this early experience was not being replicated in other ethnic minority groups e.g. the Turks. Policy was reviewed and research was started, with an emphasis on ethnic variations in mortality and morbidity and utilization of health care. The results of recent research by Vivian Bos and colleagues (2002) examining mortality data indicate substantial variations that can, in large part, be accounted for (statistically) by differences in socio-economic status. Studies of quality of care have pointed to some challenges in delivering equity in services, although in many respects these are satisfactory. Agyemang and colleagues's study (2005) gives typical findings. It examined blood pressure in Black Surinamese, South Asian Surinamese and White Dutch people in Amsterdam (as a comparison), in the period between 2001 and 2003. Blood pressure was, comparatively, higher in both minority groups. There were no differences between study populations in awareness of the problem or the utilization of treatment, but the most important issue was the level of control, which was worse in Black Surinamese, and there was a suggestion this might also be so for the South Asian Surinamese. The study is not untypical of findings for many countries, that is, utilization of services may not result in outcomes of equal quality in minority groups.

Unfortunately, just as a major programme of work in the 1990s was leading to discussions on policy and strategic actions the political climate changed. At the turn of the century the Netherlands saw new and negative attitudes towards some ethnic minority groups. The assassination of a prominent right wing politician (Pim Fortuyn) and of a film producer who portrayed Islam negatively (Theo van Gogh) have created a shockwave through the country. Fortuyn argued on a political anti-immigration stance, stating that the Netherlands was full and describing Islam as a backward culture. Within the first few years of the twenty-first century, the country has moved from a liberal attitude to an exploration of needs, and to a less understanding perspective. The current attitude is that while special efforts may be required for the foreign-born, rapid integration and assimilation should occur such that the descendents of migrants ought to require no special services. At the time of writing numerous policies have been imposed or proposed that restrict the freedoms of ethnic minority groups and that are mostly targeted at Muslims: apart from those from USA, Canada, Australia, the EU countries and Japan, immigrants must take an exam on Dutch language and culture, and a Dutch language course at their own expense; and there are proposals to restrict the wearing of the burqua in public on the grounds of public safety. These are, at least arguably, racist policies e.g. what logic is there to exempt immigrants from some countries from the need to take the exam? Why single out the burqua rather than generalize to forms of clothing that are associated with religion, or cover the face? On 12 October 2005 *The Times* quoted Rita Verdonk, a Dutch minister, who said that 'time of cosy tea drinking' with Muslim groups had passed (Browne 2005).

4.3 A pattern of response—derivation of principles

From the above, and other accessible accounts (see also Chapters 6 and 8), it is clear that the study of health and health care differences by racial and ethnic groups will be influenced by the prevailing ethos in society. If our society is a racist one, the study of racial/ethnic difference is likely also to be racist in effect, even if not in intent. Second, the act of seeking differentials by race and ethnic group is both essential and a great danger to the people studied: the outcome is dependent on the interpretation and use of the data. While racist attitudes and behaviours persist the danger of misuse of research for racist purposes will remain.

Over the last 200 years, sciences have made key 'contributions' to the eugenics movement, immigration policies and the practice of medicine. Some of these were referred to in Chapter 1, and others will be discussed in Chapter 9. Essentially, differences in health status were attributed to biological or social inferiority and this was used to justify discriminatory policies and practices, which were sometimes explained as being in the interests of the race being discriminated against. The greatest of all abuses, by Nazi Germany, is discussed in Chapter 6. One major change has undoubtedly occurred in the last twenty years which distinguishes the research and scholarship of the 1990s from that of the 1890s. The current focus is not only on the description of disease patterns for the sake of science but also so the information can be used for the betterment of the health of ethnic minority groups. This subtle change, which reflects a change in society's attitude, is all-important. The strategy in science has, however, remained unchanged with the basic method being the comparison of the health of the minority population to a majority population with the health status of the latter acting as the norm or standard for comparison. This ethnocentric view, which is potentially misleading and damaging, remains the paradigm for scientific inquiry in this century as in the last. In Chapter 9 I will offer alternatives to this approach.

A resurgence of racial science is underway as we enter the new millennium, which is coincident with the hardening of immigration and welfare policy in both Europe and North America, and adverse media publicity for ethnic minorities. The proposed denial of education and health care rights to 'illegal' immigrants (most of whom are non-White ethnic minorities) in California is the logical and extreme effect of such new thinking. As of April 2006 these proposals were rejected, a result that almost certainly reflects the power of Hispanic and other minorities in the state. This power derives from their numbers and contributions to the economy.

In seeking understanding on why societies and institutions either respond or fail to respond to the challenge of equity across ethnic groups, one is reminded of the question 'which came first—the chicken or the egg?' (Or, in our context, the awareness or the data?) Clearly, a social and political awareness will generate the impetus to collect research data and undertake case studies, and will provide the willingness to interpret the information evenly and take appropriate actions. Equally, such information can be used to generate social and political awareness. As the same data can be interpreted in many ways, the social and political milieu is clearly vital in guiding such interpretation. Those aspects of race and ethnicity—colour, language, dress etc.—that may stimulate prejudice, discrimination and racism also lead to inequalities in the quality of, and access to, health care. In societies that foster justice, equity and equality, strategies to tackle such inequalities are needed, and in turn, these need to be based on data that quantify the inequalities, set targets for achievement and monitor progress to the agreed goals. In addition, opportunities for the advancement of understanding in the social, public health and biological sciences ought not to be lost. In societies that are hostile to ethnic minorities data collection is likely to do harm rather than good.

As a simple example of what would be lost without race and ethnicity data we reflected in Chapter 3 (Table 3.1), on data on smoking in South Asian populations. Smoking is the foremost controllable causal factor for an array of killing and disabling diseases including cancers and cardiovascular diseases. Smoking is a socially patterned habit, and the interventions required to inhibit people from starting up and promoting giving up, have to be tailored to the needs of the specific population. Do smoking habits vary by ethnic or racial group? By how much do smoking patterns vary? Are the differences enough to matter? These are important questions. How are they to be answered if race and ethnicity are to be rejected? There were massive differences between ethnic groups, and between men and women in the minority populations but not between European origin White men and women. The way ethnic groups are defined clearly matters. For South Asian men combined the presence of smoking was virtually identical to that for European men. No doubt some subgroups within the category European also differ, but as no data were collected to explore them, such potential variations cannot be examined. Boxes 4.2 and 4.3 show the heterogeneity of the South Asian populations in the UK. It is safe to say most immigrant populations are highly heterogeneous.

Box 4.2 Country of birth of 1,036,807 people classified as Indians in the UK census

478,017	Born in UK
309	Born in Republic of Ireland
1,923	Born in Western Europe
167,610	Born in Africa
357,632	Born in South Asia
3,078	Born in North America
2,110	Born in Oceania

Box 4.3 South Asians' religions, languages and origins

Sikhism		Punjabi
Islam		Urdu
Hinduism		Hindi
(Jainism)		Gujerati
(Christianity)		Bengali
(Buddhism)		Pushto
	Punjab	
	Mirpur + NW Frontier	
	Gujerat	
	Bengal	
	East Africa	

Such differences are of paramount importance and it is hard to imagine how we can develop effective public health responses without data on them. There are other questions that need answering before we can proceed to action e.g. on the cross-cultural validity of self-report data, on the beliefs, attitudes and social conventions that underpin such variations, and the effectiveness of public health programmes. The immediate need, nonetheless, is for data for discussion and consideration. Try the following exercise before reading on.

Exercise 4.2 Assessing the health needs of a minority group that has not been studied (invisible minority)

- What do you think of the phrase 'invisible minority'?
- Why are some groups not studied or noted and hence become, effectively, invisible?
- Given the challenge of reporting rapidly on the health needs of an invisible minority group, how would you feel?
- Thinking about an invisible minority e.g. White Irish, Polish or Bosnian people, what can you do to make progress?

This exercise, asking you to report on a difficult question, ought to provoke anxiety, because the dangers of misinforming policy-makers and planners are very high. Even the phrase 'invisible minority' is a charged one though highly descriptive. Some populations' specific needs have never been studied though there is usually some awareness, e.g. few high-quality research data exist on the Polish immigrants in Scotland and gypsy travellers. They are little studied for reasons including that they have little political power, they have not asserted their needs, they have few champions for their cause, and they are not captured in census or health statistics. Without data, a report is likely to be based on stereotypes and general impressions that may well be wrong. It is quite possible that the general principles derived from general population research and policy development may not apply to the minority groups you are asked to report on. For example, there may be a social distance between the group and the service and its professionals, leading to problems of inequitable access and poor quality of care. This may be specific to a small number of issues or general. You can make progress, nonetheless.

Your population may be similar to other populations studied elsewhere, whether in other parts of your country or internationally. You may need to learn from the country of origin, e.g. what are the issues facing Poles in Poland or the Irish in Ireland? At least some of them are likely to be pertinent to the situation in your country. A close examination of publications internationally, both in academic journals and in other sources such as government reports might give very useful insights. The third approach would be to do a rapid needs assessment, which would be based mainly on a dialogue with health service providers and representatives of the population on which you are reporting. Direct observation might be helpful e.g. of the living conditions of some members of the population. Given a small budget and prioritization, you would probably recommend an assessment of the size and characteristics of the populations (possibly including a more detailed analysis of existing census data e.g. by country of birth, or failing that a new mini-census focused on this population), and acquisition of data on mortality, major causes of hospitalization and use of general practice services, and major aspects of lifestyle that are relevant to health. Even the simplest of data, despite their limitations, can be the foundation for health needs assessment (see Chapter 5).

4.4 **Conclusion**

Contemporary and enlightened multi-ethnic societies ought not to ignore the issues raised by racial/ethnic variations in health and health care, and ought to be particularly conscious of the effects on society as a whole of immigration. Historically, the response to rising ethnic diversity has usually been, initially at least, a negative one, with a tendency to blame the minority populations for innate or cultural 'defects' that underlie their health problems. Spurred by rising global and national movements for universal human rights in the late twentieth century, many countries are changing their stance, with equity of health status and health care being a central focus. The response to ethnic inequalities is, therefore, closely related to political and social trends. It is imperative that researchers, practitioners and policy-makers learn from historical and international experience.

Data on race and ethnic group have both harmed and benefited ethnic minority populations, yet without the data the need for services cannot be established. Such data underpin both policies of exclusion and of positive action. The lesson seems to be that data need to be collected within an ethical and legal framework that safeguards the human rights of minority and majority populations alike and requires their use to improve the welfare of populations. This does not, of course, guarantee that data will not be abused but it does impose obstacles to that. The goals of equality and equity, and monitoring of progress towards the goals, cannot be achieved without data on race or ethnicity. There is, therefore, little choice but to work with the concepts and the resulting classifications, but with the goal of continuous improvement in the quality of the data and their uses. The scale of the challenge is great and none of the five countries considered here has demonstrably achieved the goal of narrowing in meaningful and substantial ways ethnic inequalities in health status. Careful health needs assessment, the topic of the next chapter, is a prerequisite for thoughtful action.

Summary

Generally, ethnically diverse societies are conscious that the health status and health care needs of their population vary by ethnic group. These variations draw the attention of researchers, professionals and policy-makers. Once noted, such variations are not easily ignored. The responses range from merely studying the differences, blaming the minority population for their health problems, excluding them from services, setting up special initiatives, adapting services to meet needs, and a general policy of equality and equity–service to meet need. The response depends on the social context and political and public views on race and ethnicity. This chapter outlined the response in five countries.

In the UK the health focus has been on immigrants and their descendants. Each group of immigrants, whether Irish, Jewish or Indian, has been associated with raising the risk to the wider society of infectious diseases and environmental hazards. Since the 1970s there has been an appreciation of the potential value of studying epidemiologically the substantial variations in disease patterns, which has increased attention on ethnic minority groups. This has been followed by a policy response to tackle health problems seen in excess in minority groups. The 1990s and early twenty-first century has seen the rise of a social justice agenda accompanied by powerful anti-discriminatory legislation to promote equality in Britain's multi-ethnic society.

In the USA attention in the field of race and health has focused on African origin populations. Until the latter half of the twentieth century the response was generally unsupportive or openly discriminatory. Following the civil rights movement the aim of narrowing the gap between the health of African-Americans and White Americans has come to the fore. This has not been achieved, and inequalities may even be increasing. More recently, attention has turned to a wider range of minority populations.

Australia is a country of immigrants but, surprisingly, ethnicity and race have not loomed large in the health response. Rather, the focus has been on the indigenous populations, especially the aborigines. The late twentieth century saw an awakening to the appalling health and health services they have and a resolve to improve matters. Efforts to date have paid little dividend.

South Africa under apartheid exemplified the damaging effects of a policy promoting separate services for different racial groups, the results being excellent service for the country's White population and inadequate ones for the other groups, especially the Black African majority. Vigorous efforts are being made to redress these injustices in post-apartheid South Africa.

The Netherlands became a multi-ethnic society in the late twentieth century. Its policy response has been unstable in the light of recent political change. The current attitude is that while special efforts may be required for the foreign-born, rapid integration and assimilation should occur such that the descendents of migrants ought to require no special services.

The variety of responses in these countries is striking. Nonetheless, some pattern is discernible: first, an awareness of health problems and especially of a risk of infections disease harming society as a whole; second, formal study of health status and health care by ethnic or racial group; third, articulation of policy and plans sometimes backed by legislation; fourth, a move from policies of exclusion of minorities to the promotion of the welfare of minorities; fifth, specific actions to redress inequities; and, finally, an attempt to adapt general service to meet needs. The scale of the challenge is great and none of the five countries considered here has achieved the goal of demonstrably narrowing health inequalities or achieving equity of service.

Chapter 5

Defining health and health care needs using quantitative and qualitative data

Although this may be put down to a certain naivety on our part, we were surprised to find an attitude prevalent, particularly among health care professionals, which failed totally to recognise any necessity to provide special facilities for an ethnic minority within the population. This attitude was summed up very nicely in a questionnaire which was returned to us by an administrator, who, at the end had made the following, unsolicited, comment: 'Asians shouldn't be singled out for anything special.' We would like to take issue with this statement on the grounds that we believe the only possible path towards the provision of satisfactory health care to the Asian community, in the immediate future, must inevitably lie in the adoption of a policy of positive discrimination.

Murphy *et al.* Working paper No 45,
1981 Health Care Provision for the Asian Community, p32

Contents

Objectives

On completion of this chapter you should be able to:

◆ In outline, appreciate the purpose, principles and methods of health and health care needs assessment
◆ Understand the difficulties in undertaking health needs assessment in minority ethnic groups when there is a lack of data
◆ Given data, be able to devise and utilize frameworks to set out and interpret information, both using approaches where the minority groups are compared against a standard, and where data are examined for each group alone, i.e. relative and absolute risk approaches
◆ Be able to explain how qualitative data can help to strengthen quantitative work, so increasing the validity and value of the health needs assessment
◆ In outline, know the outcomes of key health needs assessment in terms of health and demographic status, services needed and service gaps

5.1 Health needs assessment: an overview

Health needs assessment requires the collection and use of a wide range of information, and hence it overlaps considerably with research, the subject of Chapter 9. Unlike research, however, its purpose is practical and specific, rather than the extension of theoretical and generalizable knowledge. This chapter also builds upon the material in Chapters 2 and 3 and places special emphasis on understanding the ideas behind health needs assessment; the uses of epidemiology; making use of existing information, whether statistics, specific reports or general principles; the acquisition and interpretation of both quantitative and qualitative data; and taking advantage of the experience of others. If the view of the administrator in the quotation opening this chapter were to prevail, there would be no value in health needs assessment focusing on ethnic minority populations. The position that this chapter follows reflects some of the principles of the Report of the National Association of Health Authorities (NAHA) of the UK.

Basic principles (extracted from a longer list)

◆ NHS provision should be sensitive to the needs of all groups in society;
◆ If service provision in the NHS is to become flexible and responsive to the needs of black and minority ethnic groups, positive action is needed at all levels particularly the participation of members from black and minority ethnic groups in management planning;
◆ Historically, NHS provision has been based on the needs of a white, culturally homogeneous population. Britain is now a multi-racial and multi-cultural society and the NHS needs to adapt to its changing population;

(NAHA 1998)

5.1.1 **The concepts of health and health needs in a nutshell**

The ideas of health and health needs, are like beauty, to a very large extent in the eye of the beholder. Before reading on, you may wish to reflect briefly on these concepts by trying Exercise 5.1.

Exercise 5.1 Health and health needs

- What definition of health do you prefer and use?
- How would you measure health?
- Do you think definitions and concepts of health might vary by ethnic group? If so, in what way?
- What do you understand by the phrase 'health needs'?

There are many definitions of health, and most of them agree that health has physical, social and psychological components and that it is not a static but a dynamic concept. The most famous, but sometimes derided, definition of health is that of the World Health Organization, that health is not merely the absence of disease or disability but a state of complete physical, mental and social well-being. Some people would argue that a spiritual dimension should also be added, and this might be highly relevant to those groups whose identity is closely linked to religion, as often applies to ethnic minority populations. The main purpose of such a definition, which is self-evidently unrealistic, is to broaden thinking away from what is often described as the biomedical definition of health (the absence of medically defined disease) to embrace a psychosocial model. A more realistic working definition of health might be that health requires that people are alive, free of disabilities in so far as this is possible, and in the presence of disabilities are able to function well enough to achieve their potential and personal and social obligations.

Many tools exist for measuring aspects of health, and there are detailed discussions of this difficult concept, particularly well described by Ann Bowling (1994). From the point of view of this book and chapter, which is based on a public health approach, measures are needed which provide a summary of health status within communities or populations. The best perspective for this purpose is an epidemiological one whereby the health problems are assessed in terms of their actual and relative frequency within the population or community, expressed either as a prevalence or incidence, or other summary statistics derived from such data (see glossary for definitions).

The phrase 'health need' is difficult to define. Stevens and Raftery's (1994) book provides detailed discussion. One interesting classification of need is 'Bradshaws taxonomy of social need'. This classification is a useful starting point because it illustrates that, like health, the perspective of the beholder is crucial. Four types of need are identified:

1. *'Normative need'* is that defined by an expert or professional

2. *'Felt need'* is what people want

3. '*Expressed need*' is what people want put into action. Within the context of providing a service this is equivalent to the demand made upon that service

4. '*Comparative need*' is identified by comparing populations.

In epidemiological and public health settings comparative and normative needs tend to dominate. In an ideal world all needs, arguably, would be met. It is possible, however, that in meeting all needs the recipients of the service are actually harmed. For example, experts and lay individuals might be wrong about a need, even one which was normative, felt, expressed and comparative. Over the last 20 years there has been a great demand for hormone replacement therapy after the menopause, at least partly driven by a professional view that this would protect against cardiovascular disease and the lay view that the hormone keeps women youthful. Recently, large-scale clinical trials have concluded this is not true and this therapy increases the risk of cardiovascular diseases. The potential to provide benefit, is therefore, a crucial component of health needs. In publicly funded health care systems, therefore, felt and expressed needs tend to be de-emphasized.

Even in an ideal world it would be desirable, and perhaps even necessary, to recognize a hierarchy of need. For example, fundamental needs include air, water, food, clothing, warmth and shelter. Within the field of health care, most people, both health care professionals and lay, recognize a hierarchy of need. They may not, however, find it easy or comfortable to make it explicit. As resources available to provide health care are limited it is not possible to meet all needs, so those that are met should be more important than those that are not. Clearly, one's perspective on needs changes with circumstances, over time and with experience. A healthy person may extol the virtues of preventative medicine, but the person with breast cancer may extol the value of high-technology and potentially very costly health care directed at diagnosing, managing and caring for diseases. Concepts of health and need are shaped by culture and experience, and are likely to differ by ethnic group, particularly as the patterns of disease vary. That said, there are likely to be many similarities too.

5.1.2 **Health needs assessment**

The purpose of health needs assessment in public health is to assist in the planning and provision of health care (in our context for minority ethnic populations). The definition that is most suitable here is the one taken from Stevens and Raftery's book: *The assessment of a population or community's health status and health care utilization patterns in relation to its ability to benefit from health care.* The emphasis is, therefore, on health care based on preventive or treatment services that have the potential to remedy health problems, whether the health problems are diseases, disease risk factors, disabilities or lack of wellbeing. This does not imply a narrow clinical focus. 'Benefit' can include benefit beyond the person with the health problem, such as benefit to carers; and 'health care' can include health promotion, rehabilitation and palliative care. Some of the nuances of this definition are given in Table 5.1.

Table 5.1 The need for health care: the population's ability to benefit from health care (with this author's footnotes)

◆ The population's ability to benefit from health care equals the aggregate of the individual's ability to benefit.*

◆ The ability to benefit does not mean that every outcome is guaranteed to be favourable, but rather that need implies the potential to benefit which is on average effective.

◆ The benefit is not just a question of clinical status, but can include reassurance, supportive care and the relief of carers. Many individual health problems have a social impact via multiple knock-on effects or via a burden to families and carers. Hence the list of beneficiaries of care can extend beyond the patient.

◆ Health care includes not just treatment, but also prevention, diagnosis, continuing care, rehabilitation and palliative care.**

---

*Sometimes the population benefit exceeds the sum of individual benefits e.g. immunisation may stop an epidemic spreading even to unimmunized people (so-called herd immunity).

** Health care can also include advocacy for social and environmental change e.g. research and practice to bring about a ban on smoking in public places.

Reproduced from Stevens, A., Raftery, J. NHS Executive publication: Health Care Needs Assessment: the epidemiologically based needs assessment reviews (1994) with permission from Ratcliffe Medical Press, Oxford.

Health needs assessment requires a systematic, comprehensive overview of both quantitative and qualitative data on a population or subgroup of the population. It then needs to be applied to creating or adapting policies, strategies and services to improve population health, through better health care. Health needs assessment in relation to ethnic minority groups is often problematic because of the lack of data by ethnicity, particularly at local level, and at the level of subgroup detail that is often required. Its application to improve ethnic minority health is difficult. For national health needs assessments data available from administrative databases, usually recording broad ethnic categories or proxies for ethnic group such as country of birth, may need to be used in the absence of better information. The limitations of such data need to be understood to avoid making poor decisions, but equally their strength and value must not be overlooked. In addition to lack of data there may be lack of time, funds, expertise, political will and means of implementing the findings. Health needs assessment of ethnic minority health is too often limited to qualitative studies or even simply consultations, sometimes only with members of the ethnic minority communities, or only with health professionals. Such limited approaches may do more harm than good.

Without denying their many achievements, modern health care systems, including the UK's NHS, have found it difficult to adapt themselves to meet the needs of ethnic minority groups, despite the relatively impressive track record of policy analysis and research (see Chapter 8 and 9). Health needs assessment is important to the achievement of the patient-centred and equity-oriented goals of modern health care systems in multi-ethnic societies, and to the narrowing of the inequalities in health. The task is difficult—and it needs good quality quantitative and qualitative information to underpin it.

Before reading on, try Exercise 5.2.

Exercise 5.2 Data for health needs assessment and problems envisaged

- ◆ In general terms what kind of data would help you to assess health needs?
- ◆ What problems can you foresee in relation to gaining, interpreting and using such data?

The quantitative component of the needs assessment for ethnic minority populations should start by examining the actual health status, disease patterns and health care utilization within each group. This is the so-called absolute risk approach. The findings can also be compared with other ethnic groups, and this is the relative risk approach. In most instances, at least in countries where non-White populations are in the minority, the standard comparison is with the White population. This form of comparison is done for ease, habit, ethnocentrism, availability of data, or statistical power.

An alternative conceptual approach is to set the standard comparison against the ethnic group with the most desirable level of the health indicator under study. If this was done in the UK, for example, the Chinese population would be the standard for overall mortality and many specific diseases too. That would give high-level and very challenging health targets for all other ethnic groups in the UK, including White populations. In Chapter 6 I discuss how the relative risk approach could even widen inequalities, and In Chapter 9 I consider this issue in the context of research.

The problem with quantitative information is that it is difficult and expensive to obtain, requires epidemiological and statistical skills for analysis and interpretation, and is open to abuse, as discussed in Chapters 1 and 9. Abuses include using data to show a minority group as having worse health and then to use this to denigrate, stigmatize, discriminate or even directly harm the group. The extreme example of this was in Nazi Germany (See Ch 6). The step from analysis and interpretation to beneficial implementation of the recommendations arising is a tough one and it needs an appropriate political and strategic framework for success (see Chapters 9 and 10).

Qualitative data enrich, augment and validate the health needs analysis by adding opinions, beliefs, perceptions, attitudes, self-reported behaviour, and case history material. Such data are particularly valuable when collected and analysed in a rigorous way. Having said this, we need to exercise caution in regard to qualitative data based on casual opinions and perceptions, particularly if it reinforces stereotyping. Health needs assessments using quantitative information have shown that perceptions of the needs of minorities are often erroneous e.g. on perceived levels of immunization (perceived low, actually often high), overall life expectancy (perceived as worse, actually often better or similar), availability of health education materials in relation to disease patterns (little material for the dominant fatal and serious conditions and more for conditions perceived to be important) etc. Stereotyping is easy and dangerous and health needs assessments are done to counter the problem.

Ethnicity is a complex concept and it does not allow easy assumptions that a person possesses a particular behaviour or health characteristic on the grounds that they are a member of a particular ethnic group. The usefulness of recording a patient's ethnic origin, using a simple label such as Indian, White, or Chinese, without taking account of other factors, is limited. Within every ethnic group there are significant variations in social class, culture and customs. For example, whether a person needs an interpreter cannot be judged from the label Bangladeshi, but it can from knowledge of the languages spoken and preferred. Similarly, the label Indian does not inform (and may misinform) about the need for 'halal' food in hospital but the fact that an Indian person is a Muslim indicates, but no more than that, that this is much more likely to be a need than in the average patient. This does not mean that we can always dismiss generalizations or even that all stereotypes are wrong. Some perceptions are accurate and, for example, as is generally believed: needs do vary substantially by ethnic group; minority ethnic groups are better off in some respects and worse in others; service quality, particularly for health promotion and preventive health issues requiring knowledge, is usually worse for minority groups; the cost of care for minority populations for a particular condition (but not necessarily overall) is higher; the needs of minority groups include better communication; and meeting cultural needs often requires religious and dietary preferences being met and health professionals being educated about such matters. There is, however, a fine dividing line between general principles derived from detailed observation and research, and stereotypes based on cursory examination.

The central question that drives health needs assessment for minority populations is this: in what ways are the health needs of minority ethnic groups similar to, and different from, the (usually majority) population that the health care system has evolved to serve?

Before reading on, you should reflect on how you would answer this question by doing Exercise 5.3.

Exercise 5.3 Similarities and differences

+ Is the approach of examining differences sound?
+ What, in general terms, is such an analysis going to show?
+ What are the pitfalls of emphasizing differences?

The answer to the central question is usually complex. In fact, many differences are easily demonstrated. Recent thinking shows a shift away from emphasizing differences, which are surprisingly small when compared to the even more overwhelming similarities. Differences can be exaggerated both because of the human tendency to find them interesting, and the scientific approach of using them as the starting point for research, which is of course the basis of epidemiology. Health needs assessments, as a result, tend to present data to highlight and accentuate differences at the expense of similarities. This can give a biased viewpoint on priorities. Mackintosh and colleagues' (1998) *Step-by-Step*

Guide to Epidemiological Health Needs Assessment (which I draw on extensively in this book), shows how to avoid this problem.

A comprehensive needs assessment following the step-by-step principles has been published by Gill and colleagues (2006), who have shown that the UK's major health priorities are largely applicable to the main minority ethnic groups in the UK and, in particular, that the emphasis on cardiovascular diseases, cancers, mental health and other health problems of modern societies is apt. However, this does not imply that no change in approach, or refinement of services, is needed. A few diseases and problems not figuring in the UK's declared priorities deserve a place in the context of minority ethnic health, e.g. haemoglobinopathies, and tuberculosis. This must not, however, be at the expense of the main priorities, but in addition to them. The need for a balanced and considered approach to priority-setting is well illustrated by the example of stroke and coronary heart disease in the African-Caribbean population. (The challenge of priority setting will be discussed in Chapter 7.) Stroke mortality is undoubtedly exceptionally high, and with the possible exception of Bangladeshi men, the highest of all the ethnic groups studied. In comparison with most ethnic groups CHD mortality rates in African-Caribbeans are low. Superficially, one may judge that for this ethnic group stroke services and prevention ought to take priority over CHD. A closer examination shows that CHD is actually a substantially commoner cause of death in African-Caribbeans than stroke is. Neglecting CHD in favour of stroke would miss the bigger problem and run the risk of the African-Caribbean community losing its relative advantage in regard to CHD over the population as a whole. (This has happened to African-Americans in the USA.) The remainder of this chapter concerns the methods underlying this type of analysis.

5.2 The questions driving data collection in health needs assessment

Salman Rawaf's ten steps for health needs assessment, originally applied to drug misuse, are illustrative of the process (see Table 5.2). An assessment of health need is educative for the people doing it.

The eight key questions driving health needs assessment are as follows:

1. What are the demographic and social characteristics of the minority ethnic groups in the area and how are these changing? (Section 5.2.1)
2. What is the culture and lifestyle of the ethnic minority population and how is this changing? (Section 5.2.2)
3. What illnesses and diseases affect the ethnic minority populations and in what quantity? (Sections 5.2.3–5.2.7)
4. What services are available for these conditions and how are they adapting? (Section 5.2.8)
5. How well are services meeting needs and what plans are already in place to improve them? (Section 5.3)

6. What do the public and professionals think about the services? (Sections 5.3.2 and 5.4) Are they being used? (Section 5.5)

7. How can service for minority ethnic groups be evaluated? (Section 5.6)

8. What changes are needed to match services to needs better? (Whole chapter, and Chapters 7 and 8.)

5.2.1 What are the demographic and social characteristics of the minority ethnic groups in the local area and how are these changing?

Demography is the study of the structure and change in populations based, in particular, on the census and vital registration statistics on births, deaths, migrations and marriages. Such data are most accurate around the census year (in many countries the census is decennial i.e. it occurs every ten years). Between census years, and also in some places even in the census year e.g. the inner city, information is not very accurate, especially for small areas. Despite its limitations there is no serious alternative to a census. In some countries, such as the Netherlands, there is a population register, usually held and managed at city level. Such registers have the benefit of being continuously updated, but

Table 5.2 The ten steps for needs assessment (as adapted by the author)

STEP 1:	Profile your population. Source of data: census data, health and social population surveys, specific surveys and research studies, professional and lay judgements.
STEP 2:	Measure the extent of the problem/issue. Source of data: analysis of national and local statistics on causes of illness, disease and death.
STEP 3:	Calculate the expected number of cases. Apply the best possible incidence/prevalence to the population or a group of the population in a given geographical area at a given time (year) to extrapolate the expected number of cases.
STEP 4:	Collect and analyse routine data on service utilisation (current and trends). Source of data: General and mental hospital activity statistics (A & E, inpatients, outpatients, outreach service); community service statistics; social service activity statistics; crime statistics; arrest and probation statistics.
STEP 5:	Calculate the unmet needs or excessive service provision: compare your expected number of cases with the current number of cases demanding intervention(s) and the capacity of the service to identify the size of possible unmet needs or surplus services.
STEP 6:	Segment your population into different strata (population segmentation): once the population structure is dissected and the estimate of the prevalence by various age groups, sex, etc. has been determined, it would be useful to segment the population in terms of their ability to benefit from the intervention.
STEP 7:	Review the current evidence on the effectiveness of intervention(s): as effectiveness studies by ethnic group are rare, a general review will almost certainly be needed.
STEP 8:	Measure your population's perceptions and expectations: focus in particular on people's understanding of the issues, and utilization and quality of services.
STEP 9:	Seek the opinions of professionals about the size of the problems, best practices and service delivery.
STEP 10:	Project the type and size of the action programs and services need to deal with the identified problem.

Reproduced with permission from Rawaf, S. and Marshall, F. (1999). Drug Misuse: The Ten Steps for Needs Assessment. *Public Health Medicine*, 1: 21–26.

they have very limited data on social and economic circumstances on the registrants. Also how are the data on registers to be verified? Census data can be cross-checked against estimates obtained from registers. The most reliable method of obtaining information by ethnic group is a census—for those wishing to assess needs of ethnic minority populations the highest priority is for a census that includes ethnicity as eloquently explained by Veena Raleigh.

> The 1991 census offers rich opportunities for studying Britain's multi-ethnic populations. For the first time health authorities have comprehensive data on their ethnic minority populations, which can be used to assess needs and purchase services. Furthermore, ethnic epidemiology, hitherto limited largely to analysis by country of birth and thereby resulting in the omission of about half of the Asian and black populations who are born in Britain, will be revolutionised by the availability of population denominators from the census. No longer can ignorance be used as a cover for inaction or inappropriate action.
>
> Raleigh (1994: 288)

The UK censuses, in common with other countries, also incorporated questions on country of birth, religion (in 2001 for the first time), long-term illness, occupation, housing conditions, family structure, social class, etc., and so a picture of the minority population can be built up from this one source of information. Some censuses include information on languages spoken and questions on this are being considered for the UK censuses in 2011. (See Chapter 2.)

Unfortunately, members of minority ethnic groups are more likely than average to be missed by the census, which is also the case for those living in inner city areas (also characteristic of ethnic minority groups), and for younger age groups (characteristic of ethnic minority groups), and so their census-derived numbers may be erroneously low. The census offices are likely to offer estimates of the undercount. The validity of health statistics by ethnic group is based on the assumptions that ethnicity categories are valid and consistently defined and ascertained, that they are understood by the populations questioned, that participation and response rates are high and similar for all populations questioned, and that people's responses are consistent over time. These assumptions cannot be taken for granted for reasons that are discussed throughout this book, but particularly in Chapters 2 and 3.

Professionals may have knowledge of the ethnic make-up of their local population and in some instances, their understanding may be deeper and more up to date than that from statistical sources, particularly where there is a rapid change in the composition of the population, possibly through recent relocation or migration for example of asylum seekers and refugees, where change can be very rapid. However, practitioners usually do not know the numbers of people by ethnic group, and in particular, may not be able to differentiate subgroups e.g. Punjabi Indians and Punjabi Pakistanis, very accurately. Census offices usually predict changes in the size and composition of the population. Population change by ethnic minority group is usually only available at national level or in regions where the population is large. Such information is vital for the size and distribution of population is essential for health care planning.

5.2.2 What are the cultures and lifestyles of the ethnic minority populations and how are they changing?

The census usually provides information on a population in relation to population structure (age, sex, marital status etc.) and on many aspects of socio-economic circumstances (employment, housing, and so on). Local health or government authorities may have commissioned reports or even local censuses or surveys about the local population that will augment or update the census data. Usually, however, we need to examine national data and extrapolate to our locality, either qualitatively or quantitatively, from that. These data paint the background picture and help in the interpretation of information on more specific health-related lifestyles. For example, the level of physical activity for disease prevention in a population needs to be interpreted in the light of the location and fabric of the homes, the occupational circumstances, and economic well-being of this population.

Culture and lifestyle are major determinants of health. All aspects of culture and lifestyle which are important for the general population are important for ethnic minorities including smoking, alcohol, exercise, diet and stress. These will be substantially affected by cultural influences such as religion, for example, Sikkism prohibits tobacco and alcohol consumption. Of course, people may not adhere to religious prohibitions, and many Sikhs disobey prohibitions on alcohol consumption yet follow those on tobacco. These general lifestyles must not be overlooked when undertaking health promotion with ethnic minorities (there is evidence that this can happen when attention is diverted by some more specific issue). Other lifestyle issues worth noting in some communities include the use of traditional substances that may contain heavy metals such as eye cosmetics, self-treatment with herbal and other remedies, and a strong sense of modesty especially among women which may affect their health (vitamin D deficiency as a result of inadequate exposure to sunshine) and health care (reluctance in getting physical examinations). Many such traditional customs have been recorded and much attention has been given to them. However, their overall importance to health is relatively small in comparison with lifestyle matters that are general such as exercise or diet.

Information on health-related culture and lifestyle is almost invariably based on self-report. There are many difficulties in comparing ethnic groups using self-reported health and lifestyle data.

Before reading on reflect on some of the uses of self-report data, difficulties in making comparisons, and the questions to ask, by doing Exercise 5.3.

Exercise 5.4 Difficulties in comparing data on lifestyles

- Make a note of some difficulties you envisage in comparing data on the health-related lifestyles of different ethnic groups.
- Examples of lifestyles you might wish to consider include smoking, exercise, diet, alcohol.
- What uses might you make of self-reported data in health settings?

Table 5.3 Uses of self-report data

◆ As an integral part of the clinical interview

◆ As an adjunct to clinical measures, for example using standardized questionnaires such as the SF36 for the assessment of general health status, to assess degree of disability, to check for the presence and severity of symptoms, or to gather patient-assessed outcomes, increasingly included in clinical trials and other studies of treatment efficacy

◆ As a part of epidemiological studies, for example gathering data on health-related behaviour to monitor changes in personal habits, the use of diagnostic tools such as the Rose Angina Questionnaire and for periodic international data collection, such as that on child and adolescent health

◆ By the NHS in relation to health needs assessment for planning and targetting of services

◆ In studies of satisfaction with health care, for example women's views of maternity services

---

From: Hent and Bhopal, *JECH* (2004).

Some of the uses of self-reported data data are in Table 5.3.
The most important questions to ask are these:

◆ Are the populations comparable? It is common practice to draw samples for different ethnic groups using different methods, times or locations. Differences are inevitable when this happens, and may have little or no relation to ethnicity. For example, if the ethnic minority populations are inner city ones, and the comparison population is a mix of urban and rural people, differences may well reflect geography not ethnicity.

◆ Are the data collected equally well and accurately in the different ethnic groups. The concepts underpinning questions (let us say on angina) may be interpreted differently in different ethnic groups. Where questions need translating the potential pitfalls are magnified.

Hunt and Bhopal (1993) have offered guidelines on how to maximize the cross-cultural comparability of self-reported data—the primary source of lifestyle information. Some of the key principles are given in Table 5.4. Hanna and colleagues have shown how difficult it is to create questionnaires employing these principles (in press).

Collecting valid lifestyle data by ethnic group is difficult. Even if the right choices of topic are defined, the study is designed well and the data collection instruments are cross-culturally valid (all tough goals), finding a sampling frame, recruiting people, collecting data, interpreting the results correctly and using them to achieve better health and health care are all taxing challenges. These and other matters will be discussed in Chapter 9 in a research context. A number of surveys are available, nonetheless, with variable quality of data (see references and websites e.g. Erens (books p317)).

Perhaps the best example of how such data can be used is the observation of the high prevalence of tobacco use and oral tobacco in UK Bangladeshi men in particular and Muslim men more generally. Until the data became available smoking control and cessation policies and programmes paid little or no attention to the needs of ethnic minorities and especially South Asians. The revelation that the highest prevalence of

Table 5.4 State of the art translation/adaptation procedures

- Translation of items by a team of bilinguals
- Comparison of translations
- Negotiation of 'best' items
- Consultations with people who are monolingual in the target language(s)
- Item refinement
- Field testing with monolinguals
- Refinements as needed
- Testing for face, content, construct and criterion validity in each language
- Testing for reliability and responsiveness
- Statistical analysis of ratings of quality of translation across different countries

Reproduced from Hunt, S. and Bhopal, R. Self report in clinical and epidemiological studies with non-English speakers the challenge of language and culture. *Journal of Epidemiology and Community Health*, 2004; 58: 618–22.

smoking in the UK is in Bangladeshi men and that smoking cessation rates in ethnic minority groups are comparatively low has focused policy, service and research attention on the issue.

Surveys tend to paint a static picture whereas the reality is one of rapid change. In particular, the children of migrants are often growing up with strikingly different cultural influences and lifestyles compared to their parents. Keeping track of rapid change poses an additional but vital challenge to health needs assessment.

5.2.3 Which illnesses and diseases affect the ethnic minority populations and in what quantity?

Most illnesses and diseases that needs assessors will be interested in are fairly rare, and fortunately, this is especially so for deaths—just over 1 per cent of the population dies in any year. Except in some regions with very large ethnic minority populations, usually those containing major multi-ethnic cities such as London, local information on causes of death will be hard to make sense of, because the numbers of deaths per year will be small and disease rates will be estimated imprecisely.

Knowing the make up of the local ethnic minority community, it should be possible to describe the major health problems by applying the findings from national data by ethnic group to the local population. Even in the extreme case of the complete absence of any data on the causes of death in the ethnic group of interest remember that disease patterns are likely to be similar to the general population, e.g. coronary heart disease and strokes are among the top-ranking fatal diseases for all ethnic groups in the UK, and this applies to most industrialized countries. Usually, however, there are some data nationally. It is possible to extrapolate from national data on mortality in ethnic groups and say with some confidence what are likely to be the health problems of the local ethnic minority population.

Another set of insights applicable to an ethnic minority group come from the disease patterns in the country of ancestral origin. In some cases the insights are obvious e.g. haemoglobinopathies are common in Africa, the Middle East and India and these genetic problems are likely to be important in ethnic minority groups who originate from these places wherever they live. Genetic diseases are a relatively fixed feature of a population. The knowledge gained may, however, be much more subtle especially for environmentally acquired problems. An appreciation that oral cancers are common in the Indian subcontinent, and nasopharyngeal cancers common in China, would alert the needs assessors to these problems in the overseas Indian and Chinese origin populations, respectively. There is, however, no substitute for real data that pertain to the population under assessment. Again, this is because of the rapid change in the disease patterns. It is likely that over time the ethnic minority groups' disease pattern will converge towards the pattern seen in the population as a whole.

Information on the pattern of non-fatal ill-health (morbidity) by ethnic group is very difficult to obtain. You may have to do your own local survey. First, however, check whether your requirements can be met from other sources of data such as registers of people with particular conditions e.g. people with diabetes. In Scotland, the NHS requires every health board to maintain a register of people with diabetes. The local diabetes centre (or other specialist centre) should have a list of all people with known diabetes and it may be possible to identify people from the ethnic minority community - perhaps on the basis of name (although this will only apply to specific groups, as discussed in Chapter 3), or better, by the recorded ethnic code. Cancer registrations in the UK include country of birth.

Information on diseases, on its own, is of limited use, but used with the census for the denominators (population at risk) it will be possible to calculate disease incidence rates by country of birth, or ethnic group, or both. Data on ethnicity should, in theory, be available in hospital statistics in countries that have implemented ethnic coding. English hospitals have been required to collect the ethnic background of patients since 1995 as part of the minimum data set, although this has not been properly achieved yet—in recent years efforts to do this well have been redoubled. With improvements in ethnic monitoring, reliable data on numbers of people with specific illnesses ought to be available from hospitals. (Ethnic monitoring was discussed in Chapter 3, and policies underpinning it will be discussed in Chapter 8.)

General practitioner records in the UK and primary care/family practice records in other countries may be a useful method of obtaining numbers of people with specific conditions. Although GP records in the UK do not routinely state ethnicity, it is common for people from certain ethnic minority groups to be registered with a small number of GPs who may be able to both identify people and describe their needs. In practice, however, this is often not achievable. The case for ethnic monitoring of GP records is very strong, particularly as then the ethnic group and other relevant data can be forwarded to specialists on referral. Small-scale studies have demonstrated this is feasible. In the UK, shortly, there will be a small incentive payment to general practices that collect ethnic codes on their newly registered patients. (This topic was discussed in Chapter 3.)

There may have been some research carried out into the health and disease patterns of ethnic minority groups locally and so reports and scientific papers may be available. In most instances, however, local estimates will need to be obtained by applying national rates to the local population—for example, approximately 20 per cent of South Asians aged 35–64 have diabetes, therefore it can be estimated that 20 per cent or 1 in 5 of your local South Asian population within this age group will probably have this disease. This simple procedure can be applied to any condition. Where there are no national studies, it is necessary to apply data from local research studies carried out in other areas. For example, data on the health of the Chinese population are rare. However, it would be possible for someone working in, say, Manchester, to use data from a study in Newcastle reported on by Nigel Unwin and colleagues and apply it to their population. From the age-adjusted figures in Table 5.5 the disease rate for men from the Chinese community in Newcastle who have diabetes is almost twice that of the European origin (Europid was the preferred term of the investigators) population. (Overall, glucose tolerance is similar.)

The figure for Chinese women is also higher than for European origin (Europid) women, although the difference is not as great. However, the rate for Chinese women who have impaired glucose tolerance (IGT) is almost twice that of European origin (Europid) women. (Impaired glucose tolerance is said to be present when blood glucose measurement is higher than the normal range but below the diabetic range.)

Table 5.5 The numbers, proportions, and age adjusted rates for Europid and Chinese men and women in Newcastle upon Tyne with glucose intolerance in relation to age group

	No		Impaired glucose tolerance		Diabetes		All glucose intolerance	
	Chinese	Europids	Chinese	Europids	Chinese	Europids	Chinese	Europids
Men								
25–34	53	42	2(3.8)	3(7.1)	0	0	2(3.8)	3(7.1)
35–44	51	77	3(5.9)	7(9.1)	3(5.9)	1(1.3)	6(11.8)	8(10.4)
45–54	43	81	3(7.0)	9(11.1)	3(7.0)	5(6.2)	6(14.0)	14(17.3)
55–64	32	104	6(18.8)	19(18.3)	3(9.4)	6(5.8)	9(28.1)	25(24.0)
All	179	304	14(7.8)	38(12.5)	9(5.0)	12(3.9)	23(12.8)	50(16.4)
Age adjusted			8.0	10.7	5.0	2.9	13.0	13.6
(95% CI)			(4.0,12.0)	(7.2,14.2)	(1.8,8.2)	(1.0,4.8)	(8.1,17.9)	(9.7,17.5)
Women								
25–34	64	38	5(7.8)	0	0	1(2.6)	5(7.8)	1(2.6)
35–44	65	67	10(15.4)	7(10.4)	2(3.1)	1(1.5)	12(18.5)	8(11.9)
45–54	43	83	7(16.3)	12(14.5)	3(7.0)	4(4.8)	10(23.3)	16(19.3)
55–64	24	118	7(29.2)	21(17.8)	2(8.3)	8(6.7)	9(37.5)	29(24.3)
All	196	306	29(14.8)	40(13.1)	7(3.6)	14(4.6)	36(18.4)	63(17.3)
Age adjusted			16.1	9.7*	4.1	3.6	20.2	13.3*
(95% CI)			(11.0,21.2)	(6.4,13.0)	(1.3,6.9)	(1.4,5.6)	(14.6,25.8)	(9.4,17.0)

p values, Chinese vs. Europid.   * <0.05. Figures in brackets indicate 95% confidence intervals

Reproduced from Unwin N, Harland J, White M, Bhopal R, Winocour P, Stephenson P, Watson W, Turner C, Alberti KGMM. *Journal of Epidemiology and Community Health*, 1997; 51: 160–166

These findings are likely to be relevant outside Newcastle. Detailed data of these kind are only available in expensive research projects and it is important to use them, but how can we increase confidence that the findings can be generalized? First, we can check whether the Newcastle Chinese population is similar in its characteristics e.g. age and sex structure, region of origin in China, religion, height, weight, etc., to that in the other places where the information is to be applied. Some of this (age, sex structure) can be done using census data. Second, we can see whether the findings on a more easily obtained data item e.g. self-reported diabetes, are comparable between the research report and other information sources, say, national data. If so, confidence on generalizability is increased.

Once the data are obtained describing and interpreting disease patterns is based on epidemiological approaches. This is vital to health needs assessment and is discussed in detail below.

5.2.4 Epidemiological approaches to presentation and interpretation of data

Epidemiological approaches to health needs assessment present data to show actual and relative morbidity and mortality rates, calculate years of life lost, and assess the impact and loss of social functioning. In assessing the health needs of ethnic minority groups, the most popular approach has been to compare their health status to the population as a whole or the ethnic majority i.e. in Britain the White population. Essentially, in this way a disease that is commoner than in the White population is declared a problem and a relatively higher priority than one that is less common than in the White population. This comparative perspective, which is intrinsically ethnocentric, has some merit but it can also be misleading. By concentrating on issues where the problem is in excess, attention may be given to a narrow range of issues and drawn away from ensuring that all health services are equitable and available to all. This approach may lead to some needs of ethnic minorities being sidelined in relation to their importance—in the UK this had happened with respiratory diseases and lung cancer. The principles are illustrated with mortality data from the UK. (You may wish to re-read Section 3.6.3 in Chapter 3 on mortality data by country of birth.)

The SMR (standardized mortality/morbidity ratio) is a summary measure of the rate of disease or death in a population that takes into account differences in age structure of populations. The standard or reference population is given a value of 100. A SMR exceeding 100 means an excess of the health problem in the study population, and a value of less than 100 means a deficit. Table 5.6 contains data originally presented by Michael Marmot and colleagues.

As in this table, SMRs relative to the majority or whole population are almost invariably provided in reports on ethnicity and health (which sometimes present disease ranking by SMR) and are usually given emphasis in text. Try Exercise 5.5 before reading on.

Table 5.6 Deaths and SMRs among a male immigrant population (aged 20 and over) to England and Wales by cause

Cause of death	Rank (top 5)	Deaths	SMR
Ch I Infective and parasitic diseases A6–10 Tuberculosis—all forms	3	64	315
Ch II Neoplasms		722	69
Malignant neoplasm of:			
A45 Buccal cavity and pharynx	5	28	178
A46 Oesophagus		30	110
A47 Stomach		50	45
A48 Intestine		38	55
A49 Rectum		27	57
ICD 155 Liver and intrahepatic ducts	2	19	338
ICD 156 Gall bladder and bile ducts		9	139
A50 Larynx		12	127
A51 Trachea, bronchus and lung		218	53
A53 Skin		8	73
A54 Breast		0	—
A55 Cervix uteri			
A56 Uterus (other)			
A57 Prostate		48	105
ICD 183 Ovary, fallopian tube and broad ligament			
A59–60 Leukaemia and other neoplasms of lymphatic and haematopoietic tissue		74	96
Ch III Endocrine, nutritional and metabolic diseases			
A64 Diabetes mellitus	4	55	188
Ch IV Diseases of blood and blood-forming organs		8	92
A73 Multiple Sclerosis		2	22
Ch VII Circulatory diseases		2,377	111
A81 Chronic rheumatic heart disease		46	86
A82 Hypertensive disease		85	128
A83 Ischaemec heart disease		1,533	115
A84 Other forms of heart disease		134	96
A85 Cerebrovascular disease		438	108
A86 Diseases of arteries		101	99
A87 Venous thrombosis and embolism		37	102

Table 5.6 (*Continued*)

Cause of death	Rank (top 5)	Deaths	SMR
Ch VIII Respiratory diseases		494	86
A90 Influenza		22	80
A92 Other (non-viral) pneumonia		214	100
A93 Bronchitis emphysema and asthma		223	77
Ch IX Digestive diseases		111	106
A98 Peptic ulcer		37	105
A102 Cirrhosis of liver		25	145
Ch X Diseases of the genito-urinary system		93	151
A106 other (non-acute) nephritis		39	160
A107 Infections of kidney		20	176
Ch XI Complications of pregnancy, childbirth and puerperium			
Ch XVII Accidents, poisonings and violence		333	102
AE138 Motor vehicle accidents		134	110
AE140 Accidental poisoning		15	118
AE141 Accidental falls		24	76
AE147 Suicide		69	90
AE148 Homicide	1	21	341
AE149 Injury undetermined whether accidentally or purposely inflicted		28	147
All causes		4,352	98

Data from Marmot *et al.* (1984) extract of table A14.3, p. 132.

Exercise 5.5 Tables of mortality by SMRs and case numbers

◆ What is your reaction on being presented with a Table like 5.6?

◆ What is your eye drawn to? What facts strike you as important ones?

◆ Which diseases would you pick out as reflecting the priority needs of this male immigrant population?

◆ Examine the data in Table 5.7. Now look at the table and confirm that the right-hand column ranks diseases by their relative frequency based on SMR and that the left-hand column shows diseases among the same men ranked by number of deaths.

◆ Which cause of death killed most men born in the Indian subcontinent? (Q1)

◆ Which cause of death is greatest in Indian subcontinent-born men relative to the men born in England and Wales? (Q2)

◆ Which is a bigger health issue for Indian subcontinent-born men, ischaemic heart disease or homicide? (Q3)

Most people find tables like 5.6 daunting. It takes considerable patience to extract the key messages. The eye is drawn to summary figures. Here the summary figures are, first, the ranks (top five) and second the SMR. The raw, unsummarized data are on numbers of deaths. The diseases one would pick out depends on the readers' perspectives but most readers would be guided by the text given by the authors. In this case, as is often true, the authors emphasized the patterns shown by the comparatively high SMRs.

Table 5.7 contains a reworking by me and published with Senior, of the data originally presented by Michael Marmot and colleagues (the same as table 1.4). The two columns give radically different perspectives on disease patterns. The priority needs would certainly include ischaemic heart disease, cerebrovascular disease, and neoplasm of the trachea, bronchus and lung. In terms of impact on the population's health, homicide (21 deaths but ranked first in table 5.6) is dwarfed by ischaemic heart disease (1533 deaths). Analysis and interpretation using SMRs is grounded on the classic epidemiological strategy of generating hypotheses about disease causation by focusing on differences. However, this is insufficient for assessing health needs. Coronary heart disease was not in the top five ranks based on SMR in Table 5.6. The top-ranking conditions in Table 5.6 (homicide and neoplasm of the liver and intrahepatic bile duct) do not figure in the left-hand side of Table 5.6 but dominate the right-hand side.

Based on the actual number of deaths ischaemic heart disease is the main problem, but using the SMR, homicide seems the main problem. Thus, without examination of

Table 5.7 Deaths and SMR's* in male immigrants from the Indian subcontinent (aged 20 and over; total deaths = 4,352)

By rank order of number of deaths				By rank order of SMR			
Cause	Number of deaths	% of total	SMR	Cause	Number of deaths	% of total	SMR
Ischaemic heart disease	1533	35.2	115	Homicide	21	0.5	341
Cerebrovascular disease	438	10.1	108	Liver and intrahepatic bile duct neoplasm	19	0.4	338
Bronchitis, emphysema and asthma	223	5.1	77	Tuberculosis	64	1.5	315
Neoplasm of the trachea, bronchus and lung	218	5.0	53	Diabetes mellitus	55	1.3	188
Other non-viral pneumonia	214	4.9	100	Neoplasm of buccal cavity and pharynx	28	0.6	178
Total	2626	60.3	–		187	4.3	–

*Standardized mortality ratios, comparing with the male population of England and Wales, which was by definition 100.
Source of original data for the construction of this table was Marmot and collegues (1984).
Reproduced from Senior P, Bhopal RS. Ethnicity as a variable in epidemiological research. *British Medical Journal*, 1994; 309: 327–330, with permission from BMJ Publishing Group.

table 5.6 from these two perspectives, we get a misleading interpretation of major health problems in this immigrant group (in fact men born in the Indian subcontinent). The primary perspective of the right hand side of Table 5.7 is to compare and contrast the performance of other ethnic groups to that of the majority population. The perspective of the left-hand side is to consider the common, dominant problems of groups.

Generally, when the data are presented using the number of cases, or rankings based upon this, the major health problems for minority groups seem similar to those of the population as a whole. When presented using the SMR, the differences are emphasized. For example, while there are some differences between ethnic groups in the UK, circulatory diseases, cancers and respiratory diseases are the major fatal diseases for all ethnic groups. The comparative, relative risk approach underlying SMRs, which focuses on diseases either more or less common in ethnic minority groups, refines the analysis, so it should not be discarded but it should be seen as supplementary.

Interpretation of data has often been misguided by an excessive emphasis on differences rather than similarities, the uncritical use of 'White populations as a standard to which minority populations should aspire, and the use of data sets looking at a limited number of conditions or particular age groups. To avoid these and similar problems the following approach is recommended:

◆ Base the epidemiological component of the needs assessment on disease causes using case numbers and disease rates and rankings based on these.

◆ Refine understanding by looking at comparative indices such as the SMR, and rankings based on this, which will focus attention on inequalities and potential inequities.

◆ Draw causal hypotheses based on differences with care, and with due emphasis to social and economic deprivation as explanatory factors.

◆ Beware that inferences of biological difference between ethnic and racial groups may be particularly prone to error and misinterpretation, and may harm the standing of minority groups.

A sample 'dummy' health needs assessment data table is shown as Table 5.8.

Unfortunately, most existing reports and papers neither present analyses in this format nor provide the information to permit readers to extract it themselves. Gill and colleagues (2006) have, however, presented data in this format. Other issues that underpin the epidemiological approach are considered below.

Table 5.8 The standard table for assessment of the pattern of disease, particulary for needs assessment purposes

Disease or condition	Number of cases	Rate	Rank position on number of cases or rate	SMR/relative risk	Rank on SMR

5.2.5 **Epidemiological approaches for health needs assessment: making choices and understanding limitations**

Questions which are essential to the process of epidemiological modes of health needs assessment for ethnic minority groups include:

- Which ethnic groups are to be studied?
- Are the ethnic categories used to define population subgroups acceptable, ethical and accurate?
- What data need to be collected?
- Have we collected accurate, representative data?
- How do we derive from the data a true picture of health and health care needs and priorities (the latter is considered in Chapter 7)?

For reasons discussed in Chapter 2, the choice of ethnic groups and group categories is usually influenced by the classification used at census. For national studies reliant on census data for denominator information this is invariably the case but there is sometimes flexibility in local studies. For example, we may be interested in the pattern of health and disease in Muslims, Punjabis, Gujeratis, or Christians compared to Buddhist Chinese, but data are unlikely to be available, at least nationally. The nearest we can usually get is the appropriate category at census. We could gather data on Indians and their religions. The appropriate denominators would be available from the census. The census is the key to building a picture of the ethnic minority communities and analysing and interpreting most epidemiological data. Using pragmatic categories that cannot be linked to the census can be misleading and wasteful. For example, one ethnic category that is commonly used is 'Asian' as a label for people from India, Pakistan, Bangladesh and Sri Lanka. This label may lead to an erroneous view that South Asians are ethnically homogeneous—which may have adverse consequences for health (as discussed earlier generally in Chapters 1 and 2, and in relation to the smoking prevalence data in Table 3.1 in Chapter 3). Moreover, it may prove impossible to get an accurate denominator for the 'Asian' population, so disease rates cannot be calculated.

The limitations of census categories are discussed in Chapter 2, but as they have usually been tested in both pilot studies and in widespread community consultation they are likely to be acceptable to the populations described at the time they are devised. This generalization may not hold in societies where the power imbalance permits one ethnic group to impose its will on others. Also, categories that are acceptable at one point in time may become unacceptable (as discussed in Chapter 2 we see this with words used to describe African origin populations e.g. black, Negro; and we know that Oriental to denote Far East peoples is no longer acceptable). Where due consultation has taken place, and the purposes of data collection are fair, holding such data is likely to be ethical and legal (see Chapters 9 and 10 for further elaboration of this point).

The choice of data items depends on the underlying purpose. In health needs assessment the challenge is to provide both professionals, and ideally also members of ethnic minority communities, as quickly as possible, with balanced information to allow them to make informed choices about priority issues. The ultimate aim is to make rational judgements on the actions to be taken. The value of mortality and morbidity data is self-evident even if proxies for ethnicity are used. Reliable national statistics on hospital utilization by ethnic group or country of birth are often not available. Information on the patterns of (non-fatal) ill-health is difficult to obtain. The challenge is to balance the ideal against what is available. Data on mortality and lifestyles can be re-analysed or extracted from published documents comparatively easily so it is inevitable that needs assessments will use them. The demonstration of missing gaps is important to guide future work. To interpret data properly needs an understanding of their limitations. We have already examined the strengths and limitations of mortality variations by country of birth in Chapter 3 (Section 3.6.3 and Exercise 3.6). Nonetheless, some further emphasis and revision in the context of health needs assessment is appropriate. Many of the principles discussed here apply to other kinds of data, particularly those in large databases and collected for administrative purposes.

Before reading on try Exercise 5.6.

Exercise 5.6 Limitations of mortality data

◆ List the potential limitations of mortality data analysis by ethnic group for assessing health needs

---

The accuracy and validity of the numerator (death data) and denominator (population data) and the possibility of a mismatch in the way ethnicity or country of birth is recorded in the two data sets (numerator–denominator bias) should be considered carefully in interpreting mortality data. Death data usually include information on any person dying in a country and thereby may include deaths of visitors. Death data may include information on residents of a country dying in other countries only if these are notified to the authorities. Such reporting probably varies across different populations and thereby by ethnic group. It is evident that ethnic minority groups are both more likely to have overseas visitors and to spend time overseas. If they die overseas in the country of origin it is less likely that their remains will be repatriated—not least because of the dual nature of residency, nationality and sense of home and belonging of recent migrants.

Recording of country of birth or other indicators of ethnicity on death certificates, which is reliant on an informant (usually the next of kin), may be less accurate than on the census (recorded by head of household), when the person is still alive to provide the information. This can lead to numerator–denominator bias (i.e. where country of birth is recorded differently in census and mortality data). One answer, used in previous analyses of mortality by country of birth (e.g. Marmot and colleagues), is to group together countries where this is a particular issue (e.g. Indian subcontinent countries). This grouping approach obscures potentially important differences between people with different countries of birth, so substituting one kind of error with another. Death certificates and hence mortality statistics do not provide an accurate reflection of the importance of certain conditions in the general population e.g. diabetes mellitus, which is very common but which usually ends in death from cardiovascular diseases. Variation in accuracy of cause of death described on death certificates by country of birth or ethnic group may exist. This is likely to be especially important for deaths occurring abroad, particularly where the cause of death has not been given by a medical doctor.

In analysis of mortality statistics we need to align counts of cases and population at risk (from the census). Usually the published census statistics exclude people who are not normally residents. If so, deaths of visitors should not be included in the count of cases, the numerator. Census data is invariably incomplete. The effect of this is to overestimate the calculated mortality rates. Restricting the mortality analyses to the year of, or years around (usually three, four or at most five years), the census minimizes the effect of population change and inaccuracies in the denominator. The downside is that the numbers of deaths are reduced by this restriction. Sometimes it is possible to estimate population size and structure between censuses by using two censuses e.g. the 1996 structure might, for example, be estimated as midway that in 1991 and 2001.

At present, analyses of mortality in the UK, and some other countries, are limited to the use of country of birth because ethnic group is not available on death certificates. Country of birth provides no indication of length of stay in either the country of birth or country of residence. Mortality by country of birth is a particularly poor measure of health in children as, for example, very few ethnic minority children living in the UK were born abroad and so mortality statistics are a very incomplete measure of mortality by ethnic group. By contrast, in the UK nearly all non-White ethnic minority people over 60 years of age were born abroad. So in this age group country of birth statistics are a good alternative to ethnic group. In other countries, this may not apply.

Studies of immigrant populations show that mortality experience converges to that of the host population with time and particularly in succeeding generations. Surprisingly, the overall mortality of even very poor new migrants is usually either similar to or lower than the population as a whole, even when the immigrants are from countries with high mortality. This is probably because they are a select group of people without the health problems that would deter migration. The 'healthy migrant effect' is the term used to describe the fact that migrants tend to be healthier than the populations they leave and join. There is also the possibility that ethnic minority people emigrate, often to their country of ancestral origin (so-called salmon bias) or elsewhere, as a consequence of ill-health. There is certainly a tendency to return to the place of birth or ancestral homeland in old age. Some people probably die unexpectedly during such visits. Others may go there deliberately in the knowledge they will die there. On the other hand medical facilities are likely to be poorer in the country of origin, which is a deterrent to returning. Overall, 'salmon bias' has not been studied in detail, but the general view is that it is not very important.

Notwithstanding these and other limitations data need to be turned into information and the next section summarizes what information has accrued as a result of UK based epidemiological analyses.

5.2.6 Patterns of disease in ethnic minority groups

Armed with the cautions and principles above it is possible to draw much of value and interest from the rich and enlarging data sets on ethnicity and health internationally. The following are some of the types of conclusions that are fairly robust, and arise from a number of health needs assessments, particularly that by Gill and colleagues.

Ethnic minority groups are heterogeneous in their health, both in overall health (e.g. measured by the all-cause mortality or self-reported health) and specific causes (e.g. coronary heart disease or oral cancers). There is also great heterogeneity within the usual broad ethnic groupings (South Asian, Chinese, Black, White, etc.) although this is insufficiently explored territory. Harnessing this heterogeneity is definitely an area for future research.

There is a common assumption and frequently stated view that the health of ethnic minorities is worse than expected (judged by the standard of the ethnic majority, usually White, population). This is at best simplistic, and sometimes wrong. First, such conclusions need to be cautious in the light of the possible weaknesses in the underlying data, particularly those based on mortality statistics. Second, even on the basis of the published statistics, overall measures such as SMRs are often around and sometimes less than 100 in some ethnic minority populations. Recent analysis in England and Wales shows that Chinese and Caribbean populations have all-cause SMRs well below 100. There is the subtle question of how we judge the level of expected health. Is it right to base the expected level on the White population which, on average, has much higher economic standing? Might it be that taking into account social and economic factors the health of ethnic minority groups is about the level to be expected? Sometimes the highest all cause SMRs are not in the ethnic minority groups but in a subgroup of the White population—e.g. Irish-born and Scots-born people living in England.

In many respects the ethnic minority groups have similar patterns of disease and overall health to the ethnic majority. This is most obvious when disease rankings are based on frequency as in Tables 5.7 (L. hand column) and 5.9.

For example, coronary heart disease, stroke and cancer are the commonest cause of death, and accidents, poisonings, digestive disorders, respiratory infection and circulatory problems the main reasons for admission to hospital in the UK whichever community you consider. Health professionals caring for ethnic minority patients will usually be confronted with these common problems, and will see the conditions that are more specific to ethnic minorities comparatively infrequently. Health professionals will need to make the correct diagnosis in the face of greater communication or cultural barriers than they are accustomed to. However, both health authorities and individual practitioners need to know of the conditions that are rare in the population as a whole and yet sometimes

Table 5.9 Commonest causes of admission (in rank order) to hospitals in Leicestershire

'Asians' by diagnostic category	Number	Non-Asians by diagnostic category	Number
1. Accidents/poisonings	404	1. Accidents/poisonings	7442
Fracture	93	Fracture	2204
Burns	11		
2. Digestive system	384	2. Circulatory system	6693
Appendicitis	56	Ischaemic heart disease	2155
Cirrhosis	10		
3. Respiratory system	377	3. Digestive system	6141
Obstructive	104	Appendicitis	864
Airways disease			
4. Symptoms and signs	370	4. Symptoms and signs	5088
5. Circulatory system	352	5. Respiratory system	4606
Ischaemic heart disease	141	Chronic obstructive airways disease	749
6. Infectious disease	277	6. Neoplasms	4343
Tuberculosis	153	Lung	755
Malaria	28		
7. Nervous system	206	7. Nervous system	2887
8. Genito-urinary system	160	8. Genito-urinary system	2634
9. Perinatal	156	9. Musculoskeletal	1952
10. Congenital abnormality	126	10. Congenital anomalies	1193
11. Neoplasms	120	11. Infectious diseases	872
Lung	11	Tuberculosis	128
Oesophagus	6		

From Bhopal RS, Donaldson LJ. Health education for ethnic minorities: current provision and future direction. *Health Education Journal* 1988; 47: 137–40, with permission from Health Education Journal.

seen in minority ethnic communities e.g. typhoid fever, tuberculosis, nasopharyngeal cancer, malaria, etc. Health authorities may need to modify their service priorities and practitioners their approach to diagnosis to accommodate these differences.

Some of the conditions that are much commoner in the UK (and probably in similar countries) in one or more minority ethnic groups than the population as a whole include:

- infectious diseases including tuberculosis and malaria;
- diabetes mellitus;

- perinatal mortality;
- hypertension and cerebro-vascular disease;
- cancer of the oropharynx; cancer of the liver; cancer of the prostate
- haemoglobinopathies;
- vitamin D deficiency.

Equally, there are some conditions which are less common in one or more minority ethnic groups relative to the population as a whole, including:

- many cancers, including the common ones of lung and breast
- anxiety and depressive disorders
- suicide
- accidents
- peripheral vascular disease
- alcoholism.

The above lists are not comprehensive. For most specific conditions, the SMR is not consistently high in every ethnic group, for example, compared to the whole UK population ischaemic heart disease is relatively common in Indian, Pakistani, and Bangladeshi populations but relatively uncommon in the Chinese and Afro-Caribbeans.

Differences in disease patterns need careful attention, but not at the expense of potentially more important diseases that show no such differences (such as respiratory diseases). Conditions which are less common in minority ethnic groups than in the White population that tend to be ignored include lung cancer, the leading cancer in men in most ethnic groups, and among the leaders for women. It and similar conditions may be worth more attention than conditions which are actually rare, though relatively more common than in the White population, e.g. liver cancer.

The differences are complex and vary over time and between ethnic groups. Simplifications may easily mislead. Information is most readily available for the visible, large populations that are enumerated using specific categories at census. Some groups where the need may be great are often relatively invisible in health statistics e.g. asylum seekers, refugees, gypsy travellers and people from Eastern Europe and the Middle East. Describing health patterns is central to health needs assessment but the value of data is enhanced by understanding the factors that cause differences.

5.2.7 **How do we explain differences?**

Describing is not enough—meeting needs also needs understanding of causes of differences, and if possible causes of similarities. Epidemiological strategies for understanding similarities, however, are not well developed. (Causal interpretation will be considered in some detail in Chapter 9.)

Before reading on do Exercise 5.7.

Exercise 5.7 Categorizing the explanations for ethnic/racial differences

- List the differences between ethnic groups which could explain their different patterns of disease. (You may wish to focus your thinking using the disease stroke, or cerebrovascular accident, which in the UK is more common in most ethnic minority groups.)
- Can you put them into categories?

This question of causality poses great difficulty because ethnic inequalities are very complex—they combine cultural, socio-economic and, for a few diseases, genetic factors as underlying causes. In understanding differences we must be wary of the idea, based on the race concept, that the differences are largely or wholly attributable to genetic factors and hence are biological and physiological (which is only true for a few diseases such as haemoglobinopathies). Equally, the idea based on the ethnicity concept that differences are caused by cultural factors is too readily accepted without scrutiny (it is sometimes true but it detracts attention from the other factors).

Other underlying explanations, such as demographic and epidemiological transitions, lifestyle/economic change, migration itself, occupation, poverty, racism and economic problems, are often inadequately explored. Socio-economic deprivation, in particular, is an important and underestimated explanation of disease differences among ethnic groups. This analysis will be developed in the context of ethnic inequalities in the next chapter, and in the context of causal research in Chapter 9.

5.2.8 **What services are available and adapted for ethnic minority populations?**

Since the primary influence of a health needs assessment is on health care, and in the case of ethnic minorities, adaptation of existing services, we need to find out what services are available and how they have already been shaped to meet needs. Fortunately, information on services actually available is usually easy to obtain. What is harder to find is what adaptations have been made to accommodate ethnic minority groups and how successful these have been, particularly in terms of health outcomes.

Service utilization data by ethnic group that are reliable are also rare, for lack of high-quality ethnic monitoring. In the UK the Race Relations Amendment Act (2000) is requiring both ethnic monitoring of service use and employment practices and review and publication of policies (as Race Equality Schemes—see Chapter 8). Even given such information it is not going to be easy to judge whether the service is adequate.

To help interpretation of such information, therefore, guidelines are needed on what should be available, and the standards that are to be attained. A list of services that should be available might be obtainable from the health service (e.g. NHS), or national bodies representing particular conditions e.g. British or American Heart Foundation.

Table 5.10 Checklist of required services for management of cardiovascular disease and diabetes

Service	Availability
Lifestyle management	
Risk factor control	
Prescription for exercise	
Annual reviews for ischaemic heart disease and diabetes	
Dietetics	
Foot care	
Eye care	
Hypertension clinics	
Anticoagulation clinics	
Open access echocardiography	
Open access ECG	
Open access Holter monitoring	
Open access exercise testing	
Emergency cardiology services	
Angiography and percutaneous transluminal coronary angioplasty	
Coronary artery bypass graft	
Carotid-endarterectomy	
Renal Services (dialysis and replacement)	
Rehabilitation (post stroke)	
Rehabilitation (post MI)	

As an example, for diabetes, the service provision needed has been detailed by the charity Diabetes UK. The charity's web site sets out the standards of care, including that interpreters are to be available when needed, and gives a detailed list of checks to be made at the annual review. Such guidance can then be checked against what is actually available in the local service. The guidance may need to be adapted for the ethnic minority communities, e.g. Table 5.10 is a checklist of services for the management of heart disease and diabetes. The needs assessor checks availability.

Before reading on try Exercise 5.8.

Exercise 5.8 Questions to guide adaptation of services

◆ What questions would you ask to help adapt the checklist in Table 5.10 for ethnic minority groups?

The kind of list in Table 5.10 needs adaptation for use for minority ethnic groups by asking further questions as in Table 5.11, a sample of the kind that could be asked. The answers may not be available but they can be the starting point of ongoing analysis. The analysis needs to be infused with the insights from quantitative data, and supplemented with qualitative information as discussed below.

Table 5.11 Questions to guide adaptation of services for ethnic minority populations—examples

◆ Are there issues that are priorities for ethnic minority groups that might be missed here? For example, the need for same-sex services for exercise and other related matters.

◆ Are there services prioritized here that are not very relevant to ethnic minority groups?

◆ Have the staff been trained in delivering culturally appropriate services to ethnic minority groups?

◆ Can staff speak in the preferred languages of the local minority populations? If not,

◆ Do patients have access to appropriately trained interpreters?

◆ Are there procedures to ensure that the cultural or religious requirements of patients are recorded in patient and nursing records which can be referred to in health care decisions e.g. regarding the type of insulin prescribed? (Pork insulin is not suitable for Muslims.)

◆ Are there mechanisms to ensure that dietetic counselling and advice to minority ethnic patients is consistent with the cultural and religious requirements of the patient and the patient's dietary patterns?

5.3 What do the public and health professionals think of the service? The role of qualitative data in health needs assessment

To answer this question requires social science rather than epidemiological methods. Health needs assessment warrants 'mixed methods' blending quantitative and qualitative methods. For more information on how to do such work readers should consult reference textbooks on field methods in research, such as that by Anne Bowling and Shah Ebrahim, which introduces quantitative and qualitative methods in health research. Joan Mackintosh and colleagues' *Step-by-step Guide* also has more information on methods in the specific context of ethnic majority health. These issues are also discussed briefly in the context of research in Chapter 9.

Qualitative research is based on information in narrative, rather than numerical, form and focuses on the meanings that people place upon their experiences. It uses methods that are applied in a rigorous way to systematically study individual and group perspectives. The result is often not only complementary to quantitative research, but powerfully synergistic. Narrative can bring statistics to life and have an unexpectedly large impact. Narrative, unlike numerical data, is easy to relate to and everyone can understand it. The case history material that qualitative research produces can be particularly powerful in influencing politicians, policy-makers, managers, the public and the media. Most health care professionals, in contrast, prefer quantitative data, which gives information on normative and comparative needs.

Qualitative methods add a new dimension by answering the following kind of questions:

◆ What do the individuals in the ethnic minority communities perceive as being their health needs? This may be different from the picture from statistics and may bring to attention issues that are not captured by formal databases or structured questions.

♦ What are the experiences of members of ethnic minority communities as users of health services?

♦ How can services for minority ethnic groups be evaluated in a way meaningful to them? What kind of evidence would they wish to see?

♦ What are the perspectives of health professionals on the needs of ethnic minority groups and on their own ability to deliver services?

♦ Has the action taken to improve things been perceived as successful? Ultimately, the perception of improvement does matter.

These questions help assess felt need, and expressed need.

The people and agencies which could help answer such questions include: service users, community representatives, community organizations, volunteer networks, local primary health care/locality teams, secondary health care providers, and local politicians. A key step is finding and involving people who either have new information to provide or those who are typical of the group. Whether collecting information by self-completion or interview-based questionnaires, or by focus groups, a reliable and comprehensive (but not necessarily representative) sample of people needs to be recruited. A range of opinion is very important, rather than the average opinion.

Data protection laws restrict access to lists of names, and contact details, that are held by health authorities so finding people to study is not very easy. These laws protect data confidentiality. Some information on how to access study samples is in Chapter 9, and given this has been achieved there are two main ways of collecting qualitative data, as considered below, i.e. semi-open and open style interviewing of individuals, and focus groups. In addition qualitative researchers may use participant observation i.e. observing directly what is going on, and not relying on self-report. The participant observations method is too rarely used in epidemiology, public health and health services research.

5.3.1 Gauging the experiences of members of ethnic minority communities as users of health services using interviewing

Typically, we need to find out what people think of the service, what problems/concerns they have, and what their experiences have been? These are not the kind of questions that can be standardized easily, and they need to be tailored to each survey. Translation and cross-cultural validity of questions is a crucial issue, as already discussed above, and to be considered again in Chapter 9. It cannot be assumed either that respondents speak English (either at all or as their first choice) or, and perhaps even more importantly, that they will necessarily share common assumptions about health and well-being which underlie questions. For example, the idea that open criticism of professionals and services is a means to the end of improving them may not be widely shared outside a social elite and health service managers. In devising questions, researchers should beware of using jargon, colloquialisms and other sayings idiosyncratic to the English language. It may be more appropriate to adopt a simple descriptive approach to questions to avoid misinterpretation either in the English or in the translation. It is important for translations to be consistent across languages.

There are basically three types of questions—structured, semi-structured and open-ended, all of which can be self-completion or interview-based. Structured questionnaires underpin quantitative methods rather than qualitative ones, although they may have a part to play. The advantage of self-completion questionnaires is that people can take their time and consider questions carefully in their own time. They may also be less embarrassed about giving details about very personal issues e.g. contraception, sex, alcohol. Topics which are not sensitive in one culture may be very sensitive in another. For example, the age of a woman is not usually a sensitive topic in Chinese or South Asian cultures, as it is in modern European ones. Smoking cigarettes is a very sensitive topic for Sikh men but not for most men.

Interview-based questionnaires allow the interviewer to ask the questions and convey the meanings of questions if they are not fully understood (possibly in a translated language). The interviewer either tape records or writes down the answer for qualitative research (or codes the answer using predefined categories for quantitative research). The interview also has great advantages when the study participants do not read and write the language well, as is often the case with ethnic minority populations, but to gain quality information, the interviewer must be trained to build rapport, and ask the questions in a standardized way.

5.4 Focus groups

The focus group is a core qualitative research method used to gain insight through the interaction of a group. The group is 'focused' in that it involves a collective, directed discussion of chosen themes. Focus groups exploit group dynamics.

Focus groups extend the interview based semi-structured or open questionnaire. People might be grouped according to sex, ethnic background, professional background etc., and be asked, for example, what do you think of local hospital services? The people are then encouraged to talk, in their own language if desired, to discuss issues and exchange experiences. Through these discussions might emerge rich and vivid stories of how people have interacted with health services. These data are then integrated into the health needs assessment and used to improve health care. Box 5.1 is an example of how the focus group method can lead to practical understanding (Elliot 1997).

5.5 How many people from ethnic minority populations use the available services? What is the quality of their interaction with staff? Are the services meeting the need?

These simple questions may be difficult to answer. Front-line staff in frequent contact with patients may have a wealth of information and views on how current services address the needs of black and minority ethnic groups and these views should be accessed in

Box 5.1 CHD/diabetes focus group methods

Focus groups were used in Newcastle to explore CHD and diabetes services for the ethnic minorities. Four focus groups were set up; separate male and female South Asian groups, a mixed sex Chinese group and an ethnic minority professionals group. Participants were encouraged to talk openly about their experiences and those of their families of heart disease and diabetes. The facilitator asked the questions which were interpreted by the community workers and the answers were fed back via the community workers to the facilitator. Immediately after the meeting, there was a group discussion between the facilitator and the community workers (the research group) to go over and clarify the main points raised. This discussion was recorded and the results transcribed. The research group met on several occasions to agree the main themes which were emerging from the focus groups. The salient points made were placed under theme headings and discussed and changed until the research group was happy that what was emerging was a true record of what had occurred. Conclusions were that the minorities knew little about their conditions (as well as preventative strategies) but wanted to know more. All participants had or knew of people who had received inadequate health services. The professionals complained that they often did not have the resources to educate the community properly e.g. materials were not translated and of those that were most were not easily understandable by the community. The professionals were often inundated with calls from people who wanted help with other matters e.g. filling out social security forms.

The focus groups produced vivid first-hand accounts of problems with health care. This material was integrated with an epidemiological health needs assessment and a strategy for change was developed. This Newcastle work was itself integrated by myself and colleagues with three other projects on the same subject (London, Walsall, Manchester) and presented to a combined local authority and health authority forum called the Newcastle Health Partnership. The recommendations were considered by funding authorities. The end result was a nurse-led primary care-based cardiovascular and diabetes risk factor reduction project set in inner city general practices in Newcastle with larger than average ethnic minority populations. Given that a service is in place (and hopefully adapted) it is important to know whether it is being used—the topic considered in Section 5.5. (Extracted and edited from Elliott, 1997)

needs assessment exercises. It is likely that the only way to assess actual numbers is to go to the service provider and examine the records. This is no easy task and can be very time-consuming. Of course, to reiterate, such data should arise from routine ethnic monitoring systems. The number of people from the ethnic minority population on the list can be compared to the number expected in the light of the population size and the pattern of illness. The figures can be judged using existing standards of health care e.g. it may be that, as a matter of policy, all people with a condition, say a stroke, are to be seen by a specialist stroke service. If there are no such standards then a reference value is needed for comparison—usually in studies of ethnic minority groups this is that of the White population, admittedly an ethnocentric method.

Simply knowing the numbers of people making use of health services is, however, of limited value. What we need to know is whether people are using the available services appropriately. There are significant differences between different ethnic groups in terms of uptake of services. Interpretation of differences is complex. Service uptake may be affected by such factors as age, sex, religion, language, diet, socio-economic status and patterns of morbidity. Timing of clinics may affect the uptake of services, for example, the attendance on Friday afternoon clinics by Muslim men may be poor due to their requirement to participate in congregational prayers.

Staff in health centres and hospitals should find it helpful, in raising the quality of care and interaction, to understand the cultural and religious aspects of their patients' lives. Awareness of how attitudes to illness and treatment differ among different ethnic groups is also important. For example, some women patients, because of religious or cultural influences, would rather have the option of consulting with, and being treated by, women health professionals. South Asian women in particular prefer to be examined by a female doctor, whenever possible, and South Asian people generally tend to select South Asian GPs. What is needed is an approach that marries diversity with equity. This does not mean treating everyone in the same way, regardless of differing needs, rather that health services be adapted to be able to take account of diverse cultures, religions and health if needed.

Staff should not, however, decide from a person's name, appearance or religion what their needs are. Culture is not static but is constantly recreated as social groups respond to their historical and contemporary experiences. Culture is dependent on living and working conditions and on the broader political, economic and social scene. The socio-economic structures under which people live can shape values and behaviours in ways that have consequences for health and it is important to be aware that complex patterns of health care utilization exist. Factors such as satisfaction with the service, or discrimination perceived as racism, may affect uptake of services. A low service uptake is not necessarily a sign that the service is not meeting needs though that interpretation needs to be considered alongside others, such as a lower prevalence of disease. Equally, it cannot be assumed that a high rate of utilization of services implies excess demand since it may be warranted by a higher morbidity.

Communication is one of the main barriers to access to health care. To enable effective communication to take place, health professionals need to be aware of cultural and social factors that shape people's perceptions and behaviours. Barriers to effective communication between health practitioner and patient include differences in social class, status and culture, which are then compounded if the patient does not speak or understand the language used by most of the staff or other patients.

Some questions that address issues concerning quantity and quality of care for ethnic minority groups are given in Box 5.2.

Box 5.2 Some questions to guide assessment of quality of care

- How appropriate is the available patient information about services?
- How physically accessible are services (e.g. public transport, disabled access etc.)?
- Is the timing of clinics and nature of appointment systems suitable?
- Are the privacy and dignity of the patient and the patient's carers respected?
- Is consideration given to the individual needs of the patient and the patient's carers?
- Are cultural and religious requirements recognized and catered for?
- Are difficulties in communication responded to and catered for?
- Are dietary requirements recognized and provided for?
- Is there access to a professional bilingual and/or advocacy service?
- Is there access to written information regarding service provision in community languages?
- Is account taken of a patient's preferences to consult and be examined by a male or female nurse/doctor?
- Do patients have access to complaints and suggstions procedures?
- Is appropriate physical and personal care available to meet individual cultural/religious requirements?

If problems are identified they should be followed up more systematically. An advisory group could be formed comprising GPs, community members/groups, allied health professionals, secondary health care providers and other interested parties. The purpose of this group would be to provide direction in the formulation of the needs analysis, links to organizations and groups within the community and to ensure that all members of the community are represented in the development and subsequent recommendations formulated. The effectiveness of the changes made need to be assessed. Unfortunately, too often there is little immediate or obvious impact. In Chapter 8, I will examine policy formulation and impact, particularly with a view on what helps successful implementation.

5.6 How can services for minority ethnic groups be evaluated?

One of the early checklists for evaluation, 'Health and Race, A Starting Point for Managers on Improving Services for Black Populations', was prepared by Yasmin Gunaratnam of the Kings Fund Centre. It gave guidance on how to ensure that the health needs assessment process identifies the specific needs of local ethnic minority populations. It also provided the framework for a strategy for active community participation in service planning and review and for ethnic record-keeping and monitoring in service provision. A more up-to-date and comprehensive toolkit for evaluation of progress in the ethnicity and health field had been developed by the National Resource Centre for Ethnic Minority Health in Scotland. These and other tools will be considered in more detail in a strategic and policy context (see Chapter 8).

Change can be shown by audit. For example, if a service audit has been undertaken, it should be repeated to assess if there is any improvement in the service e.g. number of leaflets in the South Asian languages or uptake of cardiac rehabilitation services from the minority ethnic community. This will allow researchers to see the effect—has any change taken place and if so has this change been evaluated and found to be worthwhile? Such audits can help release resources for change, as illustrated in Box 5.3.

Box 5.3 Example of improving standards by audit

An audit of diabetes services was conducted in Newcastle. This project sought to compare the quality of both GP and hospital diabetes services for the South Asian population with that of the general population. Preliminary results suggested that neither group was receiving the optimum level of care but that for the South Asian population the situation was much worse. This study complemented earlier work in the area which examined levels of CHD and diabetes in the community and looked at users' views of services for these diseases. As a result of the findings Newcastle and North Tyneside Health Authority provided funding for community linkworkers to be employed with a specific remit to support CHD and diabetes care.

Audit is a powerful and under-utilized process for evaluating change, and yet it is seldom perceived as an integral part of the health needs assessment process.

5.7 Conclusions

This chapter has summarized the health needs assessment process, based on both quantitative information (such as the epidemiology of diseases) and qualitative information obtained from interviews and focus groups. The concepts of race and ethnicity can be put to practical use in health needs assessment. Effective consultation and involvement of minority ethnic groups for establishing clear objectives for collecting information and for agreeing how such information will be used is important. In this way continuing (and not ad-hoc) dialogue between health care providers and local minority ethnic communities can occur.

Health needs assessment is, however, no more than a means of collecting and synthesizing information for policy, planning and management purposes. It is, therefore, the first hurdle. There are at least three reasons why some needs assessment projects may fail. First, there is a lack of understanding of what is involved and how to do it. Second, there is lack of resources or commitment. Third, there is a failure to integrate the results with the planning and purchasing process to produce change. Multi-ethnic societies in

Table 5.12 Some sources of data for health needs assessment

- Organizations with responsibility for census and other national demographic data, in the UK the relevant organization is called National Statistics
- Organizations set up to collate, synthesize and publish information, for example in England and Wales such organizations include Public Health Observatories
- Local government offices (town hall or civic centre). Local population data analyses are usually based on national data sets but sometimes on local censuses: these organization often do detailed analysis for the locality
- Organizations that are responsible for the health of defined populations, for example Scottish Health Boards, or English Strategic Health Authorities—for collated statistic and analyses
- Epidemiology and public health departments in higher education institutions—for the latest research on ethnic minority groups internationally, nationally and locally
- Specific disease foundations, for example the American and British Heart Foundations, for risk factor prevalence.
- Organizations responsible for health education and health promotion—for a list of health-related resources for black and minority ethnic groups available in various community languages

the modern world cannot afford such failures. With the increasing availability of data, and the interest and involvement of numerous public and charitable organizations in data collection and interpretation (Table 5.12), there is an increasingly solid platform for health needs assessment.

Whatever we do and whatever the needs assessment shows there are bound to be tensions because of conflicting preferences, needs and resource constraints. These are reflected in the following quotation. The different models for meeting needs, for example separate services, special projects and integrated approaches will be considered in Chapter 8.

> There is some debate whether special clinics such as diabetes clinics should be offered to Asians separately from other ethnic groups. Such clinics have been running in a number of cities, and their protagonists argue that it is a cost-effective use of specialized dieticians, nurses and linkworkers. In addition, many patients are more 'at home' in such an environment where efforts can be made to segregate the sexes if needed, they can be seen by a female doctor if they so wish and patients are made to feel the services are working with them rather than parallel to them. Opponents argue that it is wrong to segregate people by their ethnic group or provide special services for one group and not another.
>
> Hawthorne (1994: 457)

Multi-ethnic societies need to be conscious of the wider effects on society of meeting needs by service adaptation. As discussed in Chapter 4 the response to rising ethnic diversity is, initially at least, usually a negative one, with a tendency to blame the minority populations for innate or cultural effects that underlie their health problems. In such a phase, specialist responses of the kind in the quotation above may well be resented. Spurred by rising global and national movements for universal human rights in the late twentieth century, and the changing population structure now requiring more young and economically active citizens, however, many countries are changing their stance on immigrants. Equity of health status and health care has become a central focus in this changed world.

Despite the complexities, action is likely to be required, and should be based on the following needs assessment principles:

1. Avoid the piecemeal approach to tackling ethnic health needs whereby so-called ethnic specific topics are tackled one by one. An overview is needed.

2. Base the needs assessment on ranked causes using case numbers and disease rates.

3. Refine understanding by looking at comparative indices, which will focus attention on inequalities and inequities.

4. Interpret the quantitative data in the light of the qualitative findings.

5. Draw causal hypotheses based on differences with care, and with due emphasis on social and economic deprivation as explanatory factors.

6. Beware that inferences of biological differences between ethnic/racial groups may be particularly prone to error and misinterpretation, and may harm the standing of minority groups. Even if there are biological differences these should not be interpreted as indicating superiority or inferiority.

7. Make a judgement on how the data can be best used to improve the health and health care of ethnic minority groups. This requires an understanding of the services already available.

8. Minority ethnic groups must not be excluded from major of public health and health care initiatives.

9. The needs of minority groups should be met simultaneously with the rest of the population.

10. All public health policies and plans should make explicit how the needs of minority ethnic groups are to be met. These should not be relegated to secondary documentation.

The implementation of these principles in relation to national policies is discussed in Chapter 8. In Chapter 6, on inequalities, and Chapter 7, on priorities, I consider some of the issues that underpin the policies.

Summary

A health needs assessment is a systematic, comprehensive overview of both quantitative and qualitative data on a population or subgroup of the population. Its purpose is to help to create or adapt policies, strategies and services to improve population health and health care. Health needs assessment in relation to ethnic minority groups is usually problematic for lack of data, particularly at local level, and at the level of subgroup detail that is often required. In addition to lack of data there may be lack of time, funds, expertise and means of implementation of findings. Health needs assessment, particularly at the local level, is often limited to qualitative studies or consultations. For national studies data from administrative databases recording broad ethnic categories or proxies for ethnic group such as country of birth may need to be used. The limitations of such data need to be understood to reduce the risk of making poor decisions.

Needs assessment for ethnic minority populations should start by examining the actual level of health states, disease patterns and health care utilization within each group. This is the absolute risk approach. The findings can then be compared with other ethnic groups. In most instances the standard comparison is with the White population. This is done either for ease, habit, ethnocentrism, availability of data or statistical power. An alternative conceptual approach, but one that is rarely used, is to set the standard comparison against the ethnic group with the most desirable level of the health indicator under study. These comparative approaches comprise the relative risk approach. Qualitative data enrich and help validate the quantitative analysis by giving needs assessors access to opinions, perceptions, beliefs, attitudes, self-reported behaviour, and case histories.

Health needs assessments have shown that commonly held views on the needs of minorities are often erroneous e.g. levels of immunization are high not low, life expectancy may be greater than in the population as a whole, and health education materials may bear little relation to disease patterns etc. Having said this, some generalizations also tend to hold: needs vary by ethnic group; minority ethnic groups are better off in some respects and worse in others; service quality, particularly for preventive health issues and counselling, is usually worse for minority groups; and the articulated needs of minority groups focus on communication, information, religion, dietary preferences and consent. Needs assessment is an important way of influencing the development of services.

Chapter 6

Ethnic inequalities in health and health care

> ...race implies difference, difference implies superiority and superiority leads to predominance.
> Attributed to Benjamin Disraeli (1804–1881—British politician and Prime Minister)

Contents

- Chapter objectives
- The genesis of inequalities in health status
- Forces underpinning ethnicity and race, and their relation to those generating inequalities in health, with special emphasis on socio-economic factors and racism
- Measuring ethnic inequalities in health—validity of indicators
- The dimension of, and trends in, inequalities by ethnicity and race—international examples
- Inequity in relation to inequality—a matter of justice and reversibility
- Implications of inequalities by ethnicity and race
- Strategies for monitoring and reducing inequalities
- Conclusions
- Summary of chapter

Objectives

On completion of this chapter you should be able to:

- Understand why inequalities by race and ethnicity are inevitable
- Appreciate the scale of such inequalities in a number of countries
- Be able to differentiate between inequalities and inequities
- Appreciate the importance of these inequalities both to medical and health sciences, and to clinical and public health practice
- Be able to discuss the strengths and weaknesses of several strategies for tackling such inequalities

6.1 **What are health inequalities and why are they inevitable by race and ethnicity?**

Why is a disease or health problem, say premature death or poor perceived health, more common in one group of people than another? This question lies at the heart of the debate on inequalities in health. While the observation of inequalities in health is ancient, and is an important component of the writings of Hippocrates about 2000 years ago in Greece, attempting a scientific understanding of the causes of inequality and the development of actions to counter inequality are recent and accelerating developments.

Before reading on do Exercise 6.1.

Exercise 6.1 Inequality

- What is meant by the word inequalities? What undercurrents are there to this word in industrialized countries such as the UK, USA or the Netherlands?
- What kinds of inequalities are pursued in contemporary research and which are not?
- Can you think of actions, focused around health inequalities, that were not driven by compassion?

Inequality is, strictly speaking, a lack of uniformity: synonyms for this include difference, disparity, variability, and unevenness. In the context of health and health care, however, the term inequalities is mainly used to refer to those differences that are associated with social and economic factors that are thought to be relevant in causation. Inequality is a value-laden term, one that is undesirable in modern, democratic and, at least ostensibly, egalitarian states, particularly in relation to occupational opportunities. This was not always the case. In the time of slavery and its aftermath, in the USA the idea of equality was alien, and people in power at that time could not have imagined modern thinking. The perpetuation of inequalities has been a goal of some societies e.g. South Africa based on apartheid (see Chapter 4), Indian society where occupation and social status were linked to caste and hence controlled through lineage, and of course the racist Nazi state in Germany (see below). These are only a few examples of societies where the focus on inequalities was not their reduction through compassionate interventions, but their sustenance or even their exacerbation. Inequality could also, however, be seen as desirable for promoting creativity, nonconformity and countering authority.

Most attention to inequalities in health, at least in European countries, has focused on wealth, usually measured as income, location of residence or an indicator of earning potential such as occupation (in Britain converted into a social class scale). There is no logical reason why the inequalities in health debate should not, say, focus on inequalities between men and women, by ethnic group or inequalities by age group. Some work has been done on such inequalities, but not nearly as much as on socio-economic inequalities. It is not clear why this is so, but it is probably related to social values. Europe has placed great emphasis on equal opportunities. In the USA, until recently, emphasis on race-based inequalities exceeded that on wealth-related ones, although race was recognized as an important indicator of wealth differentials. The historical importance of race in the USA was discussed in Chapters 1 and 4.

Inequality by race and ethnic group is, potentially, a powerful tool for scientific analysis and for social action in the field of health. For example, why, in comparison to the British population as a whole, is diabetes so common in people who originate in India but live in Britain, and why is colo-rectal cancer relatively uncommon? Answers to these questions should hold important information about the causes of disease and should benefit all populations because results are likely to be generalizable. Most epidemiologists who attempt to unravel the mystery in the patterns of disease in populations become intrigued by ethnicity and health research, and particularly the mechanisms by which disease differences occur. The potential value of such research is enormous, but in practice the potential for knowledge gain has been hard to realize and it has been hard to take actions to reduce inequalities.

Before reading on, reflect on the questions in Exercise 6.2.

Exercise 6.2 Genesis of ethnic inequalities in health and health care

- Why are ethnic inequalities in health and health care inevitable?
- List 5–10 broad factors that are important in generating health, preventing disease and prolonging life.
- Are any of these factors integral to the concepts of race and ethnicity?
- Which of these factors are potentially changeable within our lifetimes?
- What are the consequences, positive and negative, for health inequalities by race and ethnicity?
- What are the consequences for trying to explain, as opposed to describe, ethnic health inequalities?

Health status, disease occurrence and mortality patterns in populations are sculpted by factors such as wealth, environmental quality and protection, diet, behaviour, occupational and domestic stresses, and genetic inheritance. Varying exposures to these and other factors by ethnic group over long (in some instances evolutionary) timescales generate ethnic differences as shown in Box 6.1 and Figure 6.1.

Most of these factors are directly or indirectly related to ethnicity and/or race, e.g. globally and within most multi-ethnic societies White populations are wealthier than non-White populations. (There are exceptions, of course, as in most generalizations and, for example, Patel, a Gujerati Indian name, is said to be the commonest surname for UK millionaires.) The concepts of ethnicity and race imply group differences with, traditionally, an emphasis on culture and biology, respectively. Differences in environmental and socio-economic circumstances arise from migration and in the geographical and socio-economic segregation that is so common following migration. (Immigrants tend to settle in areas where there is cheap housing, and to take on poorly paid jobs.) Fundamental

---

Box 6.1 Major factors generating or influencing ethnic health inequalities

- Culture e.g. taboos on tobacco, alcohol, contraception etc., many of them generated by religious and spiritual beliefs
- Social, educational and economic status e.g. knowledge of biology and health influences, languages spoken and read, qualifications that are recognized and lead to occupational opportunities
- Environment before and after migration e.g. climate, housing, air quality, etc.
- Lifestyle e.g. behaviours in relation to exercise, alchol, diet
- Accessing, and concordance with, health care advice e.g. willingness to seek social and health services and adhere to advice, use of 'complementary/alternative' methods of care including the health systems of the country or origin
- Genetic and biological factors e.g. birthweight, growth trajectory, body composition, genetic traits and diseases, etc.

---

differences in culture, biology and environment, all implied by the concepts of race and ethnicity, must lead to inequalities in health. It would be rather extraordinary if they did not occur. Some of these differences are captured in Box 6.1.

Socio-economic factors are accepted as profoundly important in explaining and countering health inequalities. There may, however, be some difficulties in demonstrating the association between socio-economic status and ill health in ethnic minority groups, particularly in the period following migration, for reasons that are discussed below.

Try Exercise 6.3 before reading on.

Exercise 6.3 Inequalities, socioeconomic status and ethnicity

- Would you expect there to be important inequalities by occupation-based social class in ethnic minority groups?
- Why?
- If they did not occur why might that be so?
- What measures would you use to study the association, in an ethnic minority group, between ill health and socio-economic status?

Social class measured by occupation may be a poor measure in the period following migration, as many well-educated people in ethnic minority groups may need to hold low-paid jobs, and many immigrants in the managerial classes are in small businesses which are often struggling financially and involve low income and long and hard working hours. (The main exceptions are immigrants who are selected into the country on the basis of special skills for jobs where there is a shortage of qualified candidates.) The relationship between educational and social status, income and health may well be

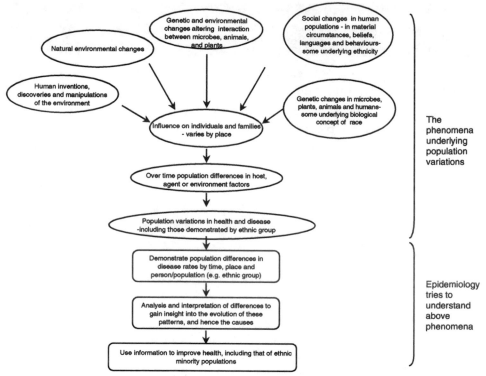

Fig. 6.1 A model illustrating the genesis of ethnic inequalities in health and how epidemiology tries to understand them (adapted from Bhopal, Concepts of Epidemiology, figure 10.1)

disrupted by these kind of changes. Over time, however, these relationships would be expected to be re-established. Other more direct and immediate indicators of socio-economic status e.g. ownership of household goods, might give a truer picture in this stage. This point, illustrated in the quotation below, is discussed in more detail in Section 6.4.

> As some minority ethnic groups are among the most disadvantaged sections of British society, measures which misrepresent the standard of living of minority ethnic groups risk not only perpetrating but exacerbating disadvantage through inadequate investment of public resources.
>
> There is therefore a pressing need to develop more sensitive indicators of socioeconomic position, particularly for use in research into the causes of ethnic inequalities in health.
>
> Davey Smith *et al.* (2000: 404)

Cultural factors are of great importance but are likely to decline in influence fairly rapidly as behaviours change across generations. Usually, there is a convergence of the minority populations towards the behaviours of the majority, which is sometimes infortunate.

The processes by which ethnic health inequalities occur, and the actions that are effective in narrowing them, need to be understood. Each specific health inequality is likely to have its own genesis, with, unfortunately for public health, no general explanation. For example, ethnic inequalities in risk of skin cancers such as melanoma are likely to have a biological basis relating to skin colour (hence relating to race), while inequalities in stroke need to take account of many factors including behaviour, biochemistry, physiology, culture and economic circumstances, and all these need consideration over the life-course, or even across generations. Fortunately, many of the powerful forces causing inequalities are amenable to change, and quickly—certainly over our lifetimes. The main exception to this is genetic influences. Genetic factors are likely to be all-important in generating inequalities in a small number of diseases e.g. haemoglobinopathies, and of substantial importance in others e.g. diabetes. Of course, the interplay of genetic and environmental factors underlies most specific diseases. One of the most contentious factors underlying inequalities is racism. It is by no means the sole or even dominant cause, but it has special importance and is given prominence in this chapter (Section 6.3).

Ethnic health inequalities are complex and rapidly changing phenomena, and only partially understood—a state that is unlikely to change greatly, because population sciences are not able to decipher such complexity. Nonetheless, there is no room for complacency as worthwhile, if imperfect, public health actions are possible with incomplete knowledge based on sound general principles of health and disease in populations. Some such actions are considered in Chapter 8: the scale of ethnic health inequalities is considered below.

6.2 What is the scale of ethnic health inequalities?

Before reading on, try Exercise 6.4.

Exercise 6.4 The scale of ethnic inequalities

♦ Estimate using the percentage scale, where 100 per cent is the value for the population as a whole, the ethnic difference in the occurrence of the following health conditions in industrialized wealthy nations such as Australia, the USA, the UK and the Netherlands:

  Tuberculosis
  Prostatic cancer
  Lung cancer
  Coronary heart disease
  Suicide
  Road traffic accidents.

♦ Assume that the value for the group with the lowest occurrence is 100 per cent, then state, as a percentage, the value in the group with the highest rate e.g. 300 per cent indicates threefold variation.

The danger of emphasizing differences is ever-present but, nonetheless, ethnic inequalities are surprisingly wide. For most of the specific conditions listed in Exercise 6.4 the variation would be at least threefold and often much bigger. Some sample data are given in Table 6.1.

Table 6.1 Extent of variations by ethnic group: examples in males in England and Wales, the Netherlands, the USA and Canada

Condition	England and Wales[1]		Netherlands[2]		Canada	
Diabetes						
Highest	Bangladeshi-born	670	Surinamese-born	5.29	Not reported	
Lowest	Chinese-born	85	Turkish-born	1.72		
Variation		788%		308%		
Ischemic heart disease						
Highest	Bangladeshi-born	151	Surinamese-born	0.93	South Asian Origin	320.2
Lowest	Chinese-born	44	Moroccans	0.40	Chinese Origin	107
Variation		343%		233%		299%
Lung cancer						
Highest	Whole population of England and Wales	100	Turkish/Antillean/ Aruban-born	0.68	European Origin	129.5
Lowest	Pakistani-born	34	Surinamese-born	0.38	South Asian Origin	22.1
Variation		294%		179%		586%

1. Gill *et al.* (2006) Standardized mortality ratios.
2. Bos *et al.* (2004) Mortality rate ratios.
3. Sheth *et al.* (1999) Death rates.

We do not usually see such big variations with most other socio-economic epidemiological variables. Variations of this magnitude, or even greater, are seen in international comparisons by country. Such international variations are, of course, partly reflecting underlying ethnic variations (or vice versa). In ethnic minority groups some diseases are more common, others less common, and the balance in terms of overall mortality and morbidity can, surprisingly enough, be hard to predict, particularly in populations that have migrated relatively recently. Mostly, overall rates are close to the average.

Migration may alter or exaggerate inequalities e.g. inequalities in diabetes have been increased by migration of South Asians, African Caribbean and other groups to affluent industrialized societies. This is an example of the contradiction of the general expectation of convergence of disease patterns following migration, for the migrants' levels of diabetes greatly exceed those of the receiving population. As already discussed, including in Chapters 3 and 5, there are complex factors such as the healthy migrant effect and 'salmon bias' that make interpretation of data difficult.

In long-settled minorities and particularly in populations that have been conquered by colonists, however, there is generally a health deficit. African-Americans and Native Americans in the USA, Maoris in New Zealand and indigenous people in Australia (aborigines) are among groups that fit this generalization. Some general points on such populations were made in Chapter 4 in the discussion of Australia's response to ethnicity and health.

The causes of inequalities are, as already stated, complex and difficult to disentangle even with careful research. Of the numerous inequalities, the one that has been studied most carefully is that between African and White Americans. African-American men live 7–8 years less on average than White American men. The deficit arises from excess mortality in many causes but particularly from chronic diseases such as CHD and stroke and is partly explained by income differentials. This inequality increased over the twentieth century even in the face of improvements in civil rights and a move to political and social equality. A legacy of slavery followed by a long period of open discrimination is proving hard to overcome. Economic status, social conditions, and social status are changing for African-Americans with the rise of affluence, although far from uniformly. This ought to improve health status and reduce inequalities in the long run.

African-Americans receive less health care, especially for high technology procedures, than White Americans: this is at least partly explained by the financial burden of health insurance, which cannot be met by poor people. The USA experience over the twentieth century, which has seen widening rather than narrowing inequalities, teaches us that racial and ethnic inequalities may worsen even as they are studied and even though they are socially and politically deplored. Despite much research there is no consensus on the causes of Black/White health disparities in health status and health in the USA, but racism is one of the proposed explanations. Naturally, this is a highly controversial topic, with many people, particularly politicians, unwilling to admit that racism could cause such effects. I will consider in Section 6.3 why it is necessary to look into the history of racism in science and medicine to help overcome disbelief about the potential importance of contemporary racism, to generate the moral drive for action, to provide insight on how the powerful groups in societies may abuse data on racial differences, and to learn that individuals and institutions act according to the ethos of the era.

An emphasis on disease differences, so appropriate to the analysis required in science, has spilled over to the health policy and management arenas, where it is not always appropriate. Because the overriding interest of scientists, and of scientific journals, is on disease causation, hypothesis generation and hypothesis testing, the presentation of data generally emphasizes relative risks using summary measures which compare one population with another. Such presentations under-emphasize disease numbers or rates. (The principles were discussed in Chapter 5.) Such research may then be used in making policy on disease priorities. Uncommon diseases which are, nonetheless, more common than in the general population may receive emphasis at the expense of common diseases which have comparable or lower frequency. For example, lung cancer in Indian-origin populations rarely receives attention, yet it is the commonest cancer in Indian-origin men. One outcome is that health education for Indian-origin populations about smoking, the principal cause of this disease, is not given due priority. This matter is considered in more detail in Chapter 7.

6.3 Perpetuation and augmentation of ethnic health inequalities: the role of racism

Try Exercise 6.5 on racism before reading on.

Exercise 6.5 Racism

- What do you understand by the term racism?
- What kind of racism can you envisage in a health care setting?
- In what way might information on ethnic differences in health worsen racism?

6.3.1 Defining racism and assessing its importance

Racism is the belief that some races are superior to others, which is then extended to justify actions that create inequality by favouring the supposedly superior groups to others. In practice, as was done by the House of Lords in the UK, the definition of race is broadened to include ethnic, religious and other similar groups, so that discrimination on such grounds is also termed racism. Various kinds of racism are discussed later in this chapter.

While racism is usually ideological in that it is not based on research evidence, it can both be initiated and made more potent by research. Paradoxically, differences caused by racism can then be used to justify it, for example if the rate of homicide is high in a particular ethnic group, or performance on IQ or school tests is poor, perhaps as a result of racism leading to economic deprivation, this information can be used to make claims about the inferiority of such an ethnic group. In this way further racism is justified and a vicious cycle is created. For more general health inequalities arguments might be based upon pseudo-Darwinian-type notions of survival of the fittest, as illustrated by the following quotation.

> By the turn of the century, Darwinism had provided a new rationale for American racism. Essentially primitive peoples, it was argued, could not be assimilated into a complex, white civilization. Scientists speculated that in the struggle for survival the Negro in America was doomed. Particularly prone to disease, vice, and crime, black Americans could not be helped by education or philanthropy. Social Darwinists analyzed census data to predict the virtual extinction of the Negro in the twentieth century, for they believed the Negro race in America was in the throes of a degenerative evolutionary process.
>
> The medical profession supported these findings of late nineteenth- and early twentieth-century anthropologists, ethnologists, and biologists. Physicians studying the effects of emancipation on health concluded almost universally that freedom had caused the mental, moral, and physical deterioration of the black population.
>
> Brandt (1978)

Some people deny that racism is commonplace in modern, industrialized, multi-ethnic societies, but research shows it is very important. In a national representative survey in the 1990s in the UK by the Policy Studies Institute 20–26 per cent of the White participants admitted at interview to prejudice against Asian, Caribbean, or Muslim ethnic minorities (Modood *et al.* 1997). In truth, the figure is likely to be larger, for some people do not give publicly unacceptable answers at interview. While racism in modern society is perceived to be a pervasive problem being brought under control, the charge that a health care system is racist is hard to bear by proud health professions governed by ethical codes emphasizing their humanitarian duties.

While racism in health care is often evoked as the explanation for inequalities, empirical research is surprisingly hard to find, interpret and act upon. Much anecdote and analysis, however, puts racism at the hub of ethnic and racial disparities in health and health care. A rapid rise in ethnic minority populations in Western cities, easy international travel, pressures increasing migration from developing countries, and a rise in the number of refugees are among factors likely to fuel racism in health and welfare services in the twenty-first century.

When research implies genetic factors as the cause of racial differences in health, racial minorities tend to be perceived as biologically weak. In these circumstances biology and medicine become the servants of racism. We have already discussed in Chapter 1 the potential harms of the race concept. Racism can cause death and despair in ways that are, with the exception of disease epidemics, almost unparalleled in human history, as in the massacres in Nazi Germany, Bosnia, Serbia, and Rwanda. Racism can be compounded by other forms of discrimination, for example, on the basis of sex or disability. Anti-racism activity, therefore, sits squarely in the wider arena of the struggle against oppression. A historical perspective is useful in shedding light on what is happening and what could happen, and provides a sound if not essential basis for thinking through the arguments for and against positive discrimination. The following account builds upon the foundation laid in Chapter 1, and will be considered in the context of research in Chapter 9.

6.3.2 **Historical racism**

Hippocrates contrasted the feebleness of the Asiatic races to the hardiness of the Europeans, but his concept of race was of human groups shaped by ancestry in different geographical conditions, especially climate, which he saw as a powerful influence on character. The following quotation from Montagu illustrates the kind of thinking there was in earlier eras.

> From the earliest times, the emotional attitude that one's own ethnic group, nation, or culture is superior to others, has been a concomitant of virtually every culture. Within any society, in earlier times, men might be persecuted or made the object of discrimination on the grounds of differences in religion, culture, politics, or class, but never on any biological grounds such as are implied in the idea of racial differences.
>
> Montagu (1998: 59)

The scientific and popular idea of races as distinct species, which was against the teachings of most religions including Christianity, gave way to races as biological subspecies of a single species in the eighteenth century (see Chapter 1). In the nineteenth century differences in anatomical, physiological, behavioural and health status in these races were avidly sought. The central tenet of racism, that some races are superior to others, was widely believed and vigorously supported by influential scholars and researchers in the nineteenth century (for more details see Chapter 9). Genetics undermined the biological concept of race in the twentieth century and Nazi racism generated the widespread disgust that fatally undermined eugenics. In the next section I introduce Hitler's views on race and health as an example, admittedly extreme, but still informative, of why racism is a central public health issue.

Remarkably, although the concept of races is now considered to be based on a few physical features (such as colour and facial features) that are of small direct importance to health, but which serve important social and political purposes, the idea of the biological basis of health differences by race and ethnicity remains strong. The resurgence of the biological race concept is highly likely, and there is new genetic research that is re-exploring old territory with novel methods. Some of it is perpetuating the traditional racial classifications. Again, see Chapter 9 for more information.

According to Krieger *et al.* (1993) much research has supported, albeit unwittingly, the four assumptions needed for racism: distinct races, racial features linked to other important attributes, the differences between races being genetic, and the view that some races are superior to others. Krieger *et al.*'s charge is that racism is important because it leads to socio-economic inequalities, which underlie health inequalities; and that there are unexplained inequities in health care, including treatment for heart disease, renal failure, bladder cancer and pneumonia.

I believe that few health professionals and researchers in the field of ethnicity and health research are racist, and that most hold humanitarian, anti-racist views. However, scientists and policy-makers of the nineteenth century, when the prevailing attitude was that White races were superior and had a right (indeed responsibility) to subordinate coloured people, also did not perceive their views and actions as immoral and justified them as in the interest of society and all racial groups. The current thinking is that the basis of inequality is complex and we need to demonstrate and quantify the specific effect of racism so that rational action can be taken. In time, will this viewpoint be judged in the same harsh way we judge nineteenth-century thinking? Will our successors judge current health care to be racist, and our institutions to be trapped by the prevailing ethos of *our* times? Will they judge that knowledge about racism was more than ample to justify action?

As the research record does not permit an unequivocal quantitative answer to the question of whether current disparities in health and health care are created and main-tained by racism, should we do more research until its distinct contribution becomes clear, or should we accept the consensus of scholarly and political analysis as the basis for action? The answer is unclear. Guinan questioned the value of researching racism:

> I do not think there is any question that racism is a partial cause of the morbidity/mortality gap. Now, how much more research do we need to do to describe the problem? Do we need to define the attributable risk of racism? Should we move forward by studying the precise mechanism by which racism causes the problems? I do not think so.
>
> Guinan (1993: 193–195)

In contrast Warren (1993), advocated that racism is researchable and should be researched.

In Britain, empirical research evidence which directly supports the case for racism being important to the health and health care of ethnic minority groups is rare except for discrimination in health care employment and training. This was discussed in a wider context in Chapter 4, and the NHS's response will be considered in Chapter 8. Research has demonstrated that the race or ethnicity of doctors, even the name, and not the place of graduation or qualification, was a key factor in obtaining entry to medical school and subsequent employment opportunities, and rewards. As a *British Medical Journal* editorial proclaimed: 'Equity for patients is unlikely if we don't treat doctors fairly' (Smith 1987). Negative or prejudiced beliefs, attitudes, and behaviours of professionals and services are worrying. The book *Racism in Medicine* provides evidence, particularly in relation to equal opportunities, that racism in medicine matters (Coker 2001). This book's essential message is that reliable testimony and qualitative and quantitative research confirm racism in medicine, and that it must stop. Professionals need to be aware of the dangers of prejudice, stereotyping and racism, and that insensitivity may be interpreted by patients, and society at large, as racism.

The USA leads, by a very long way, in the examination of inequalities in health care by ethnic group, as illustrated in the next section.

6.3.3 Differences between Black and White patients in the management of disease in the USA

Numerous studies have documented that in the USA the intensity of medical care activity for White patients exceeds that for non-White, especially Black, ones. Commenting on Gornick and colleagues' (1986) research, showing inequalities in the uptake of a range of health services by Black compared to White people in the USA, Geiger wrote:

> With major confounding factors increasingly controlled and adjusted for, investigators tend to invoke unspecified cultural differences, undocumented patient preferences, or a lack of information about the need for care as reasons for the differences. The alternative explanation is racism, that is, racially discriminatory rationing by physicians and health care institutions. We don't yet know enough to make that charge definitively. Furthermore, if racism is involved it is unlikely to be overt or even conscious.
>
> Geiger (1996: 815)

The consistent and repeated findings that Black Americans receive less health care, particularly expensive new technology, than White people is becoming an indictment of the USA's health care. The disparities have been observed across geographical areas and times and are not simply due to differences in socio-economic circumstances, but are undoubtedly strongly influenced by the capacity to purchase medical insurance in the USA.

A study by Escarce and colleagues (1993) was typical of the genre (for others see next section). They examined 32 procedures and found that White patients were more likely to receive 23 services while Blacks were more likely to receive seven. Four main hypotheses were considered: different disease patterns; differential contact with physicians, especially specialists; financial and organizational barriers e.g. caused by the fact that Medicare and Medicaid still require patients to pay some costs; and patients' preferences. The authors emphasized the possibility that physicians managed their patients differently on the basis of race. Gornick *et al.* (1986) showed Blacks had fewer mammograms, immunizations and ambulatory care visits but more mortality and hospitalization.

In Chapter 8, we will briefly examine some of the policy documents that review the evidence, and the recommended responses. A great deal of work has studied heart disease, and for this reason I have focused on it. For example:

+ Wenneker and Epstein (1989) reported that Black patients had fewer coronary angiography tests and coronary artery bypass grafts than Whites even after adjustment for a range of confounding factors.
+ Hannan *et al.* (1991) showed that Blacks had fewer cardiac procedures than Whites even after adjustment for disease severity.
+ Goldberg *et al.* (1992) reported that coronary artery bypass rates varied by race with Black men having one-quarter of the rate in Whites and Black women a little over a third.
+ Whittle *et al.* (1993) showed inequalities in invasive cardiac procedures, concluding: 'We believe that inadequate health education, differences in patients' preferences for invasive management, delivery systems that are unfriendly to members of certain cultures, and overt racism may all play a part.'
+ Ayanian *et al.* (1993) demonstrated that Black patients had less coronary revascularization than Whites but they were not clear whether Whites had an excess or Blacks a deficit of intervention.
+ Carlisle *et al.* (1995) showed that in Los Angeles invasive cardiac procedures were less common in Latinos and Blacks but not in Asians.
+ Peterson *et al.* (1994) showed Blacks had less cardiac procedures yet better short-term survival and equivalent intermediate survival rates.

The literature on disparities in the management of heart disease by race in the USA is exceedingly difficult to interpret. The studies focus on quantity, not quality, of care and the one study examining outcomes by Peterson and colleagues does not evoke a sense of inequity unlike those which only examine quantity of care. The increasingly common interpretation that racism has a part to play surely has some truth in it, but how much? Can the distinctive contribution of racism be disassociated from the many interacting factors, including patients' preferences? For example, one explanation of the findings on medical care procedures which links historical racism to the current disparities is this: that due to the legacy of racism Blacks distrust invasive diagnostic and therapeutic procedures which inhibits them accessing care and accepting it even when offered. In this climate of distrust, physicians may be inhibited from advising invasive procedures. If so, even if patients' preferences are judged to be partially responsible for the disparities, racism will not be exonerated. This explanation is over-simplistic because given the opportunity, African-Americans are enthusiastic users of the USA's health care system.

These kind of questions require the continuing use of data by ethnic and racial group, as even the critics of these concepts generally accept. Such critics emphasize, however, that the focus of the investigations must be maintained on reducing inequalities. Bringing health and health care inequalities to public attention, however, has risks, as discussed below.

6.3.4 Inequalities, stigma and the social standing of ethnic minority groups

Before reading on, do Exercise 6.6.

Exercise 6.6

◆ Consider the inherent dangers of publicizing ethnic inequalities
◆ Consider the dangers for public standing, priority setting, policy formulation, the type of research done, and media portrayal

---

The perception that the health of ethnic minority groups is poor, as opposed to different (in some ways better, in some ways worse), can augment the popular belief that ethnic minorities are a burden particularly on health care systems, but also on society generally. An influential example of writing which created this impression was the Annual Report of 1991 of the English Chief Medical Officer (CHO 1992). The perception is at least partially false and some migrant groups, especially men, as shown in Table 6.2, show a healthy migrant effect. There are variations by disease cause but overall SMR's hover around the average for the population of England and Wales.

By contrast, variations in specific diseases are very considerable, as we have already discussed in association with Table 6.1. The perception of poor health arises from a focus on differences where there is an excess of disease in the ethnic minority population, while ignoring differences were there is lower risk of disease. In fact, for many causes morbidity and mortality rates are lower in ethnic majority groups.

Most research studies (including most of my own) are based on the comparative paradigm and present data using the White population as the standard against which to compare minority groups. Attention is then focused on those diseases which are more

Table 6.2 Standardized mortality ratio for all causes of death by country of birth and gender in the age group 20–69 (20 plus years for Wild[4]).

Country of birth (First author)	Gender	
	Men	Women
Indian subcontinent/India		
♦ Marmot[2]	99	111
♦ Balarajan[2]	106	105
♦ Wild[3]	106	100
♦ Wild[4] (India only)	96	104
Caribbean /West Indies		
♦ Marmot[2]	95	131
♦ Balarajan[2]	79	105
♦ Wild[3]	77	91
♦ Wild[4]	102	98
Africa/West Africa		
♦ Marmot[2]	133	144
♦ Balarajan[2]	109	114
♦ Wild-West Africa[3]	113	126
♦ Wild-West Africa[4]	117	121

[1] Mortality in the period 1970–1972.
[2] Mortality in the period 1979–1983.
[3] Mortality in the period 1989–1992.
[4] Mortality in the period 2001–2003 (unpublished—personal communication).

common in ethnic minority groups than in the White population, thereby displacing such problems as cancer and respiratory disease, which are very common but less so than in the White population (Gill *et al.* 2006). Cancers are, indeed, one of the central priorities of ethnic minority groups as we discuss in Chapter 7.

Racial prejudice is fuelled by the selective emphasis of facts, particularly in the media, which generally portray ethnic minorities as inferior and the majority as superior. Infectious diseases such as AIDS and tuberculosis are a common focus for such publicity. A glaring example of this phenomenon followed the analysis by the UK's Central Statistical Office in August 1995 of statistics on single mothers as a percentage of all mothers by ethnic group. The front page headline in the popular national newspaper the *Sunday Express* (13 August 1996) was 'The ethnic time bomb' and the subheadlines 'Six out of 10 black mothers are now single parents'; 'Crisis over the meltdown of West Indian life'; and 'Taxpayers are left to pick up a bill of £130 million a year'. The 'Linford Christie syndrome' of one parent families was said by the *Sunday Express* to be disturbingly ingrained—an example of denigration of the whole group to which one of the world's finest athletes happens to belong. Researchers and public health practitioners cannot be responsible for media reportage, but they should be aware that their data may well be used to drive deep wedges between racial and ethnic groups.

In grappling with these difficult issues, we should heed two great historical lessons. First, the study of health and health care differences by racial and ethnic groups will be distorted by the prevailing ethos in society. If our society is racist, the study of racial/ethnic difference will also be racist, in effect if not in intent. Second, the act of seeking differentials by race and ethnic group, while important to reduce inequities in health care, poses potential danger to the people studied, for the outcome is dependent on the interpretation and use of the data. While racist attitudes and behaviours persist the danger of abuse of research for racist purposes will remain, particularly by the mass media. A supreme example of these lessons is the abuse of Binet's test of intelligence, designed to select children for special educational attention, but used in the 1920s as a tool for immigration control and for the demonstration of racial differences (see Gould 1984—under books).

6.3.5 Racism: some lessons from Hitler

We forget historical lessons at our peril. We have, however, the unforgettable example of racism in Nazi Germany, as summarized below.

Motivation to fight racism can be generated by studying the effect of both ignoring it, or extolling it, and the appalling impact of Hitler on the world of medical and public health is worth reflecting on, for it illustrates both. Hitler's views were published in his book *Mein Kampf* (vol. 1 in 1925) to widespread acclaim and support, acting as an inspiration to much of the German public, and the medical profession especially. Hitler built his case upon science, albeit in retrospect poor science. If the modern world were free of racism, nationalism and other forces leading to inequality and cruelty, there would be no reason to reflect on Hitler's views. Sadly, this is not the case, and there are many signs that racism as a component of right-wing political policy is making a comeback, as witnessed in parts of England, the Netherlands and France, for example. Echoes of Hitler's views, albeit much softened, are abundant in the mainstream media e.g. arguments based upon the need to increase the cultural cohesion of society, the danger of diluting national traits by immigration, and subtle versions of the concepts of cultural and racial superiority. There is evidence, worldwide, that racism is being controlled, but it is not eradicated.

Readers can access a succinct review by Silver (2003) on the central role of the medical profession—'the staunchest supporter of the Nazi regime'—in the euthanasia of psychiatric patients, eugenics, race medicine, marriage laws, killing of children regarded as defective, experimentation in concentration camps and on prisoners, anti-Semitism, and the attack on academic and professional standards. Some of the key points in Silver's article are in Table 6.3.

Hitler built upon a rich legacy of racism in medicine and science, much of it developed in Germany (see Chapter 9). The economic, social and political circumstances that allowed Hitler's policies to flourish could return. Indeed, there are numerous groups fighting to restore Hitler's policies, as the example in Box 6.2 shows. The much-abused concept of a superior Aryan race (see the note at the end of this chapter)

Table 6.3 Key events relevant to medical professions, race science and racism in Germany

1905	Racial Hygiene Society formed in Berlin
1931	SS troops' prospective marriage partners checked by a physician for racial purity over five generations.
1932	20 institutes of racial hygiene and 10 journals in existence in Germany
1933	13,000 Jewish physicians in post. Jews forbidden from publishing in German books and journals, and German doctors forbidden to quote works of Jews. Jewish students restricted to 1.5% of total. 6% of doctors have joined Nazi league
1933	Euthanasia becomes policy
1935	Marriage or sexual intercourse between Jews and citizens of German blood prohibited
1935	Widespread medical experimentation with focus on eugenics, with Dr Joseph Mengele as a leader in Auschwitz.
1937	4,200 Jewish physicians in post
1938	Most Jewish doctors decertified
1945	45% of doctors had joined the Nazi Physicians League (6% in 1933). 7% of doctors were SS members compared to 0.5% of the population.

From Silver (2003), published as a table in Bhopal (2005).

is still being promoted as the web site material in Box 6.2 shows. In the account of Hitler's views given below, the page numbers for the original quotations taken from Mannheim's translation are given so interested readers can check them in their original context.

Box 6.2 The continuing promotion of Hitlerian Views

Extract from the application form:

TABERNACLE OF THE PHINEHAS

PRIESTHOOD/ARYAN NATIONS

DECLARATION: I am of the White Aryan Race. I concur that Aryan Nations is only Aryans of Anglo-Saxon, Germanic, Nordic, Basque, Lombard, Celtic and Slavic origin, the White non-Jew race worldwide. I agree withAryan Nations' Biblical eclusions of Jews, Negroes, Mexicans, Orientals and Mongrels.

FIDELITY: That for which we fight is to safeguard the existence and reproduction of our Race, by and of our Nations, the sustenance of our children and the purity of our blood; the freedom and independence of our Race; so that we, a kindred people, may mature for fulfillment of the mission allocated us by the Creator of the Universe, our Father and God.—WE HAIL HIS VICTORY!!

PLEDGE: I will conduct myself at all times as a gentleman (or women) reflecting the superiority of the Aryan Race.

http://www.aryan-nations.org/about/htm
Accessed 24 February 2005

6.3.6 **Hitler on racial admixture**

Race science flourished in Germany in the early twentieth century. According to Silver (2003), Hitler's policies were influenced by such work. Hitler drew his arguments against the sexual mixing of races from the natural world, for example 'Such mating is contrary to the will of Nature for a higher breeding of all life' (Hitler 1992: 258). His analogies refer repeatedly to animals. He believed that such mixed unions were deleterious, because they reduced the superior breed: 'Any crossing of two beings not exactly the same level produces a medium between the level of the two parents' (1992: 258). Hitler's denigration of mating between human racial and ethnic groups, as if they were different species, was scientifically wrong. His idea that the offspring of unions of mixed race/ethnic group are inferior does not fit with modern evolutionary theory favouring outbreeding to inbreeding, or what gardeners refer to as 'hybrid vigour'.

The philosophy that Hitler promoted did not believe in equality of the races, but rather in the subordination of the inferior and weaker '... in accordance with the eternal will that dominates this universe' (1992: 348). He wrote, 'in a bastardised and niggerised world all the concepts of the humanly beautiful and sublime, as well as all ideas of an idealised future of our humanity, would be lost forever' (1992: 348). Hitler's extreme language on mixing of the races marked the emotional foundations of his arguments, despite their being presented as ostensibly scientific.

6.3.7 **Hitler on the superiority of the Aryan race, and the exploitation of inferior groups**

Hitler attributed everything worthwhile in human culture to the Aryan. While stating that it was idle to argue which race started human culture, he then claimed that it was the Aryan, without whom the 'dark veils of an age without culture will again descend on this globe' (1992: 348). His thesis was that the contribution of Aryan people stimulated foreign people to achieve. When they reproduced with the Aryans their new-found advances collapsed, with the degradation of the master race and the subjugated race alike. 'The last visible trace of the former master people is often seen in the lighter skin colour which its blood left behind in the subjugated race' (1992: 265).

Racial commissions would be required, Hitler wrote, to issue settlement certificates in newly acquired territories, after the individual's racial purity was established. Hitler proposed that evaluation of race be done on individuals using blood tests because 'the blood components, though equal in their broad outlines, are, in particular cases, subject to thousands of the finest differentiations' (1992: 402).

6.3.8 **Drawing lessons from Hitler's legacy**

The truism that those who forget history are bound to repeat it is one that applies to racism. Hitler's goal of creating a superior society is shared by most political leaders and many of his means, e.g. nationalism, control of occupational opportunities and reproduction, and immigration control are 'respectable' components of the political armamentarium. Eugenics in its open form, led by scientists and leading thinkers, is currently out of favour but its return is a likely accompaniment of the genetic revolution. Only open racism remains offside in mainstream politics. Knowing the effects of Hitler's views should stiffen the resolve of scientists and doctors to combat racism. They should ensure their professional and learned societies have constitutions and policies that will empower them to resist, rather than assist as in Nazi Germany, a future racist state. As we will discuss in Chapters 8 and 9, some ethical codes for research and medical professional conduct are already in place, so the ground is prepared.

6.4 Racism in service delivery, ethnocentrism and equity

6.4.1 Types of racism in health care

Try Exercise 6.7 before reading on.

Exercise 6.7 Racism, ethnocentrism and equity

◆ Why might ethnic minority patients get worse care in a health setting?
◆ What kinds of racism can you see?
◆ What experiences of racism can you recount, either from personal experience, or based on the experience of close friends or relatives?

Health services may offer a poorer service to ethnic minority groups for the following four broad reasons:

1. An individual member of staff treats the patient unequally because of racial prejudice.

2. The policies of the service are based on the needs of the ethnic majority population and not those of the minority populations, thus creating inequity. Health services are planned and managed largely by members of the majority population, usually on the basis of an implicit, rather than explicit, understanding of the needs and preferences of the users of the service. However, there is also a class bias and people from poorer, less articulate groups are likely to receive poorer care. Other less privileged sections of the populations are likely to benefit from new policies taking the needs of ethnic minorities into account.

3. The specialist resources required to meet the needs of minority groups simply do not exist even though they are recognized by policy-makers.

4. Employment practices in the service are discriminatory.

There is evidence that all four of these forces are in action and contribute at least in part to the finding that even when health care is, in theory, available to ethnic minorities it is not always there in the quantity or the quality that might be expected.

There are various kinds of racism (hence the use of the word racisms by some writers), including the following:

- *Direct racism*—this occurs where people are treated less favourably because of their race, ethnicity, religion etc. Most people equate racism with this type of action and in modern societies such racism is both abhorred and illegal.

- *Indirect racism*—services are provided, on the face of it, equally to all people, but the form in which they are provided favours particular groups at the expense of others. For example, provision of information by health professionals only in English indirectly discriminates against those who cannot understand or read this language.

- *Institutional racism*—the concept further develops indirect racism but as applied to organizations. Institutional racism is defined in the Macpherson report as:

> The collective failure of an organisation to provide an appropriate and professional service to people because of their colour, culture or ethnic origin. It can be seen or detected in processes, attitudes and behaviour which amount to discrimination through unwitting prejudice, ignorance, thoughtlessness and racist stereotyping which disadvantage minority ethnic people.
>
> Macpherson (1999; para 6.34, p8)

Some people are baffled by institutional racism, while others may pretend to be, possibly as part of the process of denial. A simple example would be the failure of the health care system to make accurate diagnoses because it fails to provide the training and facilities (e.g. interpreters) to achieve communication of sufficient quality to permit an accurate medical history. Sceptics may still wonder why such practices are wrong, and argue that failing to learn the local language is a problem, not for the service, but for the minority populations. There is a kernel of sense in that argument and it is wise for minorities to maximize their language skills. While counter-arguments are usually couched in terms of social justice, morality, ethics (particularly beneficence), and rights, increasingly the argument is being made on good business practice focusing on meeting the needs of the patient as a valued customer in an efficient and effective way. We will discuss this again in Chapter 8, in the context of developing health care strategy.

Ethnocentrism may well underlie indirect and institutional racism, because it may lead to inappropriate assumptions about the needs of people from minority ethnic groups based on the experience of the health professionals in serving, and being acculturated in, the majority White populations. Practitioners, policy-makers and politicians may also feel that their (ethnocentric) way is the correct one, and that minority populations ought to conform to it. Interactions between health professionals and minority ethnic service users are, of course, shaped by social conventions, whether real or perceived. It may be that White people cannot see the advantages that they have in comparison to non-White people. The following extract, from a longer list taken from a paper by Peggy McIntosh, author of 'White Privilege and Male Privilege', illustrates some of these advantages.

- ◆ If I need to move, I can be pretty sure of renting or purchasing a house in an area which I can afford and in which I would want to live.
- ◆ I can turn on the television or open to the front page of the paper and see people of my race widely and positively represented.
- ◆ I can remain oblivious of the language and customs of persons of color who constitute the world's majority...without feeling in my culture any penalty for such oblivion.
- ◆ If I declare that there is a racial issue at hand, or there isn't a racial issue at hand, my race will lend me more credibility for either position than a person of color will have.
- ◆ I can be pretty sure that standards of behaviour where I work or go to school will be set by people of my race and that I will be judged on my behaviour, not on my race.

McIntosh (http://www.dundee.ac.uk/iea/)

Explanations offered for professionals' inability to deliver an equitable service have included the social distance between them and their minority ethnic patients, the gap of culture and communication between practitioners and patients, and the complexity of many ethnic minority patients' problems, particularly as they relate to social and economic deprivation. Fundamentally, however, most professionals can only reflect the social mores of the times—a minority will be spearheading a process of change. Globally, racism is mostly deplored but still prevalent.

6.4.2 **Personal experiences of racism**

As a child born in India but raised from the age of two years in Glasgow, Scotland, being called 'darkie' or 'Paki' was a daily event for me. When I was 17 I was offered, by telephone, a summer job selling household goods door to door—that was a much coveted opportunity for earning some money for a schoolboy. When I reported for work next day the offer was abruptly withdrawn. A senior manager had overridden the person who employed me (to his obvious embarrassment). At university some much-loved friends (including my roommate) regularly enjoyed racial banter at my expense e.g. 'you're a black bastard Jindi (my nickname).' Their intention (probably) was not to hurt me, but they did, and as time went on the banter destroyed close friendships.

The house I had surveyed as a middle-ranking doctor in training in a middle class neighbourhood in Glasgow was withdrawn from sale after I put my offer in, to the embarrassment of the estate agent. It turned out a neighbour had objected to the sale to a coloured person.

My aunt was left in diabetic coma all day in a prestigious teaching hospital because the nurses could not communicate with her and so left her 'to sleep' (a mix of negligence and institutional racism).

I have also heard a great deal of racism uttered by members of my own ethnic group i.e. Indians.

These are relatively minor matters compared to some experiences such as lynching and murder, but they are on the less severe end of the same spectrum. Nonetheless, they are far from unique, and they may have lasting consequences, as indicated by a quotation summarizing research in Glasgow.

Of particular interest is the special importance for British South Asians born abroad of not having the parental generation nearby and of experiences of mugging or assault. Recognition of these two situations may alert clinicians to potential risk. The meaning of both is particularly threatening in this community, and assault, which may be played down verbally, is felt psychosomatically. Again, in Glasgow experiences of mugging or assault are not rare in the general population too, especially for men; but descriptions of the incidents experienced by South Asians often reveal racist connotations, and the knowledge that these are present—perhaps also uncertainty about whether they are present—may help to explain their particular threat.

Williams et al. (1997: 1173)

I have preferred in my life to emphasize the thousands of positive interactions, compared to the relatively few negative ones. Certainly, in schools, university and in employment I have had huge support from teachers and colleagues, which far outweighed any racism. I am proud to be a Scottish Indian, and to work to create an even better society than the excellent one we already have.

Nonetheless, I now see that I have been guilty of some complacency throughout most of my life. Until about 1990 I refused to use the word racism in my writing and in my lectures, believing that its use did more harm than good. Injustice, harassment, and prejudice on the basis of colour, religion, culture, or ancestry are not tolerable. In retrospect, I ought to have been better prepared and more ready to confront these problems, albeit in small ways.

6.4.3 Using race and ethnicity to combat racism and achieve equity

Race and ethnicity clearly serve important functions, including the development of identity, belonging, and social relations and are, naturally, the root of racism. Trying to remove race and ethnicity from the social mindset is both impossible and self-defeating. One conundrum is that a denial of difference is not the solution, mainly because the social and service norms and policies are based historically on the needs of the 'White' population. The resulting ethnocentric (Eurocentric) approach can be tackled only after an awareness of the issues, and analysis based on examination of differences. Such an analysis requires data by racial or ethnic group (for ethnic monitoring), which requires a classification, which in turn requires acknowledging the concepts of race and ethnicity—which permits their use to accentuate differences and provides the potential for abuse. So, we need a governing principle to help us.

Equity is the core ethical principle underpinning equality of health care.

Try Exercise 6.8 before reading on.

Exercise 6.8 Equity and inequality

- ◆ What is the difference between inequality and inequity?
- ◆ Why might the concept of inequity be more fitting in the ethnicity and health arena than inequality?
- ◆ Consider whether the following is an inequity:
  - the lower prevalence of smoking in Chinese women compared to White women

- the higher rate of colo-rectal cancer in White people compared to South Asians
- the lower life expectancy of African-Americans compared to White Americans.

An equitable service would meet equal needs equally, but this requires a diversity in the organization of services, to ensure uniformity in access, use, and quality at the point of delivery. An equal service, in the sense that everyone got exactly the same service, would not suffice. For example, no health professional would think about giving the medical consultation exactly the same amount of time, say 10 minutes. Some patients with complex problems, such as depression, may get 20 minutes, while others with simple problems, say the common cold, may get four minutes. In other words, the nature of the service is tailored to meet the need, so it is equitable rather than equal. The principle in relation to meeting the needs of different ethnic groups is exactly the same.

This type of goal is by no means impossible. For example, two studies in Teeside, in the north-east of England in the 1990s, led by Rajan Madhok (1992, 1998) showed surprisingly high levels of satisfaction with specific NHS services in the predominantly poor Pakistani South Asian community there. The extra challenges identified by the studies were well within the scope of the service. Improvement in services for ethnic minority groups will almost certainly benefit the whole population, for many issues are common to all—for example, the desire for health professionals and carers of the same sex for intimate (e.g. genital) examinations, and the wish for hospital food that is tasty and variable. Meeting the health care needs of ethnic minority groups needs to be seen as a key responsibility of the service, not a chore or a problem of ethnic minorities. It would be foolish to deny that there will be some extra costs and efforts required. It may be, however, that savings will also be possible. One obvious saving is that cancers are expensive to treat and they are, at least compared to the population as a whole, relatively uncommon in some ethnic groups e.g. the Pakistani population served in the study by Madhok and colleagues.

Not every inequality is an inequity. It would be foolish, for example, to argue that ethnic variations in the prevalence of smoking are inequitable. There is no injustice in Chinese women not smoking, or in White women smoking fairly heavily. There would be injustice, hence inequity, in blocking access to smoking cessation services by ethnic group. Equally, I can see no injustice in variations in colo-rectal cancer rates. There would be an injustice in the differential access to colo-rectal cancer prevention or treatment services. I perceive a serious injustice in major differences in life expectancy in different ethnic groups, because these are almost certainly a result of other social injustices, and certainly not innate. By contrast, it is hard to claim that the greater life expectancy of women compared to men is unjust, at least until we have a better understanding of the causes. At present, the causes are thought to be largely hormonal and biological or related to lifestyles. If it turns out to be stresses of life I may change my mind.

Fairness in employment is a fundamental component of equity in service delivery. Fair and open practices are needed for selecting people for study or employment, assessment of performance, disciplinary procedures, service on strategic decision-making bodies, career progression, and rewards. Talent and ability have no racial, ethnic, or cultural exclusivity.

To create equitable services needs more than legislation; it needs winning over the hearts and minds, and particularly the consciences, of service providers and managers. The ample guidance from the profession can be combined with the powers of the Race Relations Amendment Act 2000 and international human rights legislation to promote change. The professions of medicine and public health should be in the vanguard of the historical and global struggle against inequality, injustice and racism. Strategies for doing this will be discussed in Chapter 8.

The next section considers a more technical matter: measuring inequalities, using an example around CHD.

6.5 Exploration of the measurement of the relationship of socio-economic position and health: an example of ethnic variations in CHD

Measuring ethnic inequalities by socio economic status may prove difficult. The reasons include disruption of patterns of immigration; inappropriate measures of socio-economic position or disease outcomes; cross-cultural invalidity of measures; other forms of error and bias in study design and methods. The following account uses coronary heart disease as an illustrative example of special interest to me.

Social and economic inequalities are associated with inequalities in many diseases, and are particularly well studied for coronary heart disease (CHD). In South Asians the role of social and economic disadvantage in generating CHD has had modest attention in comparison with other explanations for the high rates. Yet most ethnic minority groups, including South Asians in the UK (especially Bangladeshis and Pakistanis, rather than Indians), are economically disadvantaged compared to the White populations of the UK.

The low priority given to the possibility of socio-economic factors being important in explaining the very high levels of coronary heart disease in South Asians probably stems from the demonstration by Marmot and colleagues in 1984, based on mortality by country of birth in years around the 1971 census, that social class based on occupation and coronary mortality rates were unrelated in those born in the Indian subcontinent. Also influential were observations by others, including McKeigue and colleagues (1989), that comparatively economically deprived (eg Bangladeshis) and well off South Asian communities (such as Indians) were at similar risk. The assumption was that economic factors reflected in the concept of social class derived from occupation were not important, at least at this stage of the evolution of the coronary heart disease epidemic. This assumption fitted with the idea that coronary heart disease emerges in high income groups first and the observation that the coronary heart disease epidemic in India is affecting those in the higher economic status groups.

The inference was that the epidemic in South Asians is at an intermediate stage where it is in balance in lower and higher economic status groups. The view was that social and economic factors have not been an important determinant of coronary heart disease in South Asians, but with a prediction by Williams and colleagues (1998) that 'an inverse association between social class and coronary heart disease will emerge eventually in South Asians.'

Analysis of UK mortality data by country of birth for men aged 20–64 years by Harding and Maxwell (1994) around the 1991 census years showed a social class gradient in all ethnic groups with the highest SMRs in men in manual classes. For men born in the Indian subcontinent the overall SMR was 150, i.e. 50 per cent higher than in the standard population. The SMR ranged from 132 in those in social classes I/II combined, to 223 in social classes IV and V combined. When social class was taken into account statistically, the difference between the men born on the Indian subcontinent and the standard population was not removed. The authors concluded that social class was an important factor for studying inequalities within the South Asian population. Social class did not, however, provide an adequate explanation for mortality differences between the Indian subcontinent population and the standard population.

Nazroo found that the prevalence of self-reported coronary heart disease, assessed in a national cross-sectional survey in 1993/94, was associated inversely with the standard of living (1997, 2001). In a statistical model most of the excess in coronary heart disease prevalence in Indians, Pakistanis and Bangladeshis was removed after adjustment for an index of standard of living. For example, for diagnosed heart disease or severe chest pain the overall odds ratio for Indians and African Asians (South Asians who were born/lived in Africa prior to immigration to the UK) combined was 0.95, but after adjustment for standard of living it was 0.78 (95 per cent CI = 0.6–1.01) i.e. much lower than in the White population. Nazroo emphasized the comparatively low CHD adjusted prevalence in Indians and the differences between the Pakistani/Bangladeshi and Indian subgroups of the South Asian community. He also emphasized the difference in the socio-economic standing of the three South Asian populations with Indians being comparatively affluent, and Pakistanis and Bangladeshis relatively poor. Finally, he demonstrated that there were sizeable disparities in income between ethnic minority and majority (White) populations within the same social class grouping. These studies are coherent with the hypothesis that in the 1960s/70s social/economic inequalities did not exist but emerged later.

An alternative and more recent interpretation is that socio-economic factors have always been important but the traditional occupational categories used to determine social class failed to capture social and economic status accurately. In this interpretation the process of migration is considered to have disrupted the link between indicators of socio-economic position such as occupational class and actual position, for example, an Indian with secondary schooling or more in India may be employed in a manual post after migration while another Indian with no schooling may be the owner of a thriving business.

With colleagues I explored these ideas using data from a detailed, population based cross-sectional study, designed to ascertain disease and risk factor prevalence, in secondary analyses to explore the relations between socio-economic circumstances and coronary heart disease, diabetes and their risk factors (2002). In the absence of a definitive valid measure of socio-economic status which is applicable across ethnic groups, and questioning of standard measures such as social class, we used three measures: social class divided into manual and non-manual groups, educational status, and a composite measure based on the components of the Townsend score. These three measures capture slightly different aspects of socio-economic positioning in society. Social class is an indicator of current or recent access to income and status. Educational level reflects, in particular, social standing in childhood and youth, and is linked to potential earning power and status. Education as an indicator of social standing is likely to be particularly important in societies where education is not compulsory and not free. The Townsend Score is a reflection of the level of material wealth in the population in the area a person lives in. These three measures are in widespread use in contemporary research on health inequalities nationally (social class, Townsend Score) and internationally (education).

This study provided an opportunity to assess the consistency or otherwise of these measures in demonstrating social class variations in cross-cultural research. The hypothesis under test was that socio-economic factors are associated with these diseases and risk factors alike across the four ethnic groups studied i.e. Indians, Pakistanis, Bangladeshis and White Europeans. One specific hypothesis was subject to test. Williams and colleagues and Harding had implied that the disparity between Marmot et al.'s (1984) findings around the 1971 census, and in the findings around the 1991 census can be explained by the fact that immigrants had been in the UK for a shorter period in 1971, and that inequalities emerge with settlement. If so, in the population under study inequalities by socio-economic factors should be greatest in ethnic groups longest settled, i.e. Indians, (42 per cent moved to the UK before 1962) and Pakistanis (44 per cent moved before 1962) and least in the most recent migrants Bangladeshis (23 per cent moved before 1962).

There was substantial variation in socio-economic position between the ethnic groups in this study. Indian men were, excepting overcrowding, most advantaged and Bangladeshis least advantaged. For example, 63 per cent of Indian men were in non-manual social classes compared with 21 per cent of Bangladeshis. White European women fared better in some indicators (employment, educational attainment, overcrowding), South Asians in others (housing tenure and access to a car, with a less clear picture for social class and Townsend Score). Indian women were advantaged in comparison to Pakistanis and Bangladeshis.

Most markers of lower socio-economic position were associated with more cardiovascular disease and risk factors in White Europeans but the pattern was less clear in the South Asian groups. Specifically, for glucose intolerance, CHD and related risk factors we showed that social class, education and Townsend deprivation score were more consistently associated with disease and risk factors: in Europeans than South Asians combined; in Indians than in Pakistanis and Bangladeshis, and in women than in men. The European pattern of inequalities was partly established in South Asians, but different in different South Asian populations. Emergence of socio-economic gradients may require a mix of time, acculturation and socio-economic advancement, and be influenced by factors such as sex, religion and place of origin. In view of differences in their socio-economic position, and in the pattern of associations with the three indicators, there is a case for future studies of inequalities in health separating Indians, Pakistani and Bangladeshi populations, and not to combine them as South Asians. We recommended further research to develop and refine indicators of socio-economic position appropriate for ethnic minority groups. A wide range of indicators will be needed for ethnic minority groups to capture the relationship between socio-economic position and health.

This kind of research is relevant to developing, or indeed hampering, strategies for tackling ethnic inequalities.

6.6 Strategies for tackling ethnic inequalities in health and health care

Do Exercise 6.9 before reading on.

Exercise 6.9 Strategies to reduce inequality and inequity

- What strategies can you conceive of for tackling ethnic inequalities in the health setting?
- Which facets of the underlying concepts of race and ethnicity might be amenable to change?
- What problems/conditions would you tackle first?
- How could relative and absolute risk approaches be used to devise a strategy?

Strategic thinking in ethnic inequalities needs an adjustment of the research led ethnicity and health paradigm as, for example, extolled by Henry Rothschild who saw ethnicity as the key to unlocking the secrets of disease causation. We need to see ethnicity and race as the means of assessing inequality, and guiding policy and practical action. Adding to causal understanding is a bonus. In this regard, ethnicity and race become like indicators of social and economic status. There are two separate but overlapping strategic outcomes—health care and health status.

The development and implementation of such ideas within health service strategies is discussed in Chapter 8. Table 6.4 gives my 10 point outline used in the work of a health authority (Lothian Health Board) serving a population of 650,000 people in the East of Scotland, of whom about 4 per cent were from ethnic minority populations. This table summarizes the development of my ideas, influenced by a wide range of academic and service documents, studied over the last 20 years.

The most straightforward and achievable strategic goal is equivalent quality of health care for the entire population. This will require monitoring of equity in the quality of health care. All health and healthcare policy and service development/implementation documents should contain background information on, and a plan for inclusion of,

Table 6.4 Ten key actions to reduce ethnic health inequalities

Agree health and health care policy document

Set up, resource and provide authority to a qualified ethnicity and health group

Mainstream (and monitor) ethnicity perspective in all policies, strategies and care plans

Better information systems to produce information on ethnicity and health

Acquire health-related materials available nationally for use locally, translating and developing materials when needed

Promote and monitor utilization of translation and advocacy services

Promote and monitor equity in the quality of health care for each ethnic group

Foster culturally sensitive services e.g. appropriate food in institutional care (hospital and long stay), advice that is meaningful in the cultural context in which it is to be implemented, facilities to pray and do appropriate ablutions in inpatient facilities, and choice of the gender of the health professional

Training for staff on the issue of ethnicity and health

Equal opportunities policy that leads to sufficient employment of minority ethnic people for the service to have, within the workforce, the insights and experience needed

ethnic minority populations. The key is to ensure that meeting the needs of ethnic minority groups is an integral part of the mainstream health care and public health function. The implementation of this recommendation alone would be a huge step forward.

Guidance on the health care of ethnic minority populations should promote actions to ensure their inclusion, and this issue should be a high priority for anticipated investments to develop and implement strategy in relation to ethnicity and health. Information systems should be redesigned to produce health information by ethnic group. In addition there should be an exploration of the potential for unlocking data already available by the retrospective addition of ethnic codes (see Chapter 3).

Health-related literature available nationally, providing information and advice on both available services and on the health of ethnic minority populations, should be summarized and utilized more widely. Ethnic minority populations will require health education/health promotion and service related information to be adapted and either translated or conveyed face-to-face by interpreters/advocates. Ethnic minority populations, elders in particular, will need high-quality translation, interpretation and advocacy services to ensure high-quality communications in health care.

Culturally sensitive services will be needed, and the highest priorities here will be:

- Appropriate food in institutional care (hospital and long stay)
- Advice that is meaningful in the cultural context in which it is to be implemented
- Facilities to pray and do appropriate ablutions in inpatient facilities
- Choice of the gender of the health professional for, in particular, examination of the reproductive tract
- Sensitive and appropriate support in relation to the dying and the recently deceased.

Training for all staff involved is needed on the issue of ethnicity and health, including population size and structure; living circumstances and lifestyles; languages spoken and read; religions both in terns of their tenets and as practised; and the implications of all this for modification of care. Equal opportunities policies will need to lead to sufficient employment of minority ethnic people for the service to have, within the workforce, the role models and insights to serve ethnic minority populations. This may require proactive recruitment of staff with particular language skills or cultural understanding.

Principles on the causes, consequences and control of inequalities derived from the general body of research, though largely on White populations, are highly likely to apply to ethnic minority groups. Failure to apply the general knowledge and general principles we already have while awaiting new research evidence specific to ethnic minorities, an ideal that would take several decades and hundreds of millions of pounds, is likely to be damaging. The challenge is to adapt general policies to take into account the ethnic dimension.

Health policies need to place emphasis on integrating primary care, social services, public health measures and hospital care. They need to be based on sound data that are interpreted with care to achieve a robust understanding of priorities. Data do not, on their own, help people make coherent policy, and for this a set of social values is needed to guide their interpretation. The key value is equity—equal service for equal need. This value needs to permeate society and services, such that researchers, policy makers and practitioners are united in their common perspective and goal.

Health and health care initiatives need to build on the work of community organisations, academic researchers and the NHS. Community organisations are often well placed to highlight ethnic minority populations' experience of health and illness. They are likely to perceive health in the broad way that is usually favoured in public health, to include issues like poverty, housing, employment, discrimination and violence. These perspectives are particularly valuable when combined with the insights of academic researchers examining patterns of disease and access to service provision by ethnic group.

The diversity of the population is very important in health and health care policy and delivery. Ethnicity should be considered as an important element of diversity alongside gender, age, religion/spirituality, sexuality, disability and so on. There is, of course, diversity both within and between ethnic groups. For example, Pakistanis, Bangladeshis and Indians differ in respect of religions, spirituality and languages. They also have differing patterns of disease and disability. Even within a group that is relatively homogenous, for example Pakistanis, there will be considerable diversity. Heterogeneity of ethnic groups is a massive problem for effective policy and practice, but needs to be accounted for as best as possible. Lumping disparate groups together can mislead policy and planning e.g. as shown earlier South Asians have a low prevalence of smoking but Bangladeshi men, a subgroup of South Asians, have an extremely high one (Table 3.1).

Effective strategies will acknowledge that people from minority ethnic groups continue to experience racism in their daily lives, and this affects their mental and physical health. Refugees are likely to have suffered physical or mental torture in their place of origin, and may be particularly sensitive to the experience of racism in their receiving country.

The problem of inequity and inequality in the health and health care of ethnic minority groups has defied easy solutions. The explanation is not simply a lack of knowledge, interest or even money. Paradoxically, by focusing on differences, inequalities can widen, as will be illustrated in Chapter 7 with a theoretical example. This approach has been historically harmful and in recent decades unhelpful. The better approach, which was examined in some detail in Chapter 5, is to focus first on the important problems and diseases. Then, if necessary, refine the sense of priority using the relative approach. In this way important matters such as cancer and respiratory disease will not be ignored as is continuing to happen. This approach would also avoid the piecemeal approach to tackling so-called ethnic health issues. For example, why should we pick on cervical cancer and not breast cancer? Drawing attention to the former and not the latter does a disservice not only to breast cancer sufferers but possibly the community at large, particularly as cervical cancer is now considered as a sexually transmitted disease, and these diseases are still associated with social stigma. There are so many differences that it is difficult to find a logical way to make a selection. Coronary heart disease, stroke, cancer, haemoglobinopathies and respiratory diseases including tuberculosis would, however, find their place on any list of priorities to reduce ethnic inequalities in health status. Further discussion on priority-setting is in Chapter 7, and on the development of strategic responses is in Chapter 8.

6.7 **Conclusion**

Inequalities in health and health care by racial and ethnic group are abundant but their underlying cause, and the contribution of racism, is a complex and much debated matter (Box 6.2). Arguably, the major cause of inequalities in health, and even more of inequalities in access to health care, is inequality in wealth. Minority groups generally find it difficult to overcome inequalities in wealth, partially because of racially discriminating actions and policies. Racial discrimination in the fields of employment (including health services) and social security is well documented. Minority groups generally, but not always (particularly in the period after immigration), have worse health than the ethnic majority. Almost invariably, however, they have lower quality of health care. The difficulties are not in demonstrating differences but in interpreting their meaning and using them to benefit the population.

One major explanation, which has had insufficient attention, is the role of socio-economic status. On arrival most migrants tend to hold unskilled jobs. This legacy may be passed to their children (though there are many exceptions) and ethnic minority communities have more than their share of unemployment and low-paid work. Much though by no means all of the health disadvantage associated with ethnic minority groups may not result from their racial and cultural background, but relate to their socio-economic disadvantage. Their general health status may be comparable to the power social classes in the majority population, and the solutions to health problems may in some ways be similar. Inequalities may widen in the face of both political interest and research—the most clear-cut example being the Black/White disparity in life expectancy in the USA. This is almost certainly because wider economic and social policies are increasing inequality.

While general inequalities, e.g. overall high death rates, are unjust, specific inequalities may not be. For example, one ethnic group may have a high rate of heart disease, but low cancer rates (e.g. South Asians). Another group may have high cancer and low heart disease. Overall, the mortality or disease rates may be very similar. The differences between the two populations in cancer and heart disease would be inequalities but not inequities. Specific inequalities are, of course, important in helping set priorities and guide research.

General inequalities, such as life expectancy, have social, public health, clinical and scientific implications. They challenge the health care system to adapt policies to take into account the ethnic dimension. Heterogeneity of ethnic groups and their health status and health care needs is a massive problem for effective policy. Policies can only articulate general principles that apply to heterogeneous populations because of the complexity and changing nature of the specific issues. Policies need to be based on the concept of equity.

Ethnic inequalities in health and health care pose a formidable challenge to research. The challenge arises from a mixture of underlying causal complexity, rapid changes in circumstances, and the methodological difficulties of collecting valid, timely data across a range of ethnic groups. These research issues will be discussed in Chapter 9 in more detail. Accompanying the challenges is a promise and potential of important advances, particularly in the epidemiology of diseases. The potential has been difficult to realize, but this is not a cause for despair, but a time for reflection on and correction of expectations. Public health research describing ethnic variations in health and health care is valuable because it directs priorities, strategies and resource allocation as considered in Chapters 7 and 8. Such research brings evidence to bear on preventative care, health promotion and health care for ethnic minority populations.

Summary

Health status, disease occurrence and mortality patterns in populations are sculpted by factors such as wealth, environmental quality and protection, diet, behaviour and genetic inheritance. Most of these factors are directly or indirectly related to ethnicity and/or race e.g. globally and within multi-ethnic societies White people are usually richer than non-White people. It is, therefore, unsurprising that there are stark health inequalities by race and ethnicity. The questions of interest are why they occur and what needs to be done to narrow them. Each health inequality is likely to have its own unique genesis, with no general explanation. For example, ethnic inequalities in risk of skin cancers such as melanoma are likely to have a biological basis relating to skin colour, while inequalities in stroke need to take account of many factors, including cultural, economic and biological ones over the life course.

The concept of inequity, as opposed to inequality, is central to policy and strategy. Inequity implies an inequality that is unfair or unjust. Some inequalities are unjust, for example those arising from inadequate access to knowledge or services, and these form a primary target for action, particularly if effective interventions are available. Other inequalities, for example the differences in the rate of skin cancer, are not always unjust. They pose, nonetheless, a major challenge to understanding and a focus for science and services.

Ethnic health inequalities are demonstrable using virtually all classifications of race and ethnicity, and are usually sharpened by taking account of population heterogeneity and examining men and women separately. The differences between ethnic groups are often large, particularly for specific conditions e.g. prostate cancer, and less so for general measures of health e.g. life expectancy. Even where such inequalities have been carefully studied and actions to reverse them are proposed, mostly they have not been narrowed e.g. the lower life expectancy in African-Americans compared to White Americans.

Ethnic inequalities are of value in generating research questions for the health and medical sciences, and they are vital in guiding health policy and service delivery. They may help set new more demanding targets e.g. in the UK, using the lowest rate, the target for CHD mortality could be set as the value for the Chinese population, and that for bowel cancer as the Indian population value.

Clinical services need to be adapted to counter health inequalities. Ethnic monitoring of health status, and use and outcomes of services, is necessary to achieve this. One of many dilemmas is the choice of which of the many inequalities to tackle. Selecting the priorities based on high relative risks associated with specific conditions may increase inequalities overall. The strategies that reduce overall indicators of inequalities may offer the best option.

Notes

A definition of 'Aryan'

Prehistoric people who settled in Iran and northern India. From their language, also called Aryan, the Indo-European languages of South Asia are descended. In the nineteenth century there arose a notion, propagated by the Count de Gobineau and later by his disciple Houston Stewart Chamberlain, of an 'Aryan race': people who spoke Indo-European, especially Germanic, languages and lived in northern Europe. The 'Aryan race' was considered to be superior to all other peoples. Although this notion was repudiated by numerous scholars, including Franz Boas, the notion was seized on by Adolf Hitler and made the basis of the Nazi policy of exterminating Jews, Gypsies (Roma), and other 'non-Aryans.'

From *Encyclopaedia Britannica* online (extracted). Available at http://www. britannica.com/ ebc/article?tocId=9355900&query=aryan&ct=. Accessed 25 February 2005.

Chapter 7

Principles for setting priorities for ethnic minority populations

Setting priorities is an issue for any organisation. . . . The process should be sensible; it should be founded on science; it should be based on experience and research.

Virginia Bottomley (1993, 25)

. . . there is no technological fix, scientific method, or method of philosophic inquiry for determining priorities . . . economists, ethicists and epidemiologists—all have valuable insights to contribute to the debate . . . .

Rudolph Klein (1993, 103)

Chapter contents

- ◆ Objectives
- ◆ The nature of priority-setting, and the contribution of pubic health sciences
- ◆ Social values as an underpinning force in priority-setting for ethnic minority groups
- ◆ The utility and futility of the comparative approach
- ◆ Using epidemiological data to help influence priorities for ethnic minority health
- ◆ The impact of choosing priorities on reducing and widening ethnic inequalities in health
- ◆ Framework for priority-setting for minority ethnic health within established systems in multi-ethnic societies
- ◆ Conclusions
- ◆ Summary of chapter

Objectives

On completion of this chapter you should understand:

- ◆ That setting priorities is a crucially important but very difficult activity
- ◆ That data on health status can guide priority-setting within the framework of social values, available resources and individual preferences
- ◆ That quantitative data can be used to derive understandings of absolute (or actual) and relative health states

◆ That focusing only on differences between minority and majority populations can deflect attention from hidden priorities and exacerbate inequalities
◆ The merits and limitations of a framework for setting priorities based on a set of standards for the population as a whole, and health information based on actual and relative measures

7.1 Introduction

Before reading on, try Exercise 7.1.

Exercise 7.1 Priority-setting

◆ Why is priority-setting necessary:
    (a) in general for all populations?
    (b) when considering the needs of ethnic minority groups?
◆ Why is it difficult, and particularly so in relation to ethnic minority groups?

Priority-setting is a process for making rational choices. It is an all-important activity which, in the context of health care in particular, has received insufficient debate, analysis and research, partly because of its close connections with rationing. Rationing implies restriction of the supply of a service or goods through sharing, sometimes on the basis of allocation of a fixed amount. This tends to be politically unacceptable, particularly in rich countries, not least because it is unpopular with the public. In a static or shrinking health care economy the need for a rational and just means of priority-setting becomes glaringly obvious, especially when new interventions are to be implemented. Even where the health care economy is growing, however, priority-setting is important to guide new expenditures and for ongoing review and analysis of existing expenditures. Without this process decisions will be ad hoc and swayed by the biases of the powerful individuals and groups. The quotations that opened this chapter are illustrative and come from a book called *Rationing in Action*. In it a politician, Virginia Bottomley, then Secretary of State for Health, argues for science as the key to priority-setting, and a social science academic, Rudolph Klein, for politics. All contributors to the book agree that priority-setting is important, and some, notably the physician John Grimley Evans, see it as inseparable from rationing, itself a job for politicians (1993).

Health care systems have multiple priorities that are to a great extent dictated by the disease and health patterns of the population and population subgroups, by the expectations and explicit standards of public services, and by the public and especially the users of the service. These priorities include: the prevention and management of disease, the promotion of health, health education, reduction of inequalities in health, high quality health care, cost-effective and value for money services delivered within budget, and respectful, sensitive and equitable services that win public support. Such priorities are virtually internationally applied (at least in affluent countries), lasting, core, and though the phraseology and emphasis change, they can be found in every important health policy document. Of course, the emphasis changes from place to place and time to time e.g. inequalities and inequities are high on the agenda at the moment (see Chapter 6 for a discussion of the overlaps and distinctions between inequalities and inequities).

Are these the right priorities for minority ethnic groups? Are there others that are more important to minority ethnic health, but are not on the list? Are there nuances needed for ethnic minority groups, such that the priorities need modification or a change of emphasis? These are the key questions for this chapter, which focuses on the principles and methods for answering them, rather than the answers themselves. We need also to ensure that minority ethnic groups are not bypassed when priorities are implemented, either because the priorities are not the right ones or because they are not being applied, perhaps because managers and health professionals perceive them to be inappropriate, or even lacking endorsement or validity for minorities. There is one central issue that drives our analysis of priorities: in what ways are the health needs of minority ethnic groups similar to, and yet different from, the majority population that the health service has evolved to serve? This question, the topic of Chapter 5, provides the link between needs assessment and priority-setting. Having made this link, of course, actions need to be taken, and this is the topic of Chapter 8.

Whether in research, policy or health care, the choices for actions to improve the health of ethnic minority groups are virtually limitless, especially in complex, multi-ethnic societies. Social values are important to priority-setting and in the context of ethnicity and health the most important are the values of equality and equity. An historical analysis shows a major shift away from emphasizing differences, which are relatively small at least for health care if not specific disease patterns, to similarities, which are overwhelming (see Chapters 4 and 5). In chapter 5 I introduced the needs assessment by Gill and colleagues which showed that many of the priorities are applicable to the main minority ethnic groups in the UK, in particular, that the emphasis on the prevention, treatment, rehabilitation and palliative care for cardiovascular diseases, cancers, mental health and other health problems of modern societies is appropriate. A few diseases and problems that tend not to dominate health services' priorities were also found to deserve a place in the context of minority ethnic health, e.g. haemoglobinopathies and tuberculosis. A focus on the latter should not, however, be at the expense of the main priorities, but in addition to them.

The idea of additional priorities can easily be misinterpreted—as an extra or bonus that minorities enjoy at the expense of the majority. The majority population (usually White in Europe and North America) is also an ethnic group that has special needs e.g. cystic fibrosis is much commoner in White ethnic groups, and for reasons relating to age distribution, so is senile dementia, a very costly health problem. The need for a balanced and considered approach to priority-setting using epidemiological data was briefly illustrated in Chapter 5 (Section 5.1.2) by the example of stroke and coronary heart disease in the African-Caribbean population in the UK. We showed there that neglecting CHD in favour of stroke would miss the bigger problem and run the risk of the African-Caribbean community losing its relative advantage in regard to CHD over the population as a whole (thereby repeating what happened to African Americans in the USA). This general principle will be illustrated later in the chapter.

Like the population as a whole minority ethnic groups need services that are respectful and sensitive, but they have additional concerns because the services were not set up with their needs in mind, as discussed in Chapter 4. This poses particular demands on health services. Racism—overt or institutional or both—is usually present, whether in the delivery of care, or the appointment of staff (see Chapters 4 and 6). In Chapters 4, 5 and 6, we discussed some of the required service delivery responses, and we will consider strategy and policy in Chapter 8. Managers of health care systems need to ensure their priorities and policies are vigorously applied and evaluated in relation to the minority ethnic groups they serve. Epidemiological thinking can aid them.

7.2 **The epidemiological underpinnings of priority-setting**

Before reading on do Exercise 7.2.

Exercise 7.2 Information for priority-setting

◆ What kind of information would you need to set priorities?
◆ What kind of information is generally available on the health of ethnic minority groups? What is usually missing?

Priority-setting is a complex and incompletely understood activity. Epidemiological concepts and data underpin priority-setting, but decisions on consumption of resources are always heavily influenced by political matters (Figure 7.1 and Table 7.1).

Table 7.1 Some characteristics of problems given high priority*

(A) Epidemiological and clinical factors	
The problem is	common
	severe in its effects
	long-lasting
	communicable
	externally, or iatrogenically, acquired
	found in young people
	treatable/curable
	preventable
(B) Social, economic and political factors	
The problem is	of high public and political interest
	economically important
	lobbied for by pressure groups
	free of stigma
	socially unacceptable
	of interest to health professionals

*Problems which do not have these characteristics, or have opposite characteristics, are given low priority.
This table develops the one first published by me (Bhopal 1998) in Rawaf and Bahl (1998), Chapter 4 (table 1).

Source: The Royal College of Physicians and Faculty of Public Health Medicine. Rawaf S., Bahl V. (eds) *Assessing Health Needs of People from Minority Ethnic Groups*. London: Royal College of Physicians, Copyright © 1998 Adapted by permission.

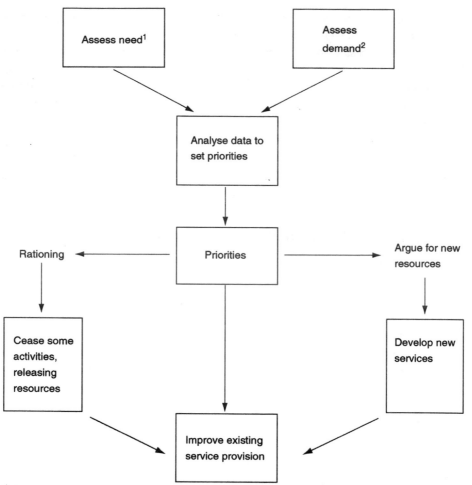

[1] Using demographic, lifestyle, sociological and epidemiological data

[2] Using the views, and patterns of past behaviour, of professionals, pressure groups, patients and the public.

Footnote: this figure develops the one published by Bhopal (1998) in Ch. 4 of Rawaf, S. & Bahl, V (fig 1)

Fig. 7.1 The place of priority-setting in relation to need for, demand for and provision of services.

Source: The Royal College of Physicians and Faculty of Public Health Medicine. Rawaf S., Bhal V. (eds.) *Assessing Health Needs of People from Minority Ethnic Groups.* London: Royal College of Physicians, Copyright © Adapted by permission.

Table 7.1 places equal emphasis on the epidemiological and medical aspects of the problem (frequency, effects, causes) and the wider social factors. While there is a shortage of epidemiological and clinical data by ethnic group the need for such information is accepted and information systems are being developed (Chapter 3 and Chapter 8). The kind of information in part B of the table is not usually available by ethnic group and methods to collect it are not well developed. So, for example, we do not know whether epilepsy has more stigma associated with it in Chinese, African or Pakistani populations than in White or Arabic ones. Nonetheless, informed judgement may help us on these matters. For example, the high priority given in health care systems (in the UK, but probably in other affluent countries also) to a diverse set of conditions such as heart disease, diabetes, obesity, childhood leukaemia, child abuse and Legionnaires' disease, can be understood in the context of the characteristics in the table. The relatively low priority for mental retardation, sexually transmitted diseases, suicide and senile dementia can also be understood.

For example, Legionnaires' disease is a very rare pneumonia, but it is externally acquired and sometimes a consequence of demonstrable negligence on the part of industries, government agencies and hospitals. If so compensation may be payable to the sufferer and the adverse publicity may be very damaging to the organization responsible. The disease can occur in outbreaks that cause panic and receive major media coverage. In principle, it is preventable, and usually it is curable. In contrast to its small public health impact this disease is a high priority. By contrast, mental retardation is not curable and rarely gains publicity unless it is caused by medical negligence. It is self-evident that the people affected are not well placed to argue the case for a higher priority, although their relatives and friends may do so. In relation to its massive public health impact this problem is given low priority. These factors and examples help us understand why some issues come to prominence and others do not.

It has been a little bewildering to many people in the ethnicity and health field that arguments for screening and good quality treatment for haemoglobinopathies have been difficult to win. By contrast, for another rare genetic disease, cystic fibrosis, similar arguments have been easy. The difference does not lie in the factors in part A of the table but in part B. Haemoglobinopathies occur mainly in ethnic minority groups while cystic fibrosis occurs mainly in White populations. There is simply more public, professional and political pressure to do something about the latter problem. Fortunately, as leaders in the ethnicity and health arena have argued the case for haemoglobinopathies, these services have gained more priority. Indeed, a national service for screening for sickle cell disease is being developed in England. The consequences of such developments are not always for the better, as the following quotation about the experience in the USA demonstrates.

> The National Sickle Cell Anaemia control act, enacted by the USA Congress on 16 May 1972, called for mandatory screening for the sickle cell trait in all people who were 'not of the Caucasian, Indian or Oriental race' and marks the start of a screening programme that is held up as the benchmark for failure. The act had a serious effect on the lives of USA citizens of African descent; in some states marriage licences were not issued to those of African descent unless the sickle cell test was taken, in others a test was a condition of entry to school. The presence of the sickle cell trait could lead to loss of employment, increased insurance premiums, inappropriate medical therapy, delay in adoption of children and sometimes problems in the revelation of 'non-paternity'.
>
> Hannah Bradby, Chapter 14, p303

The achievement of a priority needs to be well motivated and followed up by excellence in its implementation.

The entire field of ethnicity and health research can be considered in the light of part B of the table. All the factors in part B are of relevance but I would draw special attention to the role of pressure groups and freedom from stigma. As ethnic minority groups have won positions of power their voices have been heard. This combined with laws and policies that promote work on ethnicity and health has begun to free the entire field of stigma—it is no longer something to hide. In the UK, this development may have been spurred by the ideals of the Labour government which has held power for nearly ten years. Nonetheless, similar changes have occurred in the USA even as more right-wing Republican governments have come to power. In the Netherlands we are seeing, apparently, the reversal of policies favouring an interest in ethnicity and health even though the politics of the nation remain liberal. (See Chapters 4 and 8 for further discussion of the role of politics in the development of the ethnicity and health field.)

Within many new and recent health policy documents, in contrast to those of 20 years or more ago, there is an emphasis on the health and health care of ethnic minority groups. Scarce resources of time, energy and new funds may need to be found and applied to maximize the benefit of such policy statements. As funds are scarce, choosing between alternatives is invariably necessary. Setting priorities for ethnic minority populations with limited resources is an exacting challenge because they are extremely heterogeneous, and their disease patterns and lifestyles are both incompletely understood and are changing rapidly within and between generations. What principles should guide us here?

The decision to offer (or not to offer) a service is based upon a judgement on the needs of a community. Such judgements may be subjective and based on past experience or common sense. Since few decision-makers are from the ethnic minority communities the judgements based on such subjective appraisal may be inappropriate for lack of necessary insights. Of course, even people from the minority communities are unlikely to have the knowledge required to make valid and objective judgements on priorities. Their judgements should be supported by need as reflected in data on the community.

The importance of accurately interpreting data on disease patterns of ethnic minority groups is crucial to the characteristics in part A of the table. (In Chapters 3 and 5 we discussed how priorities may be skewed by misinterpretation.) It is important to attend to the factors in part B of the table. For those working on ethnicity and health there is a huge challenge in (a) maintaining ethnicity and health as a priority generally in competition with other matters and (b) deciding priorities within this theme. First I will provide an overview of past decision-making processes, and then offer a new approach for the future that is founded on epidemiology.

7.3 Analysis of past approaches

Past approaches to priority-setting can be examined in four ways: analysing the nature and emphasis of past initiatives; analysing the nature and emphasis of current initiatives; reading the scientific and professional literature; and assessing the opinions of decision-makers and providers. For illustration, I focus on South Asians in the UK, the topic I know best, but one that yields generalizations that apply, at least in part, to other populations and settings.

My analysis was first done in the 1990s: I found that there was no agreed sense of priority on the part of the NHS and that past approaches were largely tactical rather than strategic. The tactics had been based on grasping opportunities, themselves arising from the perspective that there were distinct, 'ethnic minority group problems' to be solved. For instance, national attention in the UK was aroused by the problem of so-called Asian rickets, and much professional, research, policy, and media attention was devoted to this problem in the 1960s and 1970s. It would be quite wrong to imply this was not important then and it remains important even now. The interesting question is how did it come to gain such prominence in relation to other problems? Other problems gaining early UK attention included the use of surma, an eye cosmetic that adorned my (and many other South Asians') eyes in my childhood, and traditional health remedies. There were fears (reasonably founded) that they contained lead and other metals that were hazardous. These problems drew attention to the cultures of ethnic minority groups as a prime consideration in their health.

The 1980s Mother and Baby Campaign run by the Department of Health in England remains to this day one of the biggest ever national initiatives concerning ethnic minority issues in the UK—its emphasis was also around culture and communication. The scientific literature in the 1970s mirrored the issues to which the health service was devoting attention, with an emphasis on a number of diseases and health problems, particularly nutritional and infectious ones. Tuberculosis, for example, received focused attention and publicity. What little evidence there was on professional opinion at that time indicated that there was no clear, agreed view on priorities. However, professional views seem to have been deeply influenced by the focus of the scientific literature. How did this focus match to quantitatively demonstrable health needs?

At the same time as attention was focused on such matters as rickets and surma (1960s and 1970s) 45 per cent of deaths in men born on the Indian subcontinent, but dying in Britain, were due to cardiovascular and cerebrovascular disease, as shown in the second

Table 7.2 Deaths in male immigrants from the Indian subcontinent (aged 20 and over; total deaths = 4,352)

By rank order of number of deaths

Cause	SMR*	No. of deaths	% of total (4,352)
Ischaemic heart disease	115	1533	35.2
Cerebrovascular disease	108	438	10.1
Bronchitis, emphysema and asthma	77	223	5.1
Neoplasm of the trachea, bronchus and lung	3	218	5.0
Other non-viral pneumonia	100	214	4.9
	—	2626	60.3

* Standardized mortality ratios, compared with the male population of England and Wales, which was by definition 100. Source of original data for the construction of this table is given in table 5.7.

column of Table 7.2 (an extract from Table 5.7), and the corresponding figure for women was 29 per cent. Yet until the 1980s this fact went largely unnoticed, although Hugh Tunstall Pedoe and colleagues published an influential article in 1975 showing that Asians in east London had higher rates of heart attack than the population as a whole. These were the first UK data but they supported similar observations from other countries, including South Africa and Singapore.

The landmark publication on immigrant mortality by Michael Marmot and colleagues (1984) placed heavy emphasis on relative mortality experience and the tables gave rankings based on standardized mortality ratios. I have discussed in Chapters 3 and 5 the importance of examining death data using numbers of deaths and actual death rates. The analyses based on SMRs may have made it difficult to see the priorities as clearly as a focus on actual numbers and rates of deaths might have done.

While some health education material had been specifically adapted for ethnic minority groups, up to 1987 none of those items in the catalogues of the Health Education Authority (England) concerned heart disease, as shown in my analysis with Liam Donaldson published in 1988. In 1987 information was available for ethnic minorities on a wide range of other matters including lice, spitting and colostomy. The emphasis of health education, however, was on birth control, infant care and feeding. In the 1990 Health Education Authority catalogue four of 179 items concerned heart disease. Clearly, the impact of epidemiological data was modest, at least in relation to health education. Understanding the underlying basis for this gap between need, as reflected in epidemiological data, and provision, as reflected in health education materials, and the implications for future strategy, is of great importance in priority-setting.

Public health practitioners such as health educators are to an extent 'demand-led': their work is partly and sometimes largely determined by the requests made to them by other health professionals, particularly health visitors, and by the officers of the health authority or health care operating units such as hospitals or primary care centres. In addition, most health education departments will have their own priorities, sometimes following the community development model, which emphasises social improvement, rather than the medical model, which puts emphasis on causes of death and disease. Thus, health education developments for ethnic minorities may be generated by health professionals who see a specific problem which requires a solution, rather than as a response to a comprehensive appraisal of the health education needs of a community. While this approach may result in satisfactory delivery of services for the majority of the community, the culture and health of which most health professionals have considerable knowledge, it may not suffice for ethnic minority communities because of lack of knowledge about them.

Demand for health education services may also come, directly or indirectly, from individual members of the public, community groups and politicians. Being less vocal, less well-organized in terms of groups and less familiar with health services, the ethnic minorities' own demands for health education may be very limited. Such demands may relate to recent published research and the resultant media and popular magazines reports, which often highlight differences.

Ideally in making service improvements judgements should be informed by appropriate indicators of health status, choices of which will depend on the objectives of the service. In terms of health education services, the needs are defined by what the community knows about health, what it ought to know, what its current health status is and what improvements in health status can realistically be achieved.

There are no routinely collected data in the UK on the population's health beliefs, knowledge and attitudes and we rely upon ad-hoc surveys. In the case of ethnic minorities the few data that exist indicate that their knowledge on a range of health issues, particularly the causes and prevention of ill-health and on the value of medical procedures, is low. An illustrative study is that by Judith Rankin and I (2001) showing the extremely limited knowledge on heart disease and diabetes of Indians, Pakistanis and Bangladeshis in north-east England.

The message I derived from the above analysis is that a strategic approach, based on agreed principles, is essential. The strategic approach should meet key needs, based on an analysis of the circumstances and health status of ethnic minority groups, and not merely focus on those matters where the differences between the ethnic minority and majority groups are obvious. In short, as discussed in Chapter 5, absolute and not relative needs should dominate our priority-setting strategy. Table 5.7 showed the key causes of death, first ranked on the standardized mortality ratio (SMR), a measure of relative excess or deficit of deaths, and then the actual number of deaths. The patterns are quite different. The former pattern guides research, the latter is the focus of service planning.

In setting priorities, decision-makers' perceptions, opinions and attitudes are important, as reflected in Table 7.1 part B, though they are hard to gauge objectively. On the basis of my experience in committees and other groups asked to assess priority needs, one issue has stood out: the enhancement of the quality of communication between ethnic minority populations and health professionals. Communication refers to more than the exchange of words and encompasses mutual respect, understanding of life circumstances and culture, clear use of language, and empowerment of the individual to say what they want and ask questions without fear or inhibition.

Little quantitative research has evaluated rigorously the impact of interventions that improve communications e.g. interpreters, link workers and patients' advocates, although there is a great deal of consultation and qualitative research which may provide useful information, though of a different kind. Most, if not all, health authorities in the UK have either implemented pragmatic interpretation schemes or have aired the issues as a prelude to doing so. This basic requirement of good communication with ethnic minority patients, fundamental to quality health care, is not an ingrained, high-quality and routine part of health services internationally.

Similarly, other basic issues such as correct recording of names, food that is sensitive to religious or cultural requirements in hospital, and the opportunity for examination by a health professional of the same sex (at least for intimate examinations) have yet to be attended to in most health services, despite a long period of education and exhortation.

This said, the UK is probably well ahead of most countries in grappling with these issues and the Migrant-Friendly Hospital Scheme in Europe is helping make rapid progress there.

The problems I perceive are a failure to agree priorities; too much of a focus on specific 'ethnic' health issues at the expense of larger-scale problems which are shared by the whole population; and insufficient quality of basic services which, on general opinion and research, are high priorities e.g. communication services. Principles, some of which are offered below, are required.

7.4 Towards a set of principles and standards

Try Exercise 7.3 before reading on.

Exercise 7.3 Using the population as a whole as a guide to standards and priorities for ethnic minority groups

- What are the strengths and limitations of using existing priorities for the population as a whole and applying them to ethnic minority groups?
- What about quality of care standards for the population as a whole?

Priority-setting for ethnic minority groups needs a principle. One principle might be that the priorities are those actions that maximally benefit the specific ethnic minority group. This is an approach advocated in health economics. It is an idealistic approach that requires a great deal of research to implement. Another principle is to prioritize actions that improve the health of the ethnic minority group either to the level of the population as a whole or to that of another ethnic group, perhaps the one with the best health. The usual principle, however, and sometimes unfortunately so, is to aspire to the standard of health of the White or majority population. The latter is a pragmatic approach. Integrating the three approaches meets the twin goals of maximizing health and tackling health inequalities, and would be the ideal.

Quantitative and qualitative data by ethnic group on health status and service utilization and quality are sparse and crude but the data that are available need to be utilized carefully to help apply these principles. In contrast, information on cost and effectiveness of interventions as applied to specific ethnic groups are rarely available—posing a formidable challenge to future research and making decisions on health economic grounds nigh impossible presently.

The concept of a hierarchy of health and health care needs for ethnic minority groups might be helpful. The hierarchy might be as follows:

1. Clinical Care of a Quality Equal to National Standards
   (a) Equal access to and quality of advice and facilities
   (b) Equal respect from carers
   (c) Equally clear and effective communication

(d) Equally suitable and culturally appropriate accommodation, facilities and services such as food

(e) Equally effective clinical diagnosis, therapy and advice

2. Preventive Care/Health Promotion of a Quality Equal to National Standards

(a) Equal access to appropriate range of information/advice

(b) Equally effective communication

(c) Equally acceptable and relevant information

(d) Focus on common and preventable diseases/health problems

(e) Focus on matters perceived as important by ethnic minority groups

(f) Equal efforts to involve the community.

The principles which are encapsulated in the above hierarchy are these: acceptance of national standards as the aim for health care of ethnic minority groups; emphasis on basic needs, irrespective of similarities or differences between ethnic minority and majority populations; and emphasis on quality of service rather than specific conditions.

Finally, for implementing a programme of work associated with given priorities the key principle is integration. Action is required at national, regional, district, service provider and community level. The policies, strategies and action plans at each level need to be harmonious. Chapter 8 examines how this can happen. This cannot happen, however, without priority-setting. In the next section we look at the use of epidemiological data around a specific example—cancer.

7.5 Setting priorities using epidemiological data; the example of cancer

Before reading on try Exercise 7.4.

Exercise 7.4 Prioritizing using data

- In terms of setting priorities what are the strengths and weaknesses of the relative risk and absolute risk approaches?
- In prioritizing conditions on the basis of difference, what is the danger?
- Similarly, what is the danger of prioritizing without regard to difference?

Since the ultimate objective of public health, including health education and health care services, is to improve health and control illness and disease, we can try to identify need on the basis of the common causes of ill-health as reflected in morbidity and mortality statistics.

Epidemiological data on disease frequency, causal and other risk factors, and the population's characteristics can play a key role in identifying needs and setting priorities. This section relies on Bhopal and Rankin's review (1996) of published epidemiological data on the frequency of cancer in UK ethnic minority populations to answer two key questions:

1. How common is cancer in these populations? and
2. Which cancers deserve special attention in terms of policy, prevention, service provision, aetiological research and health services research?

While the limitations of the published data mean that these questions can only be answered for a few of the ethnic minority groups in the UK, the principles of the approach outlined here, and possibly some of the conclusions, ought to be generalizable.

Published studies were identified that provided information on cancer frequency in a defined population, and permitted analysis of cancer frequency for a range of causes, following the approach advocated in Chapter 5 on health needs assessment, as follows:

◆ total cancer cases;
◆ rankings of cancer (top seven) by frequency of occurrence;
◆ overall standardized mortality ratio (SMR);
◆ rankings of cancer (top seven) by excess risk as indicated by the standardized mortality/cancer registration ratio (SMR/SRR) or the proportional mortality/registration ratio (PMR/PRR).

Measures of relative frequency were converted to percentages where authors had reported data differently.

The largest studies are based on mortality data, and focus on the Indian subcontinent-born (South Asian) and Caribbean-born populations, with some data on African-born populations. There were major limitations of the data which made interpretation and utilisation for priority-setting awkward:

1. The studies by Marmot *et al.* (1984), Balarajan and Bulusu (1990), and Grulich *et al.* (1992) were based on the country of birth code on the death certificate. The country of birth does not accurately identify ethnic origin. For example many people of White ethnic origin were born and lived in Commonwealth countries and returned to Britain following the independence of their country of residence. Marmot *et al.* (1984) used a names analysis to identify the South Asian group within the Indian subcontinent-born population.
2. Accurate denominators (population at risk) have not been available, making the calculation of accurate disease rates and SMR impossible, particularly between census years.
3. The assignment of ethnic origin used various approaches e.g. names analysis for South Asian populations. Two studies based ethnicity on information from medical records or asked doctors to assign it, and one study gave no information on how ethnicity was assigned. In general the categories for ethnic categorisation were extremely broad. Grulich *et al.* (1992) reported data on East and West Africans, but in other studies there was no differentiation of population by subregion.

Table 7.3 Cancer in adult South Asian males (mortality) and men and women (cancer registration): example of an overview for needs assessment

Author	Total cancer cases (overall SMR or SRR)	Cancer as % of all mortality or morbidity	Top 7 cancers % of all cancers	Top 7 cancers on SMR or SRR as % of all cancers
(A) Mortality				
Marmot *et al.* (1984)	722 (SMR = 69)	16.6	69	30
Balarajan and Bulusu (1990)				
20–69 years	1,183 (SMR = 59)	15.6	68	32
(B) Cancer registration				
Donaldson and Clayton (1984)*	251 (SRR not stated)	Unknown	53	14

* Male and female data combined by Donaldson and Clayton.

Reproduced from Bhopal R, Rankin J. Cancer in minority ethnic populations priorities from epidemiological data. *British Journal of Cancer*, 1996; 74: S22–S32.

4. The numbers of cases in several studies were very low, particularly those based on regional, cancer registry data. The precision of the estimates of frequency is low in these studies and especially so for rarer cancers.

5. The study of Powell *et al.* (1994), used data also used in the studies by Muir *et al.* (1992) (71 per cent of cases), and by Stiller and McKinney (1991) (20 per cent of cases), which means that the three studies on children were not independent.

Even given these limitations, progress was made.

Cancer was shown to be a common and important cause of death and morbidity in the three ethnic groups reported on here, causing about one-sixth of all deaths. Generally, cancer was less common in these ethnic groups than in the White population, with the overall SMR mostly being in the range 50–80 for South Asian and Caribbean populations but about 100 in African populations (higher in West Africans and lower in East Africans). Table 7.3 illustrates, using data on South Asians, how published data can be used to provide an overview of the importance of cancer overall, and for top-ranking cancers.

Clearly, a strategy focused on the commonest cancers captures a much higher proportion of all cancers (here 53–69 per cent) than one focused on the cancers which are relatively common in relation to the standard population (14–32 per cent).

7.5.1 **Caribbean origin populations**

Table 7.4 summarizes data from Balarajan and Bulusu (1990).

The commonest seven cancers, which include lung cancer, stomach cancer, and leukaemia, accounted for about 70 per cent of cancers. In this group four of the cancers which were common in terms of number of cases, were also relatively common in comparison to the standard population i.e. stomach, lymphatic, prostate and liver cancer.

Table 7.4 Cancer experience of Caribbean origin men: top seven based on actual and relative frequency

Balarajan and Bulusu 1990 (i) Age 20–69								Total	Total of top 7	Top 7 as % of total
Neoplasm ranked by frequency	Trachea, bronchus and lung	Lymphatic	Stomach	Prostate	Pancreas	Liver	Colon			
Number of cases	151	116	108	54	41	39	29	744	538	72
SMR	35	135	116	175	77	317	43			
Neoplasm ranked by relative frequency	Liver	Prostate	Lymphatic	Gallbladder	Stomach	Buccal cavity and pharynx	Colon			
SMR	317	175	135	118	116	78	43	744	370	50
Number of cases	39	54	116	7	108	17	29			

Reproduced from Bhopal R, Rankin J. Cancer in minority ethnic populations: priorities from epidemiological data. *British Journal of Cancer*, 1996; 74: S22–S32.

For women the seven commonest cancers contributed 67 per cent of cancers, and the ranking was dominated by the reproductive tract (breast, cervix and ovary). The cancers ranking highest on SMRs were uncommon, but those of the lymphatic system, oesophagus, cervix and stomach appeared on both sets of rankings. (Data not shown here, but see Bhopal and Rankin [1996].)

The methodological limitations of the data, as discussed above, need to be borne in mind in reaching conclusions. Patterns based on rankings, particularly when substantiated by several studies, are probably sound, even where there is uncertainty about the precision of rates and ratios, arising from the difficulty of measuring accurately numbers of cases and population at risk. Clearly, these disease data need to be interpreted alongside information on the lifestyle and behaviour of ethnic minority groups, and their access to services. Nonetheless, they are the starting point for in-depth analysis.

The sense of priority gained from this analysis differs from earlier publications. First, cancer is unequivocally a key cause of death and morbidity in the ethnic minority groups considered here. The comparative lack of attention given to cancer in the past, and the perception even amongst some informed observers that cancer is not a key issue for ethnic minority groups, is not justifiable. Certainly, the statement by Karmi and McKeigue (1993), two of the leading UK scholars in this field, that 'Although cancer is one of the key areas . . . in the Health of Nation's white paper, it is not especially relevant to ethnic groups in the UK', is untrue. Furthermore, their bibliography of research on ethnic health identified only a few papers on cancer. Hopkins and Bahl (1993) made no reference to cancer research or services in their book on access to health care and only one item on cancer was listed in a 1990 Health Education Authority publication listing health education materials. In his comprehensive book, Smaje (1995) discusses the scientific literature on cancer and ethnic minority groups in Britain in under two pages (of 151, and so less than diabetes) noting that although relatively little attention has been given to cancer research, cancer is a major killing disease in ethnic minority groups and its incidence is likely to increase.

Second, in this analysis cancers such as those of the lung, breast, cervix, stomach and leukaemia emerged as among the highest priorities. Previously, in the context of ethnicity and health, these cancers remained in the shadows, while other such as those of the liver and the oro-pharynx gained the limelight. The reason for the marked shift in perspective was simply that previous analyses had been comparing the cancer patterns in ethnic minority groups with the majority population. In the context of setting priorities such an approach is inappropriate, yet as it is so deeply rooted, the alternative and more appropriate methods of focusing on actual numbers of cases (or disease rates) is rarely used. This fundamental point is almost always overlooked. The variations between populations are, however, useful as an adjunct to disease frequency data in refining the picture of health and health care needs, and for generating hypotheses. Given this, principles for priority-setting for ethnic minorities in the field of cancer can be generated (Table 7.5) and applied as discussed below.

Table 7.5 Principles of priority-setting in the context of cancer in ethnic minority groups

Policy	Base on actual frequency
	Refine on relative frequency
	Incorporate ethnic dimension to national policy
Prevention	Primary focus on common cancers with avoidable risk factors
	Base on population attributable risk
Care	Common cancers are important
	Clinical awareness of rare cancers which are relatively common
	Education and awareness of unusual clinical history
Access, quality and outcomes research	Focus on cancer as a whole
	Relative vs actual frequency is unimportant
Aetiological research	Focus where cause is obscure and ethnic variation (relative measure show excess or deficit) provides a hypothesis or model

Reproduced from Bhopal R, Rankin J. Cancer in minority ethnic populations: priorities from epidemiological data. *British Journal of Cancer*, 1996; 74: S22–32. Table 12—lightly edited, page S31.

Policy-makers need to note that cancer is important in ethnic minority populations, and need to address the issue. UK national policy documents and national initiatives on cancer, unlike CHD, have not properly addressed the needs of ethnic minority populations. One potential explanation for this might be that the needs of ethnic minorities are perceived to be so different that priorities, principles, and initiatives for the general population are deemed by planners to be unsuitable for ethnic minority groups. This perception is, however, wrong. The analysis above demonstrated that common cancers in ethnic minority populations should be tackled as part of national initiatives.

Priorities for prevention need to be founded on the concept of population attributable risk, whereby both the prevalence of risk factors and the risk of cancer are considered, to derive an estimate of the potential amount of cancer preventable in the community by an effective strategy. Based on this concept, cancers for which the aetiology is known, those which are common, and those which are much commoner in those with known and reversible risk factors should get higher priority. Priorities for prevention are likely to lie within the top-ranking cancers. On this basis, for example, for South Asian men the priorities would be cancer of the lung, oesophagus, liver and buccal cavity. For South Asian women, cancer of the breast, lung, cervix, liver and oro-pharynx stand out. For men of Caribbean origin cancer of the lung, liver and colon are prominent, and for women those of the breast, cervix, colon, lung and liver. For African-origin men cancer of the lung, liver, colon, oesophagus, and oro-pharynx (East Africans) are priorities. For African-origin women the priorities include cancer of the breast, colon, and oropharynx (East Africans).

In the clinical setting the pattern of disease in the population is less important for each case will be diagnosed and treated individually. Doctors are more likely to see cancers which are in the top ranks on the basis of frequency, not relative frequency. However, doctors' perceptions about the patterns of disease are likely to be based on the scientific literature and will influence the process of diagnosis. For example, if there were a misperception that cancer of the lung is rare in South Asians and this diagnosis was not considered in investigating a lung mass (in favour of, say, tuberculosis) delay in diagnosis could occur. Alternatively, investigation and accurate diagnosis of a liver mass might be hastened by a high level of awareness of the relative frequency of liver cancer in some ethnic minority groups, most notably of Caribbean and African origin. A knowledge of cancer patterns by ethnic group is potentially of value in the clinical setting but the benefits can be overstated, and the dangers of false generalization overlooked. As the patterns of disease and risk factors are so complex, it would be a difficult task to educate, adequately, all doctors about all the ethnic groups. While an epidemiologist or public health practitioner can look the data up, the clinician needs to have an intuitive and internalized knowledge that can be used in the consultation. Clinicians do, however, need to be aware of unusual presentations of cancers in ethnic minority populations.

There is a paucity of research on access to, quality and effectiveness of and outcomes of health care. The priority here is a focus on cancer as a whole. The rare cancers deserve as much attention as the common ones for problems are more likely to arise with these. We already know that ethnic minority groups are less likely to use palliative care services for cancer.

The demonstration of variation in disease experience in population subgroups provides enormous opportunity for the development of hypotheses about the causes of cancer. The fact that certain cancers are common in ethnic minority populations may permit epidemiological studies otherwise impossible, because the assembling of a case-series of rare cancers may be practical e.g. oro-pharyngeal cancer studies may be possible in East London, where oral tobacco and betel leaf with areca nut is chewed commonly. Finally, hypotheses about disease causation (developed outside the context of ethnicity and health research) might be explored using the ethnicity/health model. For sparking off high-quality research we need to have unanswered questions, disease variation, testable hypotheses, and the resource and will to pursue the hypothesis until valuable observations have been made or the hypothesis is discarded. Many authors have proclaimed the potential value of ethnic variations in cancer, yet research rarely proceeds beyond the description of variation, which is insufficient to provide valuable aetiological insight. In this analysis, as in others, interesting variations deserving priority attention have been demonstrated including:

- the low SMR/standardized registration ratio for many cancers including those of the stomach and colon in South Asians;
- the high SMRs for liver and oro-pharyngeal cancers in several ethnic groups;
- the high SMRs for prostatic cancer in West African and Caribbean populations but the low SMRs for South Asian and East African populations;
- and, the surprisingly high SMR for lung cancer in South Asian women who report insignificant levels of smoking.

The priorities in relation to research are different from those relating to policy, prevention and practice. For instance, cancers which are comparatively rare in ethnic minorities may be of special research importance. I will be discussing this topic again in Chapter 9.

Priorities for policy, prevention, clinical care and research need to be analysed and stated separately. Research priorities will continue to be largely guided by relative frequency but priorities in policy, prevention and clinical care need to pay more attention to the actual, not relative, frequency of cancers, as emphasized by Amaro's quotation below.

> Collecting epidemiologic data by ethnicity and race is a highly useful undertaking; but 'benchmark' comparisons relative to majority Americans should not take priority over defining the determinants of health status within a minority group.
>
> Amaro (1995: 592)

Figure 7.1 illustrates how data may influence the provision of services. The goal is to modify, develop or even remove services. This goal is done within a context of setting priorities, whether this is explicit or implicit. The priorities themselves are based on both the values of those in decision-making positions and are influenced by two sets of complementary data: on needs and what are often described as demands. In Chapter 5, demands are considered under the headings of felt need and expressed need (Section 5.1.1). Normative and comparative needs, in particular, were discussed there. Demands are the wants in relation to services of a range of people including doctors and other health care professionals, and of course the public who use the services.

These two sets of information are brought together to set priorities which are used for modifying, or developing anew, health services. In relation to cancer we see a tension between a muffled voice for demand (see the quotation from Karmi and McKeigue on p. 197) and a clear need from quantitative data analysis. The tensions need debating in the priority-setting process. In Chapter 8 we will consider how such data and debates can be turned into strategies and actions.

One of the keys to action in modern health services is evidence of effectiveness, which is becoming an essential ingredient for fundable priorities. Yet obtaining such evidence is like searching for gold in a river bed and this applies particularly to ethnic minority populations. In Chapter 9, we will discuss what actions are needed to improve on this. In the next section we briefly consider how the case for prioritization is to be made in these difficult circumstances, with particular regard to inequalities.

7.6 Impact of priority decisions on inequalities

The choice of priorities matters for expenditure decisions on ethnic inequalities in health as illustrated here in a simplified theoretical example: Exercise 7.5.

Exercise 7.5 Effect of priority-setting on ethnic inequalities

◆ Imagine you had £100,000 to spend on one of five priorities set for health improvement in your ethnic minority population i.e. disease A, B, C, D, or E. Imagine your intervention will reduce the disease burden by 10 per cent.

◆ Using the data in Table 7.6, consider the effect on:

(a) disease burden

(b) inequalities in disease generally i.e. all-cause death rate

◆ What do we need to do to reduce inequalities?

◆ What principles are illustrated here?

Table 7.6 shows hypothetical mortality rates for all causes of deaths and for five conditions, which do not account for all the deaths. The minority population here has an overall 20 per cent excess of death. The death rates for the five conditions show an increasing inequality. The remaining causes of death are not shown here. We assume that these 5 causes have been selected as priorities for action already and a budget of £100,000 is available to tackle one of them, say, in our population of 250,000 people. Imagine that interventions are available that will reduce mortality by 10 per cent. Again imagine these interventions are specific to one condition. Which condition will you choose? Does it matter? Furthermore, does it matter whether the goal is a reduction in inequalities or a reduction in disease burden irrespective of effect on inequalities?

Table 7.7 shows the consequences of our decisions. In this table, for simplicity, we make the unlikely assumption that there is no decline in death rates in population X—the ethnic majority. It is no surprise that an intervention focused on the commonest disorders has the biggest impact on disease burden. In addition, perhaps slightly surprisingly, it also has the biggest impact on health inequalities overall—even though Cause A itself shows the least relative excess in the minority population.

It is likely that interventions are already underway to control diseases in the majority population and that the £100,000 budget is designed to help equalize services. Table 7.8 shows that a 10 per cent reduction in both populations in Cause A has no effect on

Table 7.6 Mortality data for two theoretical populations

	Majority population (X)	Minority population (Y)	Ratio of minority to majority i.e. inequality
All-cause death rate/100,000/year	1000	1200	1.20
Death rate from:			
Cause A	300	330	1.1
Cause B	200	240	1.2
Cause C	100	130	1.3
Cause D	50	70	1.4
Cause E	20	30	1.5

Table 7.7 Effect on inequalities in overall death rate of a 10% decline in death rates in the minority population

	Majority population (X)	Minority population (Y)	Ratio of minority to majority i.e. inequality
All cause-death rate/100,000/year			
At baseline	1000	1200	1.20
After an intervention on population Y that reduces the disease by 10% (see table 7.6 for actual rates) for causes A–E			
Cause A	—	1200–33* = 1167	1.167
Cause B	—	1200–24 = 1176	1.176
Cause C	—	1200–13 = 1187	1.187
Cause D	—	1200– 7 = 1193	1.193
Cause E	—	1200– 3 = 1197	1.197

* The figure is 10% of 330, the rate shown in table 7.6.

Table 7.8 Effect of (i) a 10 per cent decline in disease in both majority and minority populations on overall inequalities, and (ii) a 20 per cent decline in the disease in the minority population

	Majority population (X)	Minority population (Y)	Ratio of minority to majority (Y:X)
All-cause death rate			
Baseline	1000	1200	1.2
Overall mortality after intervention on populations			
X and Y for Cause A	1000–30 = 970	1200–33 = 1167	1.203
After intervention on Condition A for majority population and E for minority population	1000–30 = 970	1200–3 = 1197	1.234
After intensive intervention on minority populations (20% effect) and standard intervention on majority population (10% effect) Cause A	1000–30 = 970	1200–66 = 1134	1.169

inequalities. In fact they rise slightly. Imagine that a decision is taken to focus the expenditure on Condition E in the minority population (the one showing the highest ratio in table 7.6) and that, as a result, Cause A remains unchanged in them. Taking into account only the control of condition A in the majority population, with a 10% decline, the overall inequality rises substantially.

The message seems to be clear—the reduction of inequalities requires a comparatively more intensive intervention in the disadvantaged population as shown at the end of Table 7.8, where an intervention that leads to a 20 per cent decline in cause of death A is applied to the minority population.

The principles arising from this simple, theoretical exercise are that:

1. Making choices on priorities for action to reduce diseases impacts both on disease burden (obvious) and on inequalities (not so obvious)

2. An equal reduction of disease in two populations that start from an unequal position does not reduce inequalities (which actually widen in relative terms)

3. Choosing to focus on conditions that have the greatest relative excess in minority populations can widen inequalities overall

4. The reduction of inequalities requires that the disease burden declines faster in the disadvantaged group than in the advantaged one.

These principles require that we have effective interventions.

7.7 Evidence base for interventions in the field of minority ethnic health

The question of what works is always problematic in the case of complex initiatives. For many interventions, the evidence is inconclusive (and sometimes non-existent) in any population. The controlled trial, and its most strict variant, the placebo-controlled, randomized, double blind trial, undeniably provides the most solid evidence for effectiveness of initiatives. These trials are difficult and expensive to conduct, particularly for complex interventions. The question is whether we need evidence from such studies to recommend that an initiative is a high priority in minority ethnic groups. Smoking cessation services are, for example, a major priority nationally. Are they a priority for ethnic minority groups? On the basis of data on prevalence this is so for many minorities e.g. Bangladeshi men, Pakistani men and Afro-Caribbean men and women. But will the interventions work? We should look for evidence. If so, what do we do when there are no specific relevant studies? Indeed, in the UK setting there are no data and internationally they are sparse.

Clearly, it would be excellent to have such trials on minority ethnic groups and a research programme needs to be encouraged. As a minimum, studies on general populations ought not to exclude people from minority ethnic groups (as some do, often by excluding those who do not speak English). Building up a valid database of this kind for a range of important issues will be a multi-billion-pound endeavour, which needs to take place internationally, and will take 10–20 years. In the meantime, we cannot permit paralysis in relation to minority ethnic health. The principles that could be adopted here are as follows:

1. In planning an initiative for ethnic minority groups, start with a systematic review of the evidence in all ethnic groups.

2. If an initiative works in one or more populations, it may work in the minority group of interest. If it does not work elsewhere it is less likely to work in minority populations. The essential principle here is this: human populations are more alike than different.

3. If the intervention is based on physiology and biology e.g. folic acid supplementation for pregnant women to prevent congenital abnormalities, one can have a high degree of confidence that it will work across ethnic groups. This is, nonetheless, a matter for

evaluation. As a minimum there should be monitoring both of the uptake of the intervention, which may well differ by ethnic group, and the outcome, which is less likely to differ.

4. If the intervention is complex, and likely to be affected by social, economic, cultural or environmental factors, then we need to take special care. For example, brief advice from the general practitioner helps smokers quit. Will this work in Bangladeshi or Chinese men and women? It would be wrong to assume it will. This intervention may be better implemented in the context of a formal trial so it can be evaluated rigorously. If this is not possible, go ahead with the intervention, but in a questioning manner and with a pragmatic evaluation.

5. In most instances, at least for the foreseeable future, health services will need to modify interventions proven to work in one ethnic group (very often White populations) to make them cross-culturally effective. This field of study is in its infancy, but needs to be promoted.

7.8 **Conclusions**

We can conclude, on the principle that similarities between human populations tend to outweigh differences, that the general priorities of health care systems are of great importance to minority ethnic groups. Public health and health care initiatives must, therefore, cater for the ethnic majority and minority populations simultaneously, with work of equal potential effectiveness and sensitivity. To do otherwise promotes inequality and inequity. It is surely unethical and institutionally racist, and in some countries illegal, as discussed in Chapters 6 and 8.

Pending the development of a solid evidence base for effectiveness of initiatives to improve minority ethnic health (a long-term goal), interventions effective in other populations need to be carefully adapted, implemented and evaluated. In Chapter 9 there will be further discussion of how we achieve more and better research that provides data by ethnic group. Even when the effectiveness of interventions by ethnic group is known, however, it is likely that priorities will not change greatly.

Getting the priorities implemented in practice is difficult but it requires a continuation of past approaches (education, exhortation, research, taking opportunities to influence management and influencing policy documents). Increasingly, we need to promote the vigorous mobilization of an increasingly informed community voice. Stories from the community are very powerful in bringing about change and sometimes more so than statistics (which have been described as tragedies without the tears). Nonetheless, better information systems are needed, particularly to foster audit of quality of care.

Evidence showing that the quality of care for ethnic minority populations is inferior is particularly effective in bringing about change, as it goes against policies and laws promoting equality. Ethnic coding of health care records (see Chapters 3 and 8) probably holds the key for both audit and new programmes of research.

All health care and public health policies and plans should make explicit what the priorities are and how the needs of minority ethnic groups are to be met. These should not be relegated to secondary documentation. The health care system must ensure its current priorities and policies are evaluated in relation to minority ethnic groups. Services need to make appropriate modifications to ensure they meet the needs of minority ethnic groups. The health care system must not make the mistake of imagining, assuming, awaiting or expecting a different set of priorities. The next chapter discusses how this is to be achieved.

Summary

Whether in research, policy or health care, the choices for actions to improve the health of ethnic minority groups are virtually limitless, especially in complex, multi-ethnic societies. Priority-setting is a process for making rational choices from multiple alternatives. Social values are important to priority-setting and in the context of ethnicity and health the most important of these are equality and equity (discussed in detail in Chapter 10). The public health sciences, particularly epidemiology, can underpin priority-setting, which follows the process of health needs assessment. Quantitative and qualitative data on health status and service utilization are often available (though they may be crude) but need to be utilized carefully. In contrast, information on cost and effectiveness of interventions as applied to specific ethnic groups are rarely available posing a formidable challenge to both priority-setting and future research.

Priority-setting benefits from principles. One principle is that the priorities are those actions that maximally benefit the health of a specific ethnic minority group. This is an approach advocated in health economics. Another is to prioritize actions that raise the health and health care of the ethnic minority group to the level of the population as a whole or, preferably, to the level of the ethnic group with the best health. In practice the target standard is usually the health status of the White or majority population. Integrating the three approaches, each of which has strengths and weaknesses, will meet the twin goals of maximizing health and tackling health inequalities. Reductions of inequalities can only be achieved if health improvement occurs faster in the disadvantaged population. Health improvement requires demonstrably effective interventions that are cost-effective. Evidence of that kind, by ethnic group, is sparse. Pending an international programme of research to rectify this all health policies should state the priorities by ethnic group and mandate strategies and actions to achieve them.

Chapter 8

Strategic approaches to health and health care services for ethnic minority groups

More than one-third of the excess total death rate of blacks relative to whites could be explained by the excess of potentially preventable deaths. Our findings suggest that inequalities in health services reinforce broader social inequalities and are in part responsible for disparities in health status. Improvements in the health and longevity of blacks and other oppressed groups might be achieved by improved access to existing medical, public health, and other preventive measures.

Woolhandler *et al.* (1985: 1)

Despite significant achievements, the black and minority ethnic groups work of the HEA has been, to a large degree, marginalized. This is due to three main factors:

* The reluctance of the Department of Health to fund HEA's black and minority ethnic groups work has resulted in regular cuts to the programme budget culminating in a zero budget for the current financial year.
* The health of black and minority ethnic groups has not been a significant feature of Department of Health contracts across the HEA.
* The health needs of the populations has been seen as the sole responsibility of the black and minority ethnic groups programme rather than as an integral part of all HEA work

The separation and marginalisation of black and minority ethnic groups needs is a feature common to many organisations. This point is made forcibly in the Acheson report.

Unpublished HEA Paper R10/99 pp. 2–3. (Rehman *et al.*)

Contents

* Chapter objectives
* The nature of policy, strategy, tactics and service delivery

- Exemplars of strategic documents on ethnic health—England, Scotland and the USA
- Approaches, principles and effectiveness of the exemplar strategies
- An idealized strategy
- Practical limitations to ideal strategy, and the imperative to action
- Making progress in the face of constraints
- Conclusions
- Summary of chapter

Objectives

On completion of this chapter you should be able to:

- In outline, appreciate the nature of strategy in relation to policy and tactics
- Using examples of key strategy documents on ethnicity and health internationally, develop an understanding of the approaches and principles applied
- In principle, be able to articulate the content of an ideal strategic document, but to accept compromises in the light of constraints of data, expertise, resources and political circumstances

8.1 Introduction to policy, strategy and models of service delivery

Ethnic diversity is increasing in many countries primarily as a result of migration linked to globalization of trade and the movement of refugees. This offers formidable challenges in the development of policies and strategies promoting the reduction of inequalities in health and health care. Challenges in health and health care include:

- Understanding and responding to varying health behaviours, beliefs and attitudes
- Responding to differences in the pattern of diseases, and in particular reducing inequalities where this is possible
- Maintaining high quality communications in the face of language and cultural barriers
- Delivering a service that is sensitive to cultural differences, e.g. in relation to modesty among women especially, and the preference for same-sex health carers
- Overcoming both personal biases, stereotyped views, individuals' racism, and institutional inertia and racism
- Ensuring equal opportunities in employment at all stages from recruitment to retirement

These challenges have, of course, been faced by health policy, medical research and health care institutions over many decades, but recent landmark reports and legislation e.g. the UK's Race Relations Amendment Act 2000 strengthening the 1976 Race Relations Act, are mandating a rapid and sustained response. These challenges require effective policy and strategy that can underpin specific plans and local actions.

Before reading on, try Exercise 8 .1.

Exercise 8.1 The nature of policy, strategy and planning

♦ In the health context what is the difference between policy-making, strategy and health planning?
♦ Why are these necessary?
♦ In the ethnicity and health field how are policies to be reconciled with tactical opportunities?

A policy is a statement, usually issued by a governing body, on its intentions over a relatively long timescale. A policy sets high level directions and goals. A policy also sets the tone that influences a broader audience and this may be the entire nation, continent or the world. The importance of tone will be considered later in the section on the USA with an example of the controversial effects of editing.

Policies are usually written but it is common to announce them in political speeches or political manifestos (or their equivalent). Such a verbal announcement may be enough with no explicit document. It is generally understood that policy will be backed by political, legislative, managerial and financial support as appropriate. In practice many policies are never implemented and are either changed, forgotten or postponed. It is not uncommon for new leaders to sweep aside previous policies and start afresh, often merely reinventing what was there before. Policies need to be institutionalized and operationalized rapidly if they are not to be forgotten. (Admittedly, such a fate is appropriate for poor policies.)

A strategy is a general plan to make a course of action promised in a policy actually happen. Strategies are invariably written. As anyone organizing a party knows, success requires intentions (policy), foresight (vision), general ideas on the type of party and the activities (strategy), detailed planning on menus, music and other such matters and meticulous execution including sending out invitations and then being a good host (delivery). On the grand scale of health care delivery to ethnic minority and whole populations alike, policies and strategies need accompanying detailed plans that outline actions, responsibilities, timetables and costs. In practice, actions to improve the health and health care of ethnic minority populations are not always taken according to policies and strategies but on a tactical or opportunistic basis. There may be, for instance, some surplus funding that needs to be used for a good purpose before the end of the financial year. Or, alternatively, there may be an urgent perceived need to avert attention from negative publicity or criticism from some important person or media organization. Usually, there are a number of outstanding and well-recognized needs of ethnic minority populations that can be attended to in such circumstances. Long-term policies and strategies will make it easier to identify the highest priority needs when such opportunities arrive.

Health services for ethnic minority groups are usually delivered within the scope of policies and strategies for the population as a whole, which in practice this means the majority population. Traditionally, such policies and strategies have made no mention of any special needs of ethnic minority groups but this is changing. There are a number of approaches to meeting the needs of ethnic minority groups, and you should consider the strengths and weaknesses of them.

Before reading on, try Exercise 8.2.

Exercise 8.2 Strengths and weaknesses of various models of service delivery

What are the strengths and weaknesses of the following policy options for health services for ethnic minority groups?

1. One service for the whole population—all individuals and groups expected to adapt to use it
2. One service supplemented by special projects to meet special needs
3. One service adapted to meet needs of all population subgroups
4. One service purpose-designed to meet diverse needs
5. Separate services for separate ethnic groups

Ideally policies, strategies and plans for the whole population would address the needs of ethnic minority, and majority, groups in an integrated way. This concept is known as mainstreaming. In Exercise 8.2 this would mean model 4, but since designing services anew is not usually possible, model 3 is the nearest alternative. In practice this level of adaptation of services to meet diverse needs has rarely happened for reasons including one or more of lack of time, lack of understanding of need, the complexity of the task, lack of expertise or lack of publication space within the key policy and strategy documents. Mostly, individuals from ethnic minority populations are expected to adapt themselves to benefit from the available services i.e. model 1. Professionals delivering the service may make appropriate adjustments on an ad-hoc basic, hopefully with the backing of health service managers. Medical professionals, generally, have made changes and adaptations as illustrated in the following quotations. The quotation of Clyne, however, displays a somewhat simplistic view of immigration that does not acknowledge how dynamic a process it is.

> On the whole, Indian patients, at least in my practice, are 'good' patients. Their children after a few years of stay and schooling in England seem to be no different in their physical and mental make-up, complaints, and illnesses, from the native population. Within a generation or so, this article will thus probably have completely lost its relevance.
>
> Clyne (1964: 199)

> The perinatal mortality rate for our immigrant Bengali patients, who constitute about half of our obstetric population, has been lower than that in our indigenous population in recent years. These figures are the result of the changes that have occurred in the maternity service in recent years, which may well provide a model for other services with large immigrant populations. They include

the appointment of more midwives with greater flexibility for deployment into the community and Bengali speaking maternity aides.

Grudzinskas (1987: 503)

Increasingly, we see two further policy responses—setting up specialist services for ethnic minority groups, i.e. model 2; and the development of separate strategies to help re-shape existing services, i.e. to move to model 3.

Whatever the service model there is a great danger that initiatives to prevent, control and treat diseases and promote health do not provide their full benefits to minority ethnic groups. First, as discussed in Chapter 7, those responsible may wrongly assume that the service under their control is not a priority in one or more minority ethnic groups. An example of this is a perception that in South Asian populations cancers, and some of the risk factors including smoking, are not a high priority. This perception and its refutation on the basis of a systematic analysis of cancer data in Britain's major minority ethnic groups are discussed in Chapter 7. The second danger is that any steps that are taken are inadequate, e.g. a media campaign video may be dubbed with the minority group's languages, when it might be more effective to include in the original video some actors from minority groups, to convey cross-cultural relevance. The third danger is that the planners are aware of the issues but decide that the strategy for the minority groups should be separate from the main one, and in practice this is the common, perhaps even the usual, response. Such a decision should be carefully justified and implemented. There is a danger that if it is not it could be construed as institutional racism, and counter to the duty to promote racial equality under legislation such as the UK's Race Relations Amendment Act 2000. Such a decision might be undesirable on pragmatic grounds too. Pragmatically, the bulk of the required knowledge, expertise, energy, momentum and finances will lie with the architects and managers of the main strategy. The strategy for minority ethnic groups may, therefore, be of a lesser impact, so accentuating existing inequalities. Mostly, it is better for minority groups to be included within the main initiative.

Model 5 is largely deplored in modern, democratic, multi-ethnic societies as both unworkable and undesirable, if not illegal. Of course, this model has been the preferred one of openly racist states such as South Africa under the policy of apartheid. In theory, if separate services could be achieved to the same standard model 5 might be acceptable from a health care perspective, but it goes counter to be idea of integration. We will return to these models as we examine some policies and strategies.

This chapter focuses on the UK and particularly on Scotland, and within that the Lothian Health Board. The reason is that I am familiar with these policies and that the UK is highly advanced in policy-making in the ethnicity and health field. It is important that I record a conflict of interest that might have led to an over-optimistic assessment of the situation in the UK. I have served on a number of committees working to improve the health and health care of ethnic minority populations, including the NHS (England) Ethnic Health Unit, and chairmanship and/or membership of committees in the Lothian

Health Board, the Scottish Executive and the National Resource Centre For Ethnic Minority Health (Scotland). These experiences, however, have given me access to the decision-making processes. The situation is compared and contrasted to other places, mainly the USA, to draw more general lessons.

8.2 **Examples of policy and strategy**

Before reading on try Exercises 8.3 and 8.4.

Exercise 8.3 The importance of political and legal background

+ Why is the political, legal and policy environment particularly important to the task of meeting the health needs of ethnic minority populations?
+ Can you think of places where health care for ethnic minority groups has been:
  (a) Obstructed by political and legal actions
  (b) Promoted by political and legal actions?

Exercise 8.4 Idealized policy

+ What might be the principles of an ideal policy and strategy?
+ Given political and resources constraints what compromises might be needed to create an achievable policy/strategy?
+ How will we know our policy/strategy is being effective?

8.2.1 **General—the UK and the USA**

The UK policy response to ethnicity and health over the last 50 years, as in many other countries, has been intermittent and fragmented, with a mixture of stand-alone projects and modifications to mainline services. This is not surprising as the issue is complex and subject to many external influences, particularly political and financial ones. Progress has been made in the UK on key practical requirements of ethnic minority populations such as equality in employment, interpretation services and dietary needs in hospital.

The Race Relations Amendment Act 2000, coupled with explicit or implicit policies from government health departments, is currently driving more widespread changes based on a positive duty to promote racial equality. The Scottish Executive Health Department's Fair for All policy is detailed and being implemented, as evaluations have shown (2002). These national initiatives are being translated, often with great difficulty, into local action plans and ultimately service changes. Ethnic monitoring in employment and service is an example of a policy that was difficult to achieve until the law came into place, despite excellent intentions and substantial efforts. The combination of a national health care system, law and policy has been instrumental in achieving change in the UK setting.

There has been considerable frustration in the UK among those working to improve the health care of ethnic minority populations. To a large extent this has arisen because of the stop-start nature of policy. One acute observer of the UK scene is quoted below. (In 2005 he wrote again in somewhat pessimistic terms.)

> The assumption has been that the passage of time and the experience of living together would serve to reduce racial prejudice and discrimination in the United Kingdom. This has not happened. Racial inequality has become institutionalised in many organisations which are apparently 'multi-racial'. The NHS is a case in point. The situation in the Service has been made worse through neglect by health authorities, the DHSS and successive politicians. Racial equality in the NHS will not be easy to achieve, nor will it be easy to define in all circumstances. The strategy proposed in this chapter should assist in working toward this goal.
>
> McNaught (1985: 71)

I intend to show that the infrastructure is in place in the UK, and particularly Scotland, to surmount the formidable challenges.

Unlike the UK, the USA has had a long-standing programme for affirmative action based on human rights principles that aims to redress historical wrongs. A racial and ethnic classification, of the Office of Management and Budget, was explicitly designed to help achieve this goal (see Chapter 2). Despite the country having the most expensive health care system in the world, more than 40 million people in the USA have no health insurance and many people distrust health services because of their commercially driven ethos. The pluralistic nature of the health care system of the USA, based on private health care principles even though it is highly reliant on Government funding, has made a cohesive national strategy problematic to enact. There are powerful policies in place but their effectiveness seems to be limited. By law and explicit policy based on legislation minority groups cannot be excluded from research using federal government money without good scientific reason, and this has spurred a substantial research programme. In the quantity of research on ethnic minority populations the USA leads the world, and this is another example of policy and law combining forces to lever change. These points are developed later in this chapter.

8.2.2 Scotland—a late starter, making rapid progress in the context of social justice

8.2.2.1 Health inequalities are a priority for the health service in Scotland

The 1999 White Paper 'Towards a Healthier Scotland' of the Scottish Executive identified the reduction of inequalities as a key priority and suggested that research effort 'must focus on the causes of health inequalities and practical means to tackle them'. There has been recognition for some time of ethnic inequalities in health in Scotland, but a lack of information. There is no information that allows a description of the present level of ethnic inequalities in health in Scotland or allows progress to be monitored. The Race Equality Advisory Forum report, 'Making it Real; A Race Equality Strategy for Scotland' highlights the importance of better information in getting ethnic minority health into the mainstream of service provision, and as the basis for prompt, effective action.

Ethnic coding and other means of getting information were discussed in Chapters 3 and 5. In Scotland, information on ethnic status is not consistently recorded in primary care service settings although a small financial incentive of about £100 in total is now offered to practices that record their patients' ethnicity on first registration. Scottish diabetes and CHD registers do not comprehensively and accurately record ethnic status but there are plans for them to do so. Routine hospital discharge data is collated centrally in Scotland. There has been provision for the recording of ethnic status in NHS hospital discharge data, but this has usually been omitted. A new strategy for collecting these data is being implemented with earmarked funding to coordinate the process. Information collated by the General Register's Office for Scotland from death certificates includes country of birth but not ethnic status. For older people, country of birth has been used as a proxy for ethnic status, but it is becoming less useful as the number of people from ethnic minority groups born in the UK increases.

The prospective development of ethnically coded information systems is a high priority for Scotland. Scotland's health information system provides excellent opportunities including record linkage schemes that provide information about the outcomes of care. One project in a collaboration between Edinburgh University, the General Register Office for Scotland, and Information Services Division (ISD) has linked census-derived ethnic codes to health databases (see Chapter 3). The major spur to such action has come from two directions—the law and national policy, as discussed below.

8.2.2.2 The Race Relations Amendment Act and race equality schemes

The 1976 Race Relations Act with the 2000 Amendment intends to remove all racial discrimination, direct or indirect in the UK. Racial grounds are colour, race, nationality, ethnicity or national origin. Indirect and direct discrimination were discussed in Chapter 6. The Amendment Act came into effect in April 2002 and is a powerful and very ambitious piece of legislation that mandates actions that are open to public scrutiny (Home Office, 2001). According to the Amendment Act all public organizations, including the NHS, have a statutory general duty to work to eliminate unlawful racial discrimination, and to promote equal opportunities and good race relations. The size of the ethnic minority populations they serve is not relevant.

The CRE (Commission for Racial Equality) is the body responsible for overseeing the implementation of all legislation and it published explicit guidance in June 2002 on the nature of the required output, to be reported in a public document known as the race equality scheme. The scheme is to show that a health organization is meeting the duty. There was, of course, a requirement for a Race Equality Scheme for the Scottish Executive, which implements the will of the Scottish parliament. So, the political leaders and political institutions are subject to this legislation and are publicly accountable.

The anticipated outcomes for the organization of meeting the duty include the following:

- Community satisfaction and equal opportunities
- Staff satisfaction and equal opportunities
- Confidence and respect is increased
- Leadership is evident
- Services and policies are better
- Evidence of meeting the duty is clear
- Published annual reports
- Information about its services in various languages
- A race equality scheme as a three year plan, publicly available, in printed and electronic form
- Race equality objectives for partnership work, and for work carried out under contract
- All staff receive training on the Race Relations Act, and on how to prevent discrimination
- Monitoring of employees by ethnic group.

The Scottish Parliament approved the legislation and noted in its guidance the dangers of adverse consequences e.g. 'introduction of ethnic monitoring of staff may assist a Board to identify and eliminate unlawful discrimination and promote equality of opportunity, but if staff does not understand its purpose it might actually inhibit good race relations. . . . etc'. Responsibility for success lies with the Chief Executives of organizations.

This danger is well understood as the following quotation eloquently illustrates.

> In the quest for building an organisational infrastructure—one that can reflect the values, and meet the needs, of distinct ethnic communities—there is a reality of competition for resources— both economic and political. Where some ethnic communities are minorities the pursuit of these resources can result in inter-ethnic competition and hostility. Where the legitimate pursuit of ethnic self-interest is understood through the language of 'race', it is very likely to be defined as a threat to the interests of the majority. Mutual respect for ethnic diversity is undermined by the superiority claims built into 'race thinking'.
>
> The mobilisation of minority ethnic communities can, in such circumstances, be seen as both threatening and illegitimate to the dominant majority population. The idea of the 'victimisation of the majority' encapsulates exactly this sentiment. It is the unreasoned cry of a resentful majority that their interests are being neglected in the pursuit of minority ethnic self-expression.
>
> Communication and Health Care Practice: Politics of Diversity, Section 2 p14
> (See Websites Royal College of Nursing Online Course link—p 348)

To help organizations to achieve the challenge Scottish Executive funded a National Resource Centre for Ethnic Minority Health (NRCEMH-see below). Progress with Race Equality Schemes and the Fair for All plans (see below) was both supported and monitored by this Centre. The CRE and NRCEMH recognized that integrating the requirements of the Race Relations Amendment Act and Fair for All policy objectives was essential and a joint monitoring and reporting structure was created.

The key point is that race equality in Scotland is not an isolated issue. It cannot be swept away without dismantling the entire edifice of equality because it is integral to it. Other strategies for equality in NHS Scotland include:

♦ The Sex Discrimination Act (1975)
♦ The Disability Discrimination Act (1995)
♦ The Human Rights Act (1998)
♦ The Scottish Executive's Equality Strategy (2000)
♦ The Patient Focus/Involving People Strategy (2001)
♦ Spiritual Care policy in Health Department letter (2002)
♦ The NHS Reform Bill (2004)

Within this challenging context the Fair for All policy, which provided guidance, could only be welcomed.

8.2.2.3 Health Department letter (HDL) and stock-take: Fair for All

In 1998, the Scottish Minister for Health, Mr Sam Galbraith, gave a speech challenging the National Health Service in Scotland to meet the health and health care needs of ethnic minority groups in Scotland and outlined a new vision. Unfortunately, little action was evident as a result. This was, however, one of the events that triggered change, not least because questions were raised about the promises made in the speech. The Scottish Executive supported the effort to reduce inequalities in health by developing several policies with a strong emphasis on social justice. A Scottish Executive policy document called Our National Health (1999) laid down NHS Scotland's commitment to ensure that 'NHS staff are professionally and culturally equipped to meet the distinctive needs of people and family groups from ethnic minority communities'. A culturally competent service was defined as a service which recognizes and meets the diverse needs of people of different cultural backgrounds. With this background of enabling policy yet little strategy the Scottish Executive commissioned an assessment of ethnic health policies of the 15 NHS Boards that are responsible for the delivery of health care to the Scottish population. The assessment was commonly known as the Fair for All Stocktake. The stock-take found positive attitudes, but insufficient actions, expertise and resources across Scotland. It made many recommendations, as summarized in the quotations in Box 8.1.

Box 8.1 Some quotations illustrating the findings of the Fair for All Stocktake

The need for a strategic approach

'A more strategic approach to ethnic minority health issues is a key area for development within NHS Scotland ... This will involve securing commitment at executive and non-executive levels, the integration of these issues into Board or Trust strategies and planning processes (including partnership arrangements), and development of implementation plans.'

Managerial responsibility

'Managers and professionals at Board level need to be active in both setting priorities and targets for ethnic minority health improvements and monitoring performance against objectives and standards.'

Assessment of health needs and translating knowledge into action

'(NHS organizations have) little collective knowledge of the ethnic minority populations for whom they were responsible'and 'Even where work has taken place, there is a need for effective processes to translate the knowledge gained into priorities and actions for delivering services that meet the needs of these communities.'

Recruitment/development and retention of ethnic minority staff

'Recruitment and selection processes may need to be reviewed to ensure ethnic minority applicants are not unintentionally discriminated against. More positively managing race equality and equal opportunities issues should be an element of person specification and be tested as part of the recruitment process'.

Dialogue with ethnic minority communities

'More needs to be done to extend consultation beyond those groups and individuals that have traditionally been consulted, in particular to involve young people and women from ethnic minority groups'.

(*Source*: Website of National Resource Centre for Ethnic Minority Health—link on p 345—adapted)

The recommendations focused on the need for a strategic approach, clear lines of responsibility, assessing needs and planning appropriate actions.

The Scottish Executive Health Department used the stock-take and extensive consultation to formulate a comprehensive policy, issued in the form of a draft Health Department Letter (HDL), subsequently finalized as a missive for action in 2002. Box 8.2

Box 8.2 Fair for all: working together towards culturally competent services (extracts of the letter sent to all key NHS organizations)

Summary

1. This letter accompanies guidance which sets out the responsibilities placed on NHS organizations by legislation, by policy, and by the results of a recent 'Stocktake' exercise undertaken on behalf of the Scottish Executive Health Department.

Background

2. The Race Relations (Amendment) Act 2000 develops the responsibilities previously laid down by the Race Relations Act of 1976 and outlaws race discrimination in relation to functions of public authorities not previously covered by the 1976 Act.

3. The Scottish Executive has made equal opportunities for all a key element of all its work, as demonstrated by its Equality Strategy (http://www.scotland.gov.uk/library3/social/wtem-00.asp).

4. In addition, the Health Department has underlined its commitment to this agenda by encouraging Chief Executives to follow the example of Mr Trevor Jones (Chief Executive of NHS Scotland) in signing the Commission for Racial Equality's Leadership Challenge.

5. The Health Department has also funded an Ethnic Minorities Resource Centre to provide support to the service.

Action

6. Chief Executives are asked to circulate the attached guidance to executive colleagues and to appoint a senior member of the Executive Team to coordinate and be the point of contact on matters relating to the responsibilities contained within the attached guidance.

7. It is anticipated that local progress in adopting the final guidelines will be assessed on the Scottish Executive Health Department's behalf by the Ethnic Minority Resource Centre after 31 March 2003, as part of the Performance Assessment Framework.

Assessment will be carried out on the basis of relative progress made by organizations.
Yours sincerely
TREVOR JONES
Chief Executive
Dr E M ARMSTRONG
Chief Medical Officer
ANNE JARVIE
Chief Nursing Officer
MARK BUTLER
Director of Human Resources

(*Source*: Scottish Executive. Fair for All—see p 349 for Website—adapted)

summarizes the key points made in the covering letter that accompanied the detailed guidance.

The outputs, or elements as they were called, of the HDL were as follows:

1. **Element 1—Energising the Organization.** Statement of organizational intent; executive leadership; action plan
2. **Element 2—Demographic Profile.** Surveying the local population; needs assessment; commitment to research
3. **Element 3—Access and Service Delivery.** Access audit; personal care; food; spiritual care; translation and interpretation; advocacy; gender issues; bereavement
4. **Element 4—Human Resources.** Equal opportunities; improvement policies; bullying and harassment
5. **Element 5—Community Development.** Collaborative mechanisms; developing the community

These ideas are not dissimilar to those expressed earlier in Yasmin Gunaratnam's checklist (1993), Jeff Chandra's Toolkit (1996) and later by the Chief Executive of the NHS in England (Table 8.1).

This commonality seen among these documents is a strength as it shows the principles are both lasting, generalizable and consistent across time and place.

Each organization was required to prepare a detailed, dated and costed action plan outlining how it intended to respond. The Fair for All policy placed emphasis on population profiling, needs assessment and research e.g. upon completing the initial demographic survey and needs assessment, each organization had to actively consider further research on more detailed levels, regarding incidence of disease, service utilization, and other topics as appropriate. Each organization was expected to utilize the results of its assessment to measure how effectively its service provision was meeting the needs of minority ethnic communities.

One of the structural requirements, seen as essential to the specific tasks, was the development of a forum in partnership with the community to guide the health organization. The guidance included that:

- The forum should be jointly chaired by the named member of the executive team and an appropriate member of the local minority ethnic community.
- The forum should be used to consult the local minority ethnic community on service delivery issues.
- This forum must draw sufficient membership from within the NHS organization it is attached to and local external agencies and groups to ensure that it can accurately be described as multidisciplinary.
- This forum should be considered to be an informed voice on local service provision.

Table 8.1 The Chief Executive of the NHS in England's ten-point plan
This action plan has been developed with the help of staff from ethnic minorities within the NHS, building on the advice from leaders in other sectors, and the Commission for Race Equality. It has the full backing of Ministers, the Department of Health's Management Board and the NHS 'Top Team'.

Action	Responsibility
1. Health services and outcomes	
Strategic direction: Through the forthcoming planning guidance, embed race equality into future Local Delivery Plans to enable more personalized care, reduced chronic disease and health inequalities, increased capacity and community regeneration	DH (Department of Health) and all NHS leaders with national and local partners
Align incentives: Build race equality into the new standard and target setting regime, into local performance management systems and into the new inspection model	DH and all NHS leaders with national and local partners
Development: Provide practical support to help NHS organizations make service improvements for people from ethnic minorities	NHS Top Team and NHS Modernisation Agency
Communications: Encourage fresh approaches to communications to engage people from ethnic minorities more effectively in improving outcomes	All NHS organizations and DH
Partnerships: Work with other national and local agencies to promote the health and well being of people from ethnic minority communities	DH and all NHS leaders in concert with national, regional and local partners
2. Developing people	
Mentoring: Senior leaders to show their commitment by offering personal mentorship to a member of staff from an ethnic minority	All senior leaders in DH and NHS
Leadership action: Senior leaders to include a personal 'stretch' target on race equality in their 2004/5 objectives	NHS Chairs and CEs (Chief Executives); DH Board members
Expand training, development and career opportunities: Enhance training for all staff in race equality issues. Develop more entry points for people from ethnic minorities to join the NHS and take up training. Improve access for black and minority ethnic staff to the full range of development programmes, support networks and professional training. Encourage appropriately qualified leaders from ethnic minorities in health and other sectors to consider and apply for executive positions	Local WDCs (Workforce Development Confederation) and HR (Human Resources) networks, NHS Leadership Centre, NHSU (NHS University) and other training providers
Systematic tracking: Build systematic processes for tracking the career progression of staff from ethnic minorities including local and national versions of the NHS Leaders scheme	All senior leaders and NHS Leadership Centre
Celebrate achievements: Acknowledge the contributions of all staff in tackling race inequalities and promote opportunities for staff from ethnic minorities to celebrate their contribution to the NHS	DH and all NHS leaders

(Department of Health—see p 347 for website—adapted)
Reproduced under the terms of the click-use licence.

At the time of writing (April 2005) only two of the 15 Health Boards have established such forums but most have strengthened consultative mechanisms or made plans to follow the guidance.

Three years on reasonable progress with these aims has been made, according to reports of independent consultants, though there is a great deal to do.

The Fair For All HDL, therefore, took the prior policies into a new, strategic realm. The strategy was seen as needing ten years to implement. The leadership in relation to the HDL was taken on by the Patient Focus Public Involvement Programme in the Scottish Health Department. A patient-focused service was defined as a service that ensures that the service exists for the patient, where individuals are treated according to their needs and wishes. This Patient Focus Programme also funded the National Resource Centre for Ethnic Minority Health.

8.2.2.4 National Resource Centre for Ethnic Minority Health (Scotland)

The National Resource Centre for Ethnic Minority Health was set up in 2002 to help NHS Scotland deliver a quality service that addresses the needs of minority ethnic communities. The NRCEMH is, intentionally, a small organization. It has a catalytic role, aiming for change through mainstream organizations. It does not deliver any services to patients or the public, but supports those who do. In 2002 its priorities were agreed with the Scottish Executive as refinement of policy and assistance with its implementation and monitoring; assessing need for and galvanizing the development of training programmes; and supporting the development of information systems that supplied data about and for ethnic minority groups. The demand for these and numerous other challenges was considerable and the Centre has broadened its scope (see list of web sites, p 345). It works through extensive networking, thereby achieving far more than its small size suggests. The account of functions in Box 8.3 is taken from the Centre's web site and presented with minor editing. There was verbal agreement that the Centre's work would take ten years, but funding was for three years in the first instance. It has now been extended for another three years to 2008. The success of the Centre depends on the regional and local NHS services—as discussed in the next section.

8.2.2.5 Meeting the health needs of minority ethnic groups in Lothian NHS Board

The NHS in Scotland funds 15 Health Boards that are responsible for all services to their geographically defined populations. Lothian NHS Board is responsible for health care for about 675,000 people in and around the City of Edinburgh in the east of Scotland. In the NHS Lothian area, as in the remainder of the UK, numerous attempts have been made to improve health care for ethnic minority groups over several decades.

Community organizations concerned with the health and welfare of minority ethnic groups in Lothian have worked with service providers, including the Lothian NHS and local government councils, to raise the issues, and to improve services and access, for example interpretation and translation services. Consultations have been done on several occasions and reports have been produced identifying areas where action is needed. These

Box 8.3 The main functions of the National Resource Centre For Ethnic Minority Health are

- Sending explicit and consistent messages about why race equality matters to NHS Scotland.
- Providing specialist guidance, support and advice to the NHS organizations at local, regional and national levels.
- Contributing to the development of race equality champions in NHS Boards.
- Developing tools that can assist NHS Boards in their work in race equality and cultural competence.
- Identifying and sharing good practice and encouraging learning for staff that will achieve change for patients and carers alike.
- Creating a framework of indicators of progress for performance management.
- Contribute to the analysis and interpretation of information about ethnicity of patients in the NHS and about their health needs and health differences (in partnership with ISD Scotland).
- Auditing progress by NHS Boards in the development and implementation of Fair for All and Race Equality Scheme action plans.
- Addressing multiple identity issues by working on specific common areas of interest with other diversity strand teams, for example for disability, lesbian, gay, bisexual and transgender (LGBT) issues, age, gender and religion.
- Ensuring that NHS Boards respond to population changes and increasing diversity within and between communities—taking account of the inward migration policy of the Scottish Executive.

(*Source*: National Resource Centre website—see p 345—adapted)

reports cover a wide variety of issues including the needs of particular groups such as children, carers of the sick and disabled, older people, men and women; appropriate acute health services; particular diseases (such as coronary heart disease, diabetes, mental ill health); and many other issues like housing and domestic abuse.

Initiatives funded and established within the NHS in Lothian in the 1990s designed to improve services include a Minority Ethnic Mental Health Project, with a worker based in the Royal Edinburgh Hospital, and the Minority Ethnic Health Inclusion Project (MEHIP) which is an advocacy service. Other projects include action to improve services for refugees and asylum seekers and gypsy travellers. More recently in the north-east of Lothians an innovative heart disease prevention project called Khush Dil was set up with short-term funding. All these activities were achieved largely in the absence of a strategic framework, and by widespread testimony, were very difficult to set up and sustain.

The collective experience of these projects testifies to the need for enormous energy, commitment and effort to set up limited initiatives. These initiatives have struggled around one or more of the issues of resource constraints, multiple demands exceeding available resources, short-term funding and vision, insufficient managerial or peer support, insufficient cross-coordination, and difficulties in moving from project to mainstream service status even when success was demonstrable. The outstanding, impressive feature of all these services is the gratitude and support of the ethnic minority groups served and the dedication of the staff.

In the mid-1990s a strategic document on ethnicity and health was prepared by a senior public health practitioner in the Health Board's Public Health Department. For reasons that are unclear, this document was not progressed, even though many of its recommendations were later to be echoed in the Board's strategy. We can only assume that the issue was not perceived to be a sufficiently high priority at that time.

In the late 1990s and early 2000s the Lothian Health Board noted that the need to tackle health inequalities experienced by minority ethnic people was recognized in the Scottish Executive's White Paper, Towards a Healthier Scotland (1999), the Acheson Report on Inequalities in Health (1998), the Scottish Executive's Equality Strategy, a Management Executive Letter in 1999 asking Scottish health boards to improve health services for minority ethnic communities, in the stocktake of action in Scottish Health Boards and in the HDL of 2002 (Fair For All). Further, it noted a new emphasis on the active involvement of people and communities in planning of health-related services. A chief executive—Trevor Jones, later chief executive of the whole of the NHS in Scotland and signatory to the HDL 2002—was appointed who had experience of the challenges of serving multi-ethnic populations in England and a proactive approach to this agenda. He convened and chaired an informal interdepartmental group to galvanize action across the Board. I was appointed in 1999 to Lothian Health Board as honorary consultant. For this informal group I prepared a brief ten-point plan (see Chapter 6) to guide action.

The next stage was to move from specific projects and initiatives to integrating the needs of minority ethnic groups. The Scottish Executive Equality Unit's definition of mainstreaming was the guiding one i.e. making sure that concern for equality is built-in from the start to the development of policy, to the design of services and in the monitoring and evaluation frameworks.

Lothian NHS Board, and specifically its Chief Executive, was a signatory to a pan-Lothian declaration to root out racism. This document signified a public commitment to work to promote equal access to all citizens, regardless of skin colour, race, culture or religion, and to make this part of Scotland a safer place for people from minority ethnic communities.

Within such a supportive context the task of preparing an ethnicity and health strategy for Lothian NHS health care delivery services was made much easier. Lothian Health developed a strategy (that preceded the 2002 HDL and developed by a committee chaired by me) on the health needs of minority ethnic groups (Lothian NHS Minority Health Group, 2003), which was summarized and embedded in the Health Improvement Plan for 2000–2005. The challenge of the strategy was to get all NHS Lothian's health policies but particularly those on inequalities to take into account the ethnic dimension. We foresaw that the implementation of this recommendation alone would be a huge step forward, particularly for mainstreaming. We also emphasized that the health of people from minority ethnic groups in Lothian is affected by their relative levels of disadvantage due to socio-economic factors including poverty, poor housing and unemployment, and by their experience of racism reducing employment prospects and career success.

Such broad issues could only be addressed in partnership with minority ethnic communities and other service providers, including local government councils. Monitoring and evaluation needed to be set up, including ethnic monitoring of primary care and hospital services.

The process of agreeing and producing the strategy was a collaborative exercise involving staff from health services, representatives of local communities, the local government and the voluntary sector. The draft strategy was focused around four principles and a ten-point plan shown in Box 8.4. The draft was widely disseminated for consultation with ethnic minority individuals, institutions, and community organizations. The draft plan was widely endorsed with only minor changes suggested.

The plan, in turn, linked to hospital and primary care-based equivalent documents that were in more detail. Extracts from the Primary Care document include these on refugees and gypsy travellers, for example:

- services should improve links between Lothian NHS Trusts and other agencies including the Scottish Refugee Council.
- Refugee issues should be included in training for staff.
- Scottish gypsy travellers who have a nomadic lifestyle should have patient-held health records

After six years of strategic activity Lothian NHS now has an integrated Race Equality Scheme and Fair for All Action Plan, overseen by the Lothian Ethnic Health Forum. Projects are now part of policy. It would be dishonest to pretend that everything that has been agreed is being achieved but coordinated progress is being made, including the appointment of a full-time member of the management team dedicated to coordinating and performance managing the ethnicity and health agenda. One of the toughest and most important actions is ethnic monitoring, a challenge that needs national and local action simultaneously.

8.2.2.6 Ethnic monitoring

Try Exercise 8.5 before reading on.

Exercise 8.5 Ethnic coding

- What is ethnic coding? (if you do not know, have a guess, then look at the glossary)
- Why is it centrally important to implementation of policy?
- Why is it so difficult to achieve?

Box 8.4 Core principles of the Strategic Action Plan on Minority Ethnic Health

The work is based on four principles.

1. Mainstreaming of minority ethnic health so that it becomes an automatic part of all NHS activities.
2. Tackling racism. The NHS must be an advocate against racism, and work to ensure that racism does not occur in any part of its activities.
3. Providing accessible, equitable, high quality and appropriate services to all members of minority ethnic groups.
4. Partnership working with organizations, community groups and individuals so that the experience and knowledge of people from minority ethnic groups contributes to developing services.

The ten action areas

Ten action areas and aims have been listed in the draft Plan for the NHS in Lothian.

1. Mainstreaming minority ethnic health needs into the planning and delivery of all health services.
2. Advocacy and action against racism; to take action against racism in any form, and to reduce racist attacks, harassment and discrimination.
3. Appropriate, culturally sensitive, high quality and accessible healthcare, available to all people from every ethnic group.
4. Involving people and communities so that people from minority ethnic groups are involved in consultation over health services.
5. Interpretation and translation services; to ensure that interpreting and translating is available.
6. Health and health care information for minority ethnic groups; to ensure that appropriate information is available.
7. Provision of advocacy and facilitation services; so that health advocates are available, and to respond to the specific needs of particular groups, such as refugees and asylum seekers, and gypsy travellers.
8. Training for NHS staff; to raise awareness of racism, ethnicity and health, and to enable staff to provide appropriate and accessible services.
9. Employment; to ensure non-discriminatory employment practice and to work towards a workforce which reflects the diversity of local communities.
10. Patient profiling; monitoring of ethnicity; to obtain and use information about the ethnicity and health of people from minority ethnic groups.

(*Source*: Lothian Health Board Website, see p 345—adapted)

Following a very long period of debate, and numerous attempts to have ethnic monitoring implemented comprehensively (see Chapters 3 and 5), we now have a virtual consensus in the UK at policy and strategic levels that it is essential (this is also the view in the USA). In 1995 the NHS in England, through its NHS Executive, published comprehensive guidance in a volume called Collecting Ethnic Group Data for Admitted Patient Care (Shaw 1994). This itself arose from an Executive Letter issued in 1994 declaring that ethnic group is to be recorded for all hospital inpatients. The policy failed because the data collected thereafter were incomplete.

The difference, ten years later, is that policy is backed by legislation, and at the highest levels in management. *Ethnic Monitoring—A Guide for Public Authorities in Scotland* was published (website on p 345) by the Commission for Racial Equality (CRE) to help public authorities to comply with the requirements of the Race Relations Act 1976 and the Race Relations (Amendment) Act 2000 (Home Office 2001). Ethnic monitoring was seen as the process by which an authority maintains an informed view of the extent to which its race equality policy is working. In practice, it means collecting quantitative data by ethnic group. The English NHS Ten Point Race Equality Action Plan (Table 8.1) emphasizes meeting the service needs of people from ethnic minorities, ensuring a greater focus on helping people with chronic diseases and tackling health inequalities. To demonstrate success, indeed to help ensure success, information is needed to direct actions.

The Department of Health in England issued new guidance in 2005 in a *Practical Guide to Ethnic Monitoring* which promotes the standardized collection of ethnic group and related data on patients, service users and staff of the NHS and social services. It provides examples of good practice (website is on p 347). The strongest impetus towards ethnic monitoring, according to the guidance, is the business case, i.e. meeting needs cost-effectively. Other influences, for example, the Race Relations (Amendment) Act 2000, are acknowledged.

The fundamental principle for ethnic coding in the UK is self-classification, from the ethnic group codes on offer. Consent and confidentiality are to be respected with no-one forced into giving their ethnic group against their will. Collection of such data is expected to be routine. Service providers are also expected to collect data on service users' religion, language and diet, where appropriate. Staff, patients and the public should receive training, relevant to their needs, on the collection and use of ethnic group and related data. In Scotland, with earmarked funding, senior staff have been appointed to lead the initiative, and a committee has been formed to coordinate action within the broader diversity agenda, which has started with demonstration projects working with primary and secondary care staff. Already it is clear that even with all this backing the challenge is formidable and success can only be judged in the longer term. It is important that the effects of these actions are assessed. Table 8.2 summarises some of the anticipated issues.

8.2.2.7 Delivery and evaluation-checking for change

Try Exercise 8.6 before reading on.

Table 8.2 Communications Guidelines for the Introduction of Ethnic Monitoring in Health Boards in Scotland, p 4; some potential issues by audience

Audience group	Objection/barrier
White majority	No need for them to reply as their ethnic identity is obvious The end result will be preferential treatment for black and minority ethnic groups Nothing in it for me
Black and minority ethnic groups	Fear of being identified and suffering harassment or discrimination as a result Scepticism about the ability of NHS organizations to deliver real change of benefit to them If status is known, the patients may not be eligible for NHS treatment (would only apply when following the Overseas Regulations)
NHS managers	Additional burden on managers to no clear result No connection to assessment of their performance Technical difficulties in launching monitoring and managing data
NHS front line staff	Another burden that will interfere with clinical duties Will involve confrontation if patients refuse to complete the forms Procedural difficulties with the inroduction of the monitoring
Media	More bureaucracy in heath service More political correctnes NHS services being geared to needs of minorities rather than majority
All audiences	Data protection issues Raising expectations of service change well ahead of this happening in practice

Source: Ethnic Monitoring Toolkit—see website on p 347 for reports. Reproduced under the terms of the click-use licence.

Exercise 8.6 Evaluation

- Why is evaluation of policy important?
- How would you evaluate policies of the kind we have discussed?
- What difficulties can you foresee?

Evaluation is not important simply for finding out whether something works but for making it happen in the first place, and for ensuring it happens to the expected standard. Without evaluation, or the expectation of evaluation, tough jobs would not be done, or would be done poorly. It is in recognition of this basic aspect of human nature—so well known by teachers and their students and the only justification in my opinion for examinations—that the ethnicity and health field has expended considerable energy on evaluation tools.

Legislation, policy and strategy in the ethnicity and health arena is not amenable to evaluation using the gold standard of the randomized controlled trial. Even basic evaluation designs such as before and after studies are very difficult to interpret, because change is slow and the effect of one policy cannot be isolated from that of others and from demographic and other changes. These are highly complex interventions in complex political and social environments. These policy interventions are not without risks or side-effects, and they come with financial and other costs. Their implementation invariably demands an act of courage and faith that they are beneficial. Yet, it would be irresponsible to implement such important policies without assessing them. Mostly, however, evaluations are based on whether the actions have been taken rather than the effects of the actions. The approach is illustrated in the following quotation from the English Department of Health's ten-point plan lead by the then Chief Executive Sir Nigel Crisp and published in 2004 (website on p 347):

> As well as my oversight, Ministers will take a keen interest in progress. Staff in black and minority ethnic networks from the service will be encouraged to express views and keep this plan under review. And, to make sure we benchmark ourselves against the best, I have invited an independent expert panel to review our progress and report back to the September Chief Executive's conference this year.
>
> Department of Health, website 13/2/2004 (see p 347)

Expert panels need evaluation tools. Tools for both action and assessment of progress have been developed and an example is Jeff Chandra's guide *Facing up to Difference* (1996), designed to help in the creation of culturally competent health services for black and minority ethnic communities and which still remains remarkably modern and relevant. In addition to comprehensive guidance on what needs to be done, it gives a set of core standards, and targets. This kind of work sets the stage for quantitative and qualitative evaluation. Remarkably, the organization that published Chandra's work, the King's Fund, had published a *Checklist: Health and Race* by Yasmin Gunaratnam in 1993, with the subtitle 'A starting point for managers on improving services for black populations'. It starts with a set of core race equality standards on patients' rights and needs, service provision and employment. The main part of this document is a comprehensive set of questions. Other than the language on outdated service organizational structures the questions are to the point and comprehensive. This checklist points out that it concerns what needs to be in place to achieve better health outcomes and is not designed to measure the health outcomes themselves. A more recent checklist is in Box 8.5.

The Scottish National Resource Centre for Ethnic Minority Health published the toolkit *Checking for Change. A Building Blocks Approach to Race Quality in Health* in 2005 (see NRCEMHs website—URL on p 345). It is structured around the five key Fair for All elements i.e. energizing the organization (Chandra used the identical phrase in 1996), demographics, access and service delivery, human resources, and community development. The main novelty and additional strength of this toolkit, other than the fact it is tailored to Scottish policy and legislation, is that it assesses the stage (or level) that the organization is at presently, and what its next challenges are. There are four levels for each key area. It also clarifies the source of the evidence. For example, under energizing the organization level one (the lowest) is indicated by the organization having a Race Equality

---

Box 8.5 A checklist for evaluation (adapted)

Best practice checklist for planning services for Black and Minority Ethnic Groups (BMEGs)

(a) Services for BMEGs should be part of 'mainstream' health care provision.

(b) The amended Race Relations Act should be considered in all policies.

(c) Facilitate access to appropriate services by:
   providing appropriate bilingual services for effective communication
   education and training for health professionals and other staff
   appropriate and acceptable service provision
   provision of religious and dietary choice within meals offered in hospitals.

(d) ethnic workforce issues, including addressing racial discrimination and harassment within the workplace, and promoting race equality and valuing diversity in the workforce.

(e) community engagement and participation.

(f) Systematizing structures and processes for capture and use of appropriate data.

(g) asking questions:

   with what population or patients (how many and how severely ill) are we concerned?
   what services on average are currently provided?
   what is the evidence of the effectiveness and cost-effectiveness of these services?
   what is the optimum configuration of services?

   Original Source Gill *et al.* (2006). Reproduced under the terms of the click-use licence.

Scheme that is more than three years old (or none at all). Level 4 (the highest) is feedback from ethnic minority communities and other partner agencies that the organization's activities are successful.

One way of evaluating outcome is to get feedback from service users e.g. in satisfaction surveys. Gauging satisfaction is not easy. Respondents may be reluctant to admit dissatisfaction and an overall rating of satisfaction may hide dissatisfaction with specific aspects of services. There may also be cross-cultural differences in what gives satisfaction and how it is reported. Madhok and colleagues' studies in a Pakistani population in the north-east of England (1992, 1998) in the early 1990s used home interview, by a person of the same sex and ethnic group as the respondent, and in the language of the respondents' choice, to safeguard partially against such problems. Questioning on a range of services together with probing on a few, lessened the danger of finding overall satisfaction and missing specific criticisms. In this study satisfaction was generally high. One interpretation of these findings was that the expectations of this Pakistani community were low. This interpretation may hold some truth but questions the quality of the perceptions of the respondents, and the good work of the Health Authority and health professionals in meeting most needs. The alternative interpretation, and the one I favour, is that the findings reflected the good performance by the service.

Such surveys are relatively rare but an important part of the evaluation armamentarium. Another route to evaluation is to gauge the use and quality of services. The production, uptake and effects of health education and health promotion materials and services can be assessed. The acceptability of these can also be examined, as well as levels of health knowledge, and changes in attitudes, beliefs and behaviours. In the UK, minority ethnic groups (except possibly the Chinese) use general practitioner and hospital services as much or more than expected. That is an indication of effectiveness of access, though not quality. The use of other community health services tends to be lower than expected. Minority ethnic groups have, as a generalization, relatively low use of community nursing and dental and chiropody services. The pattern of service utilization can be monitored as a guide to effective access and care.

The Policy Studies Institute survey found that many service users preferred to see a doctor of their own ethnic origin (Nagroo 1997). This preference was greater in those who spoke limited or no English, and among women rather than men. However, most men from minority ethnic groups also express a preference to see a doctor of the same gender. Such preferences are greater when physical, and especially gynaecological, examination may be involved. These kinds of specific preferences can be the focus of evaluations, and lead to adaptation of services. The preference for health professionals of the same sex are also expressed, though less strongly, and usually only for intimate examinations and care procedures (e.g. cervical smears) in non-White ethnic groups. This is one of many potential examples of how attending to the needs of minorities can benefit the entire population—others include more choice in hospital foods, careful consultation with the community, and more use of symbols in signage in buildings rather than text. This point was made very well by Fuller in the quotation below.

> Firstly, improving contraceptive services for ethnic minorities will also improve services for the majority by improving skills in eliciting patients' beliefs and fears and in communicating and by leading to more flexible services. Secondly, it is no longer good enough for investigators to peer in on ethnic communities from the outside and make decisions about them. Information should come from workers who originate from the ethnic communities, so that decisions are made from within the community.
>
> Fuller (1987: 1365)

The use of complementary or alternative therapies (including, for example, use of hakims and Ayurvedic remedies) in minority ethic communities tends to be additional rather than an alternative to NHS service use—as with the population generally. It is also important to note the increasing trend to consult practitioners of alternative medicine within the general population. These are indirect indicators of the extent to which mainstream services are meeting needs.

These forms of evaluation are focused on specific health policies, but many other kinds of policies have an impact on the welfare of ethnic minority groups e.g. transport, education, housing and enterprise. Unless these also meet the needs of ethnic minority populations we will not narrow the socio-economic status gap. A new but simple idea has been implemented in Scotland and England—race impact assessment, whereby all policies are to be screened to ensure equality.

The impact assessment process is a set of questions that assesses whether the policy/strategy/programme is having or might have adverse effects on different racial or ethnic groups. If so the actions that are to be taken to remedy the problem need to be explicit. The aim is to ensure and demonstrate that we are promoting equality of opportunity and good race relations. Impact assessment is now an integral part of the policy-making/development process with guidance provided by the Scottish Executive's Equality Unit.

The challenge to come is to evaluate the outcomes in relation to health status and health care quality, and ideally even costs, cost-effectiveness and cost–benefits. It is probably true to say, certainly in Europe but probably across the world, that the worlds of race and ethnicity policy and research have overlapped too little. Researchers have focused on health status to a great extent but not in relation to testing effectiveness of policy actions. This would require much better data systems and, in particular, high quality ethnic monitoring and research. Policies would also need to be reframed in terms of expected health status and health care outcomes, which is a difficult task, not least because setting the standard is difficult both conceptually and technically. This theme will be picked up in Chapter 9. A guiding policy on research and an ethical code to ensure its benefits are, however, discussed below as a prelude to Chapter 9.

8.2.2.8 Research: policy and an ethical code for researching 'race', racism and anti-racism

Try Exercise 8.7 before reading on.

Exercise 8.7 Research

- Why is research important to policy and vice versa?
- Do you see any evidence of institutional racism in research?
- What principles would you emphasize for ethical research with ethnic minority groups?

Most policy documents recognize the need for data, whether it is from the census, routine vital statistics, or research. Research on the health and health care of ethnic minorities, nonetheless, tends to be neglected in policy implementation. The reasons are not difficult to understand. Funds are always tight, the immediate tasks such as policy implementation are urgent, and funding for research is usually routed separately and is granted on a highly competitive basis whereby committees and peer reviewers choose from a range of projects on the basis of scientific quality and promise. Ethnic minority groups have been largely bypassed in the large scale and most expensive kinds of research such as trials and cohort studies (see Chapter 9). The USA is now leading in addressing the imbalance, as discussed in Section 8.3. Researchers interested and able to work in this field are few, and timescales for research are usually much longer than for policy and service change. As a local example the NRCEMH in Scotland did not prioritize research at its inception and its later efforts to raise funds for research have not been successful (as yet, though negotiations continue).

There are qualms about research that are sometimes expressed, especially by leaders of ethnic minority community organizations. One is that they cannot see the benefits of the research to the communities (except for researchers' careers, which is a gain, although it might not be seen that way). There is sometimes a view that ethnic minority groups are over-researched, which is contrary to the empirical evidence from several extensive studies showing that few trials and cohort studies report results by ethnic group (see Chapter 9). There is also a fear that researchers are drawing away scarce funding from more pressing and obvious needs. It is usually true that community organizations have little access to funding while universities may have a great deal.

Even more importantly, there may be anxiety that research may do harm rather than good. The history of racism in research has been referred to throughout this book and will be considered again in Chapter 9. Currently, however, it is the lack of inclusion of ethnic minority groups in large-scale research that is causing most concern, with a gathering consensus that this might reflect institutional racism in the research world. Indeed, the USA has enacted legislation and policies to counteract this problem and the debate has lately been ignited in the UK. It is likely that research on race and ethnicity is going to grow rapidly, both in response to research and health policy, and it behoves us to agree a governing code of conduct. Scottish researchers have taken action on this, as has the American College of Epidemiology (see website— p343 and Chapter 9).

The Scottish Executive Central Research Unit published *Researching Ethnic Minorities in Scotland* (SECRU 2000) which made the criticism that researchers and funders had failed to acknowledge the existence of institutional racism in research. This was seen, at least in part, to be a result of the absence of an ethical code for researching race. Subsequently, *An Ethical Code for Researching 'Race', Racism and Anti-racism in Scotland* was published in 2001 by a group of researchers called the Scottish Association of Black Researchers (SABRE). SABRE is a network of 'Black' researchers within universities, local authorities and the 'Black' voluntary sector in Scotland. The principles of the Code (available on the Internet—see organisations p342) state that ethical research on race is:

- embedded in social justice and human rights concerns and legal obligations.
- explicit in its commitment to anti-racism and to promoting social inclusion.
- empowering and actively includes black and minority ethnic peoples' perspectives.

- addresses the complex and problematic nature of concepts of 'race', racism and ethnicity.
- insures that it does not pathologize, stereotype or is exploitative, particularly of black and minority ethnic people.
- values and addresses the diversity within the black and minority ethnic population and recognizes the interconnections with colour, age, gender, disability, sexuality, culture, class, language, belief, context and other socially defined characteristics.
- acknowledges the power relations inherent in social research processes, e.g., between 'white' and 'black', 'researchers' and 'researched' and families and communities.
- ensures that the whole research exercise is underpinned by a commitment to confidentiality.

The code also gives some attributes of sound researchers, including that they:

- make explicit their respective racial and ethnic origins, principles, ethics and authority and acknowledge the potential impact that this has had.
- provide a full description of the scope, constraints and procedures for gaining access to black minority ethnic communities, the ethnic categories used and their effects on the results in terms of plausibility, validity, reliability and generalizabilty.

While policy and research have not been fully integrated that does not mean a lack of mutual influence. The influence of policy on research is fairly self-evident. The power of research in influencing policy is more diffuse and is discussed in the next section.

8.2.2.9 Interaction of health and research policies: example of coronary heart disease in South Asians in Britain

Coronary heart disease (CHD) is a dominant cause of death and disability in all UK ethnic groups (and increasingly globally) and as a result there have been well-documented efforts in policy, research and practice. The UK European origin White population is internationally notorious for its high CHD mortality. It is remarkable, therefore, that Indian, Pakistani and Bangladeshi-born residents of England and Wales, coming from countries where the disease is comparatively rare (at least in the 1950s through the 1970s when most migrated), have mortality rates 40–50 per cent above those of the population in England and Wales as a whole. Similar conclusions have arisen from work in Scotland, and in many other countries too. There is virtually a consensus that emigrant South Asians, and possibly even those on the Indian subcontinent, are highly susceptible to cardiovascular diseases. By contrast the African, African-Caribbean and Chinese/Hong Kong born residents of England and Wales have comparatively low CHD mortality. Again, such patterns have been corroborated elsewhere. Such stark ethnic inequalities in a top-ranking health problem, together with the comparatively high absolute rates of disease in all ethnic groups, compel attention.

Any policy or strategy needs to grapple with the question—why is CHD so common in South Asians? There is no simple, unequivocal answer. Assuming that the high rates are not an artefact of data collection, or differentials in diagnostic activity, and it seems they are not, there are four main categories of explanation (see Ch 1, Patel and Bhopal 2004):

1. South Asians are more exposed to the established risk factors. This explanation has usually been dismissed (perhaps too readily).
2. South Asians are more susceptible to established CHD risk factors. Mechanisms proposed include genetic differences (as yet unidentified) or a mismatch between fetal/early life metabolism and that in middle age. A related explanation might be that the incredibly rapid change in some risk factors may, itself, confer a risk beyond that expected by the actual level of the factor.
3. There are specific novel risk factors that are not yet established (or discovered) specifically explaining the high risk.
4. There are fewer competing causes of death in middle-aged South Asians, particularly as cancer rates are comparatively low.

The high rates of CHD in South Asians are likely to arise from a complex mix of these explanations.

The control of the CHD epidemic in South Asians requires a coordinated and vigorous response based on the best evidence on effectiveness, and the highest standards of care. The National Service Framework (NSF) on CHD published by the Department of Health in 2000, setting 12 standards, is the key governing policy for the UK, particularly as it gives attention to ethnic variations. The NSF requires NHS organizations to ensure that the services they provide are accessible and acceptable to the people they serve, regardless of their ethnicity. This includes accessing and meeting people's needs in ways that are culturally, religiously and linguistically appropriate. It also states that staff will need to have or to acquire the relevant skills, knowledge and experience to enable them to be sensitive to the cultural and religious needs of the individuals and communities that they serve. The Scottish document (Coronary Heart Disease/Stroke Task Force, Report, published in 2001 by the Scottish Executive) applies in Scotland but it makes no mention of ethnic variations, which is a typical omission until the last few years.

Specific evidence from clinical trials of effectiveness of interventions on South Asian populations is virtually non-existent. The actions required of health services, therefore, need to be based on first principles and include those in Box 8.5.

The Director of Equality and Human Rights for the NHS in England, Surinder Sharma, has reminded those managing the National Service Framework and working on CHD control that the National Health Service was founded on the principle of equal access for all but this has not yet been achieved (BHF/NHS 2004 p3). Sharma asks for an explicit commitment to equality, diversity and respect into everything we do. These issues are discussed in a joint NHS and British Health Foundation (a charity) publication in 2004 *Heart Disease and South Asians. Delivering the National Service Framework for Coronary Heart Disease* (2004).

Box 8.6 Some action required of health services to control CHD in South Asians

1. Adopt broadly based strategies focusing on the major risk factors, and taking account of language and cultural needs, relative poverty (especially Bangladeshis) and the heterogeneity of South Asians populations. Disease registers and practice lists may require to have a valid ethnic code so services can be targeted. An example of such a strategy is available with information on how it was developed and on the Internet (Elliot B 1997).

2. Ensure that South Asian patients are well informed about CHD (their knowledge is low).

3. Ensure that standards of care for secondary and tertiary prevention follow national guidelines with equity in the quantity and quality of care.

4. Be particularly vigilant in controlling risk factors in South Asians. Thresholds for action may need to be set lower for South Asians than in the population as a whole (a topic for new research). In Chapter 9 there is a discussion of how BMI has underestimated the proportion of Asians that are carrying too much adipose tissue (fat).

Two vital principles are illustrated in this example. First, it is important that race and ethnicity are incorporated into primary policy documents, as secondary documentation will turn to that primary driving force. Second, that research and scholarship do influence policy, albeit slowly. Until the publication of my and colleagues' paper on heterogeneity of CHD risk factors in 1999, nearly all discussions, including those of highly informed researchers such as Paul McKeigue who had demonstrated heterogeneity himself, treated South Asians as a homogenous group. The following extract from *Heart Disease and South Asians. Delivering the National Service Framework for Coronary Heart Disease* illustrates how this scholarship has had a great influence on policy (BHF/NHS 2004).

> It is generally agreed, however, that certain risk factors are more common among South Asians. These vary between communities, but include high levels of smoking, particularly among Bangladeshi men, low rates of exercise across all South Asian communities and a diet high in fat and low in fruit and vegetables in certain groups. (p6)

This emphasis on differentiating South Asian subgroups is, without question, a result of research. The following quotation from this publication shows how general policies affect specific ones:

> The NHS Plan, published in July 2000, set out ambitious goals to transform the quality of services, tackle health inequalities and deliver patient centred services that are responsive and accessible to all parts of the community. In ensuring fair and equitable access of services to all, services must take account of personal needs such as religious, cultural and dietary needs. (p8)

Finally, it is pointed out that this specific work contributes to National targets for reducing CHD and tackling health inequalities and to national standards. Again, we see how race and ethnicity can be embedded and intertwined within large-scale goals, so it is not a small component that can be easily undermined.

8.3 The USA

Try Exercise 8.8 before reading on.

Exercise 8.8 Race policy in the USA

◆ What factors might make the USA particularly conscious of race and ethnicity?
◆ What might be the barriers to improving the health of minorities in the USA?
◆ What might be the strengths of the USA in the race and ethnicity field?

The USA is one of the most race-conscious countries in the world, and as a country where immigrants in the last 200–300 years comprise the majority of the population, it is multiracial, almost everywhere. It has highly advanced policies. In the UK, even taking into account recent attempts at decentralization, the country is organized in a relatively unified way with political power underpinning extensive statutory services paid from taxation. By contrast the USA's preferred stance (though not always practice) favours the privatization of services and the slicing up of political powers at federal, state and county levels. Policy analysis, policy-making and policy implementation may well, indeed are likely to be, in separate domains of power. It is a characteristic of USA federal policy that it does not state who is to do what and when. This contrasts with the UK system where a governmental policy is rapidly followed by both plans and instructions, usually developed after consultation, but nonetheless moving from the top to the bottom of the hierarchy. The USA approach can create local energy, and local achievement, as it is not so reliant on top down leadership.

Race and health is incredibly controversial in the USA. Words matter greatly, and considerable controversy occurred when the language of a major report was changed, as shown in Box 8.7. The fear, of course, is that downplaying the magnitude of the problem will reduce funding for research and policy initiatives.

The following account gives a sample of contemporary thinking at the policy level in the USA. The work on race and ethnicity is done within the civil rights framework with legislation that protects against discrimination on race, colour or national origin. There are many documents but I have not found an overarching government policy that applies to the entire USA health care system, such as the Scottish HDL or English ten-point plan (Table 8.1) do.

8.3.1 Institute of Medicine report on unequal treatment

The Institute of Medicine is one of the most influential and respected health policy analysis institutions in the USA, and perhaps the world. In March 2002, the Institute published

Box 8.7 Importance of words in the race and health field in the USA: editing and controversy

July 2003

1. Inequality in quality persists.

2. Disparities come at a personal and societal price.

3. Differential access may lead to disparities in quality.

4. Opportunities to provide preventive care are frequently missed.

5. Knowledge of why disparities exist is limited.

6. Improvement is possible.

7. Data limitations hinder targeted improvements efforts.

December 2003

1. Americans have exceptional quality of health care; but some socioeconomic, racial, ethnic and geographic differences exist.

2. Some 'priority populations' do as well or better than the general population in some aspects of health care.

3. Opportunities to provide preventive care are frequently missed.

4. Management of chronic diseases presents unique challenges.

5. Greater improvement is possible.

Steinbrook (2004: 1487)

a report, *Unequal Treatment: What Health Care System Administrators Need To Know About Racial And Ethnic Disparities In Healthcare* (see IOM website, p345). The report recognized that health system managers worked hard to provide high quality health care services to an increasingly diverse population. The report acknowledges that, nonetheless, minorities and non-English speakers have comparatively greater difficulty accessing health care, and are over-represented in publicly funded health systems. Even when they are insured, racial and ethnic minorities tend to receive a lower quality of healthcare than White people. This report concluded that 'the sources of these disparities are complex, are rooted in historic and contemporary inequities, and involve many participants at several levels, including health systems, their administrative and bureaucratic processes, utilization managers, health care professionals, and patients' (Abstract of report, p2).

The Committee that wrote the report reviewed over 100 studies on the quality of health care for racial and ethnic minority groups, while taking into account explanatory factors such as income, which did not account wholly for differences.

The report considers whether minority patients could receive a lower quality of health care as a result of differences in health care seeking behaviors e.g. refusing recommended services and delaying seeking health care. Such issues were judged unlikely to be major sources of health care disparities. (Most likely such delay results from lack of insurance, lack of money and fear of taking time off work.) Uncertainty was also considered important e.g. when faced with patients from different racial or ethnic backgrounds, doctors' uncertainty about the patient's condition and best course of treatment is increased. Another potential explanation was that health care providers' diagnostic and treatment decisions, as well as their feelings about patients, were influenced by patients' race or ethnicity and stereotypes associated with them. The ways in which systems are organized and financed, changes in funding, language barriers, and time pressures on physicians in the face of cultural or linguistic barriers were all considered.

The report argues for a comprehensive, multi-level strategy to eliminate health care disparities. Among the suggested contents of such a strategy are: base decisions about resource allocation on published clinical guidelines; take steps to improve access to care—including the provision of interpretation and translation services where community need exists; ensure that physician incentives do not disproportionately burden or restrict minority patients' access to care; and collect and monitor data on patients' access and utilization of health care services by race, ethnicity, and primary language.

The report recommends that Federal, state, and private stakeholders should continue efforts to increase the proportion of under-represented USA racial and ethnic minorities among health professionals, to improve access to care among minority patients and to reduce cultural and linguistic barriers to care. Cross cultural curricula should be part of the training of these professionals. The report proposes that such strategies are likely to reduce health care disparities, and improve the efficiency and equity of care for all patients.

In many respects, except for the matter of health insurance and private health care, the issues are similar to those in the UK, as are the broad policy recommendations. In contrast to UK documents it is less clear who is going to see these recommendations through. One of the most important of the USA's health agencies for implementing policy is the Centers For Disease Control (CDC), and its role is considered next.

8.3.2 Centres for Disease Control—REACH programme

Healthy People 2010 is the overarching document that describes the USA's health objectives including goals to eliminate racial and ethnic disparities in health. The Centers for Disease Control and Prevention's (CDC) leadership role in this initiative includes a programme called Racial and Ethnic Approaches to Community Health (REACH) 2010 which is designed to eliminate disparities in cardiovascular disease, immunizations, breast and cervical cancer screening and management, diabetes, HIV/AIDS, and infant mortality. The groups targeted by REACH 2010 are African-Americans, American Indians, Alaska Natives, Asian Americans, Hispanics, and Pacific Islanders. In 2005 $34.5 million was available for this programme. REACH 2010 supports community coalitions comprising a community-based organization and three other organizations, at least one being a health department or a university or research organization.

In a recent major report on the REACH programme, the CDC's Acting Director, G. A. Mensah gave several examples to illustrate the health disparities in the USA:

♦ In 2001, rates of death from diseases of the heart were 30 per cent higher among African-Americans than among Whites, and death rates from stroke were 41 per cent higher.

♦ Compared with white adults, American Indians and Alaska Natives are 2.3 times, African-Americans are 1.6 times, and Hispanics are 1.5 times more likely to have diagnosed diabetes.

♦ Although African-Americans and Hispanics represent only 26 per cent of the U.S. population, they account for roughly 82 per cent of paediatric AIDS cases and 69 per cent of both AIDS cases and new HIV infections among USA adults.

♦ African-American, American Indian, and Puerto Rican infants continue to have higher mortality rates than White infants. In 2001, the black-to-white ratio in infant mortality was 2.3.

Mensah advocated culturally appropriate, community-driven programs based on sound prevention research and supported by new and innovative partnerships among governments, businesses, faith-based organizations, and communities—some examples are given below.

One REACH project is targeting the Cambodian community and its leaders, health care providers, and public health researchers. Community health educators teach people how to decrease risks and enhance protective behaviours associated with diabetes and cardiovascular disease. The number of Cambodians accessing heath care at a local health centre increased from 1,070 in 2000 to 3,080 in 2004. Of those who had attended educational workshops and peer support groups, 50 per cent reported favourable behavioural changes such as limiting salt intake. Another example is the REACH Project addressing diabetes among Puerto Rican and Dominican residents. Interventions include teaching people how to control the disease and environmental strategies that improve access to primary health care.

The REACH 2010 programme is developing a dissemination plan to help others develop and implement culturally appropriate prevention and intervention strategies. REACH 2010 will also expand policy initiatives that target environmental change, document the impact of cultural competency in coalitions, and build capacity to include social determinants research.

Although REACH clearly is linked to national policy, it seems to be project orientated rather than aiming to shift the entire health care system to meet needs of minorities i.e. it does not seem to be emphasizing mainstreaming, as in the UK. This is not entirely surprising as the system in the USA is pluralistic, and the CDC (and Federal Government) has no direct jurisdiction over health care. By contrast our third example, on research, is where the USA leads the world.

8.3.3 National Institutes of Health

Research underpins USA strategies to reduce racial and ethnic disparities—the term preferred to inequalities in that country. These actions have far-reaching consequences and need evaluation. In 2000 Congress created within the National Institutes for Health, the National Center on Minority Health and Health Disparities (NCMHD), which is backed by legislation and serves to coordinate research. This legislation mandated a strategic plan for the reduction of health disparities. This plan is the vision of The National Institutes for Health (NIH), the premier health research funding body in the USA. The budget and credibility of the NIH is so great that its policies have significance internationally.

The failure of researchers to include ethnic minority populations (and women) in research led to legislation and policy in the mid-1990s that required researchers to either ensure inclusion of racial and ethnic minority populations, or to justify their exclusion on scientific grounds. The consequence has been a great expansion of research focusing on minorities. In this regard the USA easily leads the world. Ranganathan and I showed that of 31 North-American cardiovascular cohort studies 15 provided some data by ethnic group, while none of 41 European ones did. Bartlett and colleagues reported that all eight of 47 trials that were specific on the matter of ethnicity were USA based. These are only two of such observations and I have chosen them because this is the position with cardio vascular disease, which has been long recognized as a priority matter for ethnic minority groups.

The NIH policy has been controversial. The current thinking on trials focusing on one or more ethnic groups has been captured by Taylor and colleagues in their paper 'Should ethnicity serve as the basis for clinical trial design?' Such questioning has accelerated since the publication of the African-American Heart Failure Trial that found that the drug isosorbide dinitrate combined with hydralazine was effective. This drug combination, known as BiDiL, is approved for the self-identified African-American population, and not in other Americans, as an earlier trial had shown that the same combination was not superior to alternatives in the general population. This is the first race-specific approval for a drug. In the past, virtually all large-scale trials have been done on predominantly White populations. The results have been assumed to be applicable to non-White populations, but if this assumption is not correct it has huge consequences. In the case of BiDiL an effective drug was almost discarded by this assumption.

The strategic plan of the NCMHD identifies goals for research, research infrastructure, and public information and community outreach. The strategic plan was developed with input from the public, professional and patient advocacy groups, health care organizations, academic institutions, and the scientific community. NCMHD has asked the Institute of Medicine (IOM) to assess the plan in achieving the NIH's goals and objectives. As targets for health outcomes have been set, the USA is one step ahead of the UK. Nonetheless, it seems improbable that disparities in health status will narrow without a broader, integrated, and government-led approach tackling income and wealth and environmental inequalities simultaneously. In this respect the UK is well ahead of the USA.

8.4 Conclusion

While there are many policies, strategies and action projects in existence health services internationally have struggled with the challenge of equitable health care in multi-ethnic societies. While I have focused on the UK and the USA I am on reasonably safe ground in stating that matters are not better, and probably much worse, elsewhere. New Zealand has long-standing and superb policies but the health of Maoris is poor; Australian aborigines living in one of the world's richest economies have appalling health despite targeted efforts; and many European countries have yet to confront the challenges.

To date the challenge has been tackled mostly at the level of structure and process—what systems might work and what should we do? Equity in service delivery is increasingly the central focus, with outcomes in terms of health care delivery and its quality as the benchmark. The achievement of outcomes measured in terms of health status is seldom the centrepiece of discussion, although the USA has moved to this. Intuitively, this is currently too great a challenge. Even conceptually, it is difficult to set a benchmark. What would be the goal? Ethnic inequalities in health are far more complex than socio-economic inequalities. Ethnic inequalities are very hard to predict and vary by cause of ill-health and by risk factor and are rapidly changing; social class inequalities, by contrast, are mostly predictable—on the great majority of indictors the poor are worse off than the wealthy. As considered in Chapter 9, a different conceptual approach will be needed for tackling ethnic inequalities in health status—and logically it would be based on the benchmark being the ethnic group with most desirable state of health for each indicator.

Current opinion favours mainstreaming with adaptation of general existing services, and incorporation of ethnic minorities' needs into the design stage of new services. The importance of the wider determinants of health such as wealth, housing, employment, and education for ethnic minority groups is clear. Policies and strategies to achieve better health for ethnic minorities are strengthened and sustained by their incorporation within a broader agenda for social justice and civil rights, and within wider policies to reduce inequalities regardless of ethnicity. Race equality impact assessment methods are being developed. These are being applied to a wide range of policies e.g. transport, health and safety, and employment practices. In this way there is an interconnection, and synergy, across the different sectors of social life. When everyone is speaking with the one voice, action is more likely, as we saw with the example of CHD services in England where research, policy, strategy and service delivery came together with a commonality of perspective that itself was in harmony with other national policies. These increasingly accepted ideals are constrained by lack of funds, expertise, data (particularly on what works and why) and the ongoing political controversies around immigration, asylum, race equality and human rights. These inevitable constraints mean progress is slower than ideal.

While policy, strategy and action is highly dependent on local context, many of the principles, experience and lessons are transferable internationally. Perhaps the most important of all the principles is that policies are most powerful and effective when they are supported by a legal and ethical framework. These frameworks, of necessity, reflect the values of the society and particularly those of the politicians and other holders of power. Policies to improve the health and health care of ethnic minority groups depend crucially on the value that all ethnic groups are equal.

Summary

A policy is a statement of intent that sets high level directions and goals; a strategy is a general plan to make an intended action happen; and these policies and strategies need to be supported by detailed plans that specify tasks, responsibilities, timetables and costs. In practice, actions are not always taken according to policies and strategies but on a tactical or opportunistic basis.

Health services for ethnic minority groups are usually set within the policies and strategies for the population as a whole, in practice the majority (or most powerful) population. Ideally, policies for the whole population would address the needs of ethnic minority groups in an integrated way. This concept is known as mainstreaming. In practice this may not happen for reasons including absence of understanding or agreement that this is important, the complexity of the issues raised and lack of expertise, time, and publication space within policy and strategy documents.

Mostly, ethnic minority populations are expected to adapt themselves to benefit from the available services. Professionals delivering the service tend to make some adjustments on an ad-hoc basis. Increasingly, we see two further policy responses—setting up specialist services for ethnic minority group but within the main service; and the development of strategies to help re-shape existing services to meet needs. The complete separation of services by ethnic group, as under Apartheid, is currently not in favour.

The UK policy response over the last 50 years has been intermittent and fragmented, with a mixture of stand-alone projects and modifications to mainline services. Progress has been made on key requirements such as interpretation services and dietary needs in hospital. The Race Relations Amendment Act 2000 building on the 1976 Act, coupled with explicit or implicit policies from the government health departments, is currently driving more widespread changes based on a positive duty to promote racial equality. These national initiatives affect everyone and are being translated, often with great difficulty, into local action plans and ultimately service changes. Ethnic monitoring is an example of a policy that is difficult to achieve despite evident need and good intentions.

The USA has had a long-standing programme for affirmative action based on human rights principles that aims to redress historical wrongs. A racial and ethnic classification, of the Office of Management and Budget, is explicitly designed to help achieve this goal. The pluralistic nature of the health care system of the USA, based on private health care principles, makes a cohesive strategy impossible to enact nationally to serve the whole population. There are powerful policies in place but their effectiveness seems to be limited. By law minority groups cannot be excluded from research using federal government funds without good reason, and this has spurred a substantial research programme in the USA.

While many policies, strategies and action projects exist, health services internationally have struggled with the challenge of equitable health care in multi-ethnic societies. Current opinion favours mainstreaming with adaptation of general existing services, and incorporation of ethnic minorities' needs into the design of new services. These ideals are constrained by lack of funds, expertise, data and the ongoing political controversies around immigration, asylum, race equality and human rights. While policy, strategy and action is highly dependent on local context, many of the principles, experience and lessons are transferable internationally.

Chapter 9

Research on and with ethnic minority groups: Past and future

I do feel that, with a total of more than a thousand people of Afro-Caribbean and South Asian origin now interviewed in one or other of the major studies mentioned, it would be hard to justify any further research on their needs and circumstances, at least until what has been done results—and can be seen to result—in tangible benefits for Black and Asian older people.

Jonathan Barker, April 1984, p2, in Age Concern Report

While calling for more research into this subject, the WHO report is aware of the risks. Given that minority ethnic communities are highly visible in their host societies, great sensitivity is needed as any data produced may be misinterpreted and misused.

Black (1987: 566)

Contents

Objectives

On completion of this chapter you should:

- Be familiar with a history of research that has done harm to minority ethnic groups, and hence be forewarned about the potential pitfalls
- In outline, be familiar with the range of research methods that can yield understanding of both ethnic variations in health and disease, and the health and health care needs of minority ethnic groups
- Be able to apply existing, or develop new, concepts, terminology, classifications and measurement methods appropriate to the research questions and study design
- Be able to discuss the key issues of recruitment of study populations, consent and participant information in relation to the study, response rates, validity of research methods and measurements, interpretation of data, application of research for improving the health of minority groups, and publication
- Be able to articulate an ideal approach to research with minority groups but adapt it in the light of financial and other constraints

9.1 Introduction: potential, limitations and pitfalls of ethnicity and health research

Research has permeated this book, because there is so much overlap between the practice and science of medicine, epidemiology, public health and health care delivery and also because the writer is a both researcher and a practitioner. The contents of Chapters 1, 2, 3, 5 and 6 are particularly relevant to research. In Chapter 8, I discussed aspects of the ethics of research in the context of policies and strategies. Overlap between this chapter and earlier ones is, therefore, inevitable. This chapter will draw together the challenges we face and the principles and methods that will help us overcome them. Among the challenges is the question of whether we need more or less research showing ethnic variations and this challenge is illustrated in the quotations opening this chapter.

A discussion of specific methods and how they can be utilized by ethnicity and health researchers requires a book on its own, however, many of the points incorporated in this book can be integrated with the methodological and conceptual ones in general research textbooks (though the challenges are not insubstantial). Above all this chapter aims to demonstrate the potential pitfalls in relation to the benefits of race, ethnicity and health research.

There are many motivations underlying research, and not all are laudable. Scientists aspire to discover the causes and processes of disease and such problems, while health policy-makers and planners need to meet the health and health care needs of ethnic minority groups. Additional motives for research include a wish to reverse the health and social disadvantages of ethnic minority groups, curiosity about racial and ethnic variations, and an unfortunate interest in ranking races/ethnic groups which can then be used to justify inequalities. The opportunities for research are huge, as illustrated by the migration study.

9.1.1 **The migration study**

The migration study, whereby migrants are tracked as they move from one place to another, helps separate the effects of environmental and genetic influences. Leaving aside problems of bias, and the difficulties of making comparable measurements across long distances and times, migration studies are a rich source of generating and testing hypotheses. Adding the ethnic dimension, where both the migrants and their offspring are compared to other ethnic groups within one territory, enriches the possibilities and potential. Changing circumstances within and between generations in different migrant and ethnic groups can be linked to changing health states. The message from many publications on ethnicity and health is that this wonderful opportunity must not be missed. In his book Henry Rothschild entitled a book chapter *Ethnic groups: a paradigm* and offered ethnicity as a paradigm for understanding diseases of complex aetiology (1981). Marmot *et al.*'s (1984) report *Immigrant Mortality in England and Wales* opens with the words 'Studies of mortality of immigrants are useful for pointing to particular disease problems of immigrants, investigating aetiology and validating international differences in disease.' Before we turn to the methods for achieving these goals, let us consider the pitfalls and limitations.

9.1.2 **Research, values, harm, and good**

Research of any kind, whether in the human population at large, the laboratory or on animals, is not a values-free activity. Values in research are particularly important when it is on living human beings, and arguably even more important when it compares and contrasts different human populations. Race and ethnicity, as variables that distinguish human populations, are extremely important to the structure and function of human societies, and it is inevitable that research utilising these concepts is of interest to, and has influence upon, social organization and will be interpreted to serve social goals. In the UK this is openly recognized by the Data Protection Act's recognition of race and ethnicity as sensitive data requiring particularly stringent control.

Before reading on try Exercise 9.1.

Exercise 9.1 Harm from research

◆ What kind of harm can you envisage from health research demonstrating ethnic and racial:
  (a) similarities
  (b) differences?
◆ Can you recall any examples of such harms, whether historical or contemporary?
◆ Why do you think such harm may occur? Is it inherent to the field of research or dependent on social context?
◆ Why do race and ethnicity still remain popular in population research?

Just as modern day work showing ethnic differences in the health status and health care of populations is mostly, but not always, used to further current social goals of equality and justice, much research in the past was used to further previous social goals such as the continuation of slavery, the justification of Empire, the maintenance of social and material inequality (including Apartheid in South Africa), anti-immigration policies in the USA focused on keeping out those who where not Northern Europeans, eugenics and the Nazi final solution (that included the intended extermination of Jews, the disabled, the mentally handicapped and gypsies). The most important lesson from this history is that research on race, ethnicity and health needs to be done within an ethical framework emphasizing the potential benefit primarily to the population studied. Benefits to the society at large are secondary benefits. Ethics in research was discussed within Chapter 8, and a more general consideration of ethics in relation to ethnicity and health is in Chapter 10.

Harm from ethnicity and health research is not inherent within the field, but dependent on social and political context. Just as differences can be (mis)used to bolster arguments justifying and promoting inequality, similarities can be used to ignore the needs of minorities. Researchers may find themselves in a quandary as emphasizing differences can lead to action and interest but can be harmful, while emphasizing similarities can lead to their work being ignored. The argument that past research has done harm can impede current proposals that aim to undo such harms. This argument has some value, not least in cautioning us on potential dangers, but it cannot be allowed to block ethical research.

Race and ethnicity are controversial and difficult epidemiological variables, as discussed in Chapter 1. They are, however, effective in contributing to a crucial aspect of the epidemiological and medical sociological strategy: demonstrating differences in health, disease and health care experience between populations, as discussed in Chapters 3, 5 and 6. Much research on ethnicity and health is epidemiological or sociological. Such research has two prime purposes: to describe the health status of ethnic minorities in the context of their life and environmental circumstances, and to use the information to redefine health policy and practice.

As illustrated in Chapter 8, by learning that CHD is common in migrant South Asian populations and that the relationship between the rate of heart disease and social class is both complex and shifting over time, we can develop policies to place CHD as a high priority for health care and health promotion, and target interventions by social and economic subgroups within the population. Simultaneously, we can use these observations to seek understanding of the mechanisms causing CHD. We might ask why heart disease is so high in a population originally from countries where heart disease was uncommon at the time of migration, and why it does not display the same social class gradient as in the general population. In the answers to such simple questions lie fundamental truths about the nature of disease. Clearly, description may lead to understanding of aetiology (cause); and understanding to better policy-making and practice.

Unfortunately, the two research purposes may become confused so that neither descriptive nor aetiological research are put to maximal effect. Research which cannot, on its own, lead to causal understanding, such as the estimation of disease prevalence and incidence (and the derived rates and ratios), has too often been over-interpreted to make causal inferences, and its true value in generating testable hypotheses, shaping health policy and improving practice has been ignored or overlooked in the excitement of premature causal analysis. The emphasis has been on comparing the health experience of the minority with that of the majority population, and not on the numbers of cases of disease or the derived rates. As discussed in Chapters 5 and 7, with this approach the data's power in shaping priorities and health strategies can be reduced.

Characteristically, writers of such descriptive studies on ethnicity and health have concluded by emphasizing over-optimistically the great potential of their findings for understanding fundamental causes of disease. Causal knowledge usually follows a spark of inspiration, which is pursued with detailed, painstaking and carefully planned research designed to test hypotheses. No amount of enthusiasm about ethnicity and health research can overcome this basic requirement and over-interpretation of data will impede progress.

Despite the promises of investigators, ethnicity and health studies have seldom produced novel understanding of disease causation. Very often they echo the findings of research on international variations, a field which is very well established.

9.1.3 Association and causation—black box epidemiology

Thousands of associations between racial and/or ethnic group and disease have been published with the expectation and proclamation that they will help in elucidating causation. Few variations have been explained in a way which gives new insight into causation. Most ethnicity and health research is black box epidemiology, described by the late scholar Petr Skrabanek (1994) as epidemiology where the causal mechanism behind an association remained unknown and hidden (black) but the inference was that the causal mechanism was within the association (box). The metaphor is derived from the modern electronic industry where the circuitry and components are packaged in a closed compartment. Users make no attempt to examine or understand the contents and even the mechanic is not expected to open the box and diagnose the problem. When problems occur the entire component is replaced. Skrabanek argued that science must open and understand the black box. He likened black box epidemiology to repetitively punching a soft pillow, and when the dimple refills, taking another blow, perhaps in a different place, but with the end result being the same.

Many studies, for example, have studied cancer patterns in immigrant populations internationally. Marmot et al.'s (1984) analysis of cancers in immigrants in England and Wales around the 1971 census period found many differences. Overall, immigrants had lower cancer rates although for specific cancers the picture was very varied. The authors' approach is illustrated by the emphasis on causal hypotheses. For example, they note high correlations in international data for cancers of the large intestine and female breast, and with both heart disease and fat consumption. Their observation of low rates for these two cancers in Indian immigrants, but high rates for heart disease, leads them to question the assumption that dietary fat is the common factor in cancer of the large bowel and breast, and they query whether the high fibre content of the Indian diet modifies the effect of fat on large bowel cancer. Balarajan et al.'s study (1990) around the 1981 census, of immigrant populations by region of origin also found many differences from which aetiological hypotheses were drawn. They urged that ethnicity and health data should be used to develop more.

Donaldson and Clayton (1984) found numerous ethnic differences in cancer registration patterns in the Leicestershire health district. The authors rightly concluded 'The results indicate the need for formal epidemiological study to test specific aetiological hypotheses which may account for these apparent differences.' This type of work has been repeated, for example, by Barker and Baker (1990) in Bradford, by Matheson and colleagues in Scotland (1985) and by Balarajan and Bulusu (1990) in England and Wales. Similar work has been done on children. The conclusion is almost predictable: differences exist and need detailed study. Sarah Wild and colleagues (including me) have published on the cancer data by country of birth around the 2001 census (2006). Again, we have shown marked variations. Unfortunately, the level of causal understanding is little more than in the 1971 analysis. The main difference is that the 2001 work puts more emphasis on the value of such data for policy, planning and health needs assessment.

There has been little progression in causal thinking, in my view, because few studies have explored the often ingenious and potentially invaluable ideas generated by observational epidemiology in the detail and over the very long timescales required. One illustrative exception is the study of diabetes and insulin resistance as potentially the basis of the surprisingly high rates of CHD in South Asian communities. The observation of Marmot *et al.*:

> This high rate of diabetes could contribute to the high rate of ischaemic heart disease in Indians. This explanation would then pose the problem of why immigrants from the Caribbean, with their high rate of diabetes do not also have a high rate of ischaemic heart disease.
>
> Marmot *et al.* (1984: 51)

has been pursued tenaciously. It turns out that this is probably a partial but important explanation but new avenues still need to be explored. The research effort around this question has been UK-led but has been international, and it has been ongoing for some 20 years. It will probably be another 10–20 years before we get a definitive answer.

For causal advances we need to move from the repetitious demonstration of disease variations which have previously been shown either in ethnicity and health research, or in work on international variations, or in social and gender variations and move to novel territory. Ethnicity and health studies are able to provide models and contexts for advancing aetiological knowledge if research questions are clearly articulated and pursued using sound methods. They do not provide, however, the easy route to causal understanding that some people have too often implied.

Of the medical sciences, with the possible exceptions of medical sociology and medical anthropology, the one that has grappled with ethnicity and race most seriously is epidemiology. As with other sciences epidemiology has been beguiled by ethnicity and race and has become racialized. Racialization consists of the idea that race is a primary, natural and neutral means of grouping humans, and that racial groups are distinct in other ways, e.g. their behaviours (see Chapter 10). (The equivalent for ethnicity would be ethnicisation, but racialization will do.) There are lessons to be learned from the racialized research of the nineteenth century.

9.2 **Race research and history: some lessons**

This book has been peppered with examples of research that has done harm, with some examples in Chapter 1 and Chapter 6. This chapter would be incomplete without a more detailed discussion, even at the risk of repetition.

Racialized research has an inglorious history, and many books have recorded in great detail the extent and depth of the work that has been done (see references on p316–318 e.g. Gould, Kiple, La Veist). Some important scientists of the nineteenth century, in particular, were focused on race, and their fascination was encouraged by influential and powerful politicians and social commentators. The power behind scientific racism is illustrated by the prowess of some of the researchers who included Louis Agassiz, Francis Galton, Paul Broca, and John Down (the details of their contributions are in the book The Mismeasure of Man by Gould and other volumes listed in the references). All four are men of huge scientific stature, often listed in even small contemporary encyclopedias.

In the nineteenth century, for example, Northern European scientists were ranking races on their biological and social worth, particularly using measurements of the size and shape of the head and the volume of the brain to measure intelligence (not surprisingly, the North European groups ranked high). Such research was useful to politicians to justify slavery, imperialism, anti-immigration policy, and the social status quo. After all, if this viewpoint on intelligence was true, and common sense and science seemed to coincide on this question, and North Europeans were indeed the most intelligent of humans their world dominance was inevitable and possibly even desirable and essential.

Similar arguments and data were used to analyse the role of men and women in society and justify the subordinate role of women. One underlying value of this research was that biology determined social position—biological determinism.

Medical practitioners were important contributors to racialized medical science. Diseases such as drapetomania (irrational and pathological desire of slaves to run away), and dysaethesia Aethiopica (rascality) were invented to describe the behaviors of slaves. Cartwright, who invented drapetomania, said in 1851, 'It is unknown to our medical authorities, although its diagnostic symptom, the absconding from service, is well known to our planters.'

To quote a textbook of obstetrics and gynaecology 'the pelves becomes increasingly lower and broader the more civilized the race from which it is obtained' and 'coloured children weigh considerably less than white, a fact which, in large cities at least, is indicative of the physical degeneration which characterises the race' (Whitridge Williams 1926). The words and tone (civilized, degeneration) display very clearly the writer's stance and the arrogance of the society he represented.

John Down's theory of 'mongolism' (Trisomy 21 or Down syndrome) published in 1867 was that such infants were from an inferior, Mongoloid, race. Down interpreted this in a positive and humanitarian way and proposed that this demonstrated the unity of the human species, i.e. the Europeans could give birth to children of another race. The example is an apt one because it shows the deeply ingrained thinking around race and inequality at that time.

Dr James McCune Smith, an African American but a glasgow, Scotland graduate of 1837, working in the USA argued that the environment, not innate biology, was responsible for health disparities, showing that poor White families had similar patterns of diseases as Black ones. Such challenges to biologically driven explanations for health inequalities are still needed. (See Krieger 2002).

Gamble (1993) has argued that the Tuskegee Syphilis study, discussed in Chapter 1, has left a legacy of mistrust that continues to undermine good medical practice. Gamble recounts Thomas Hamilton's experiments testing remedies for heat stroke and those of Dr J. Marion Sims on surgery for vesico-vaginal fistula, done on slaves.

Osborne's 1992 review of contemporary American health research on race and ethnicity concluded that much of it is racist in its effect if not in intention, for many projects focus on Black/White differences in diseases associated with promiscuity, under-achievement and antisocial behaviour and imply that the underlying explanation lies in race rather than class, lifestyle or socio-economic status.

The concept of a package of specific 'ethnic' diseases which are associated with ethnic minority groups, and therefore worthy of special study and exploration, has echoes in the history of medicine and racism. Negro susceptibility to particular diseases, such as leprosy, tetanus, pneumonia, scurvy, and sore eyes was, as Kiple and King argue, as misinterpreted (1981) and the differences, on which scientists' attention was riveted, led to nonsensical hypotheses on causation. Differences were used to strengthen the view that Blacks were different from Whites and that slavery was morally permissible.

Krieger *et al.*'s (1993) review of racism, sexism and class concluded that science was unable to explain a myriad of racial/ethnic differences in health. They criticized current models of ethnicity and health research which focus on racial differences but usually do not study racism.

The importance of race research and the innate inequality of races was considered self-evident in the nineteenth century. Few scientists questioned whether their work in this field was ethical. They could not be aware that such work would inspire Hitler, the Nazis and the Final Solution, but they would have been well aware of the contemporary effects and uses of their work.

With hindsight much past race-oriented science was unethical, invalid, racist and inhumane, though it was perceived to be of great importance. Moreover, there is absolutely no doubt that many medical practitioners and researchers were openly racists. In Chapter 6 I discussed how strongly the medical profession supported Hitler. The South African Medical Association colluded with the policies of apartheid in South Africa, not least through its the *South African Medical Journal*, as discussed by George Ellison and colleagues (1997). In April 2006 the Lancet published articles reopening the debate on whether racists who have distinction through eponyms should have, in retrospect, their names stripped from the disease or disorder they helped to define e.g. Reiter was a Nazi doctor known to have committed war crimes whose name is hallowed through its association with Reiter's syndrome (Woywodt *et al.* 2006).

In the last 50 or so years, the concept of race as a valid and important biological idea has crumbled under the impact of scientific and social assault. The idea of race is, however, far from extinct, and may be taking a new disguise. The application of the concept of ethnicity is often indistinguishable from that of race, with a heavy and unwarranted emphasis on genetics, which means that the same criticisms ought to apply. The recent book 'The Bell Curve' is a reminder that research which purports to demonstrate the innate inferiority, particularly in intelligence, of some racial groups continues and that race science is alive (Hernstern and Murray 1994). This is not to deny the possibility that some contemporary authors have good motives, which it seems less likely for nineteenth-century writers. The Times, one of the UK's most influential newspapers, published a letter in April 2006 from a number of distinguished scientists stating that racial differences in IQ are a matter of fact, and claiming that it is likely that the lower IQ of some races is genetic (Lynn 2006). The controversy simmers, but shows no signs of dying.

In taking their stance on these controversies researchers need an understanding of how race and health research was abused in the past. Epidemiologists who remain unpersuaded that racial prejudice could influence science in the modern era should read in detail about the Tuskegee Syphilis Study which examined the natural history of syphilis in 600 poor 'negroes' in Alabama between 1932–1972, actively denying them effective treatments and hastening many deaths. I introduced this study in Chapter 1 (Jones 1993).

I believe that few modern-day researchers in the field of ethnicity and health research are racist, and that most hold humanitarian views. Many researchers are working to a racialized research agenda (my own work is no exception). If most of the current work under way is in a future era judged as racist as well as racialized, future historians should remember that it was unwittingly so. It may be, however, that this defence also applies to much historical work, and it looks very weak now.

Our contemporary work may be seen in the future as being constrained within a framework of institutional racism in research, and as bolstering such racism. (See Chapter 6 for a discussion of various forms of racism.) Simply switching from race to ethnicity does not solve the problem. Applying these arguments to ethnicity, might our work be seen as 'ethnicized' research, and the fuel of 'ethnicism'? In a wide-ranging review of UK research through to the early 1990s, Jenny Donovan warned that we were heading this way:

> A great deal of the published research in this area has come from the medical profession, published in journals such as The Lancet, the British Medical Journal, the Proceedings of the Royal Society of Medicine, with very little contribution from the black population. Consequently, there has been a bias in the work, characterized by a concentration on illnesses and diseases that interest doctors, central Government and the health service administrators; rickets, tuberculosis and sickle-cell anaemia being examples. This concentration on 'interesting' or 'unusual' ailments has meant that the opinions of black people about their own health have been largely ignored, as have the obvious links between health and the large and growing literature on 'race relations', including levels of deprivation and racial discrimination experienced by black people in Britain.
>
> Donovan (1984: 663)

Certainly the UK's focus in the 1970s and 1980s on 'ethnic problems' such as the high birth rate, 'Asian rickets', the haemoglobinopathies, congenital defects and consanguinity, was at the expense of common problems such as CHD (now being tackled), smoking, alcohol, and cancer. Health education material for ethnic minority groups in the 1980s tackled birth control, lice, child care and even spitting but there was nothing on heart disease, and little on smoking and alcohol. In the 1990s through to the present day a better balance has been achieved.

Millions had their skulls measured by craniologists to no benefit either to themselves, their ethnic group or to society at large. As we have seen, there are many examples of abuse and harm. Yet health research based on race and ethnicity remains popular. As sizeable and potentially important differences by race and ethnicity have been easy to describe, the literature on ethnicity and health is growing rapidly. This trend will accelerate as more societies become multi-ethnic ones. Let us ensure that this accelerating research endeavour on race, ethnicity and health does not suffer the fate of nineteenth-century work.

A great deal of race, ethnicity and migration research is, in my view, unsound because the questions posed are not relevant or answerable or because the underlying theories, concepts, principles and methods are not adequate. There is a need for corrective action, of the kind documented by many scholars, but which has been too often evaded by researchers and editors alike. On pages 54 and 55 I gave guidelines produced by the *British Medical Journal*. An audit by George Ellison and colleagues of ethnicity and health research published in the *BMJ* in the years following this guidance showed that it was not followed (Personal Communication).

The remainder of this chapter will focus on good practice in research.

9.3 **Research: application of the concepts of race and ethnicity**

Try Exercise 9.2 before reading on (readers unfamiliar with research methods in epidemiology may want to read a little on that first—see Bhopal 2002, reference in Glossary section p316).

Exercise 9.2 Strengths and weaknesses of study designs

Choose a topic that interests you, and is relevant to ethnicity and health. What are the strengths and weaknesses of the following research methods in advancing ethnicity, race and health research in your chosen topic:

+ literature review and meta-analysis;
+ case reports;
+ clinical and population case series;
+ case–control studies;
+ cross-sectional studies;
+ cohort studies;
+ trials;
+ studies of genetic structure, family pedigrees and genetic associations?

There are many forms of research with distinct purposes, processes and outcomes. Neither the claims that ethnicity/race research is of great value, nor the criticisms, are likely to apply uniformly to all forms of research. My answer to Exercise 9.2 is summarized in Table 9.1.

Researchers must clarify the purpose for which the research is being done and carefully choose the research design, analysis and presentation to meet it. Sometimes there will be a need for a mix of methods and designs. Literature review is a starting point for all work, and preferably, it should be a systematic one whenever possible. Is your purpose to improve the quality of care? Then design a study around one of the priority issues such as communication between ethnic minority patients and professionals. Such a study is likely to include evaluation of the outcomes and an audit of whether standards of care are being met and improved. Perhaps you will conduct a trial as a definitive test of any intervention you recommend.

Is your purpose to measure how common risk factors or diseases are and to set priorities? Then measure their incidence or prevalence or both. The study is likely to be one based on routine statistics, or cross-sectional or cohort designs.

Do you wish to generate hypotheses about the cause of disease? Then read the literature in great depth, examine routinely published statistics and cross-sectional and cohort data for between—or within—group variations. That might be enough to develop some brilliant insight into causation, but in all probability it will not be. If not, undertake a hypothesis generating case–control study. You may, however, develop ideas from first principles and publish a data-free hypothesis paper. Now refine your hypotheses. List all your important hypotheses and gather detailed information to test or refute each one. You may need cohort study data to do this. Alternatively, test your hypotheses one by one using the experimental approach. There is no shortcut here! Expect to spend years or more probably decades before your hypotheses are accepted or rejected, though the latter result is usually much quicker.

Differences in disease patterns do not always yield testable hypotheses but even testable hypotheses have too often remained untested or been superficially examined. There are numerous disease patterns in the literature which have been little studied beyond the initial observation of ethnic difference even though they could be. Explaining them is just too difficult within the short time periods that most researchers devote to a project. One reason is the lack of long-term funding, as most projects are funded for three years.

Different forms of research may need, generate and apply different facets of the concepts of race and ethnicity. The racial and ethnic classifications required are also likely to vary according to the type of research. Finally, the type of research will determine the depth of inquiry into the specific characteristics underlying race and ethnicity. For illustration of these points, three forms of research are considered here: surveillance, health services research, and causal epidemiological research (introduced in Chapter 3 in less detail).

Before reading on try Exercise 9.3.

Table 9.1 Strengths and weaknesses of a number of methods of research in the context of ethnicity and health

Method	Strengths	Weaknesses
Literature review	Quick, brings experience from all over the world, cheap	Often no or weak literature by ethnic group for many topics; much work is unpublished or difficult to obtain; may be published in reports; may be in languages other than English so adding translation difficulties and costs; hard to generalize between studies because of different contexts and terminology; and may lead to biased conclusions and recommendations
Systematic review	As above, except that it is much more time-consuming, but in return this ensures work is comprehensive and minimizes biases	As above, and synthesis may be impossible for lack of work; lack of clarity in concepts and terminology; and heterogeneity of populations or study methods
Meta-analysis	Permits quantitative synthesis of key outcomes and relations between risk factors and outcomes	As above and may not be reported in a way that permits synthesis of questionnaire data; getting hold of original data may prove too difficult because researchers are scattered and not organized into cooperative groups
Case reports	Rapid highlighting of issues for fuller investigation	Likely to be on rare and obscure or exotic issues e.g. a case report is not going to be on lung cancer but may be on lead poisoning
Clinical series	As above, but brings together experience of a clinician. Rapid publication of admittedly selective statistics on large populations; gives overview of a clinical problem	As above, but more likely than a single report to be on matters of central importance
Population case series	As above but the series is of all the known experience in a defined area and population so less biased	The statistical summary is often not by ethnic group (for lack of ethnic coding); the information is limited; errors such as numerator/denominator mismatch
Case-control studies	Feasible at reasonable cost and timescales, particularly when based in places where ethnic minority populations are large	The number of cases (outcomes) of interest may be too small, particularly for studies of incident as opposed to prevalent cases; problem of identifying cases and controls by ethnic group in the absence of ethnic coding; recall bias may be great and medical records may be incomplete for recent migrants in particular
Cross-sectional studies	The most feasible design for new research and best for burden of risk factors and common disease	Needs a sampling frame so representative samples can be identified—these lists are not usually ethnically coded; response rates may not be consistent across ethnic groups
Cohort studies	Excellent for measuring incidence rates, survival and risk-factor outcome relationships.	Need to be large, long-term and so are very expensive. Hard to set up and maintain. Experience in such work is very limited worldwide
Trials	The definitive method for evaluation of drugs, services and public health interventions, especially if it is the placebo controlled, randomized design	For legal and ethical reasons trials are even harder to set up than cohort studies but otherwise have similar weaknesses. Multi-ethnic trials designed to compare effects by ethnic group are virtually unknown, with only two or three reported—all from the USA. The theoretical basis and need for such studies has not been agreed and is under intense debate
Genetic studies	These are necessary to quantify what we already know—that health states arise mostly from gene-environment interactions. The large family size and close family links (including consanguinity in some populations) makes ethnic minority populations attractive for such work	The techniques are evolving and the ideas are unfamiliar to all populations but particularly ethnic minority groups. There is the danger that these studies will focus on specific issues and stigmatize ethnic minority groups

---

Exercise 9.3 Applying concepts of race and ethnicity in research

◆ In what ways might the concepts of race and ethnicity be applied differently for:

monitoring/surveillance research?
research on the quantity and quality of care?
research trying to understand disease causation?

9.3.1 **Surveillance**

Surveillance is the analysis, interpretation and feedback of systematically collected data with methods distinguished by their practicality, uniformity and rapidity, particularly to detect change in the pattern of disease. In the context of race and ethnicity, the main objective of surveillance is to detect and track variations in the health of populations grouped by race or ethnicity. Of course, the data would, ideally, be used to monitor the impact of interventions to improve health and reduce variations. The idea of race is simpler than that of ethnicity and hence might be expected to be better suited to surveillance than ethnicity.

Surveillance systems do, in practice, usually use simple indicators such as colour (black/white), nationality (Indian/Pakistani), or country of birth as the foundations of their classification. In respect to self-reported race and ethnicity, current classifications in the USA and the UK are primarily based on the concepts underlying race i.e. colour and region of the world (continental grouping). We have already discussed the limitations of definition of race as a reflection of biology. These kind of categories are more a social and political statement than a biological one. Exactly the same applies to the category Hispanic, which is said to be an ethnic group. It is purportedly based on language (Spanish) but in effect it is a mix of region of origin, and history of living in a place under Spanish colonial rule. Generally, surveillance indicators, with the exception of Hispanic, are closely tied to the race concept. Other markers of population characteristics such as language or religious origin, more closely tied to the ethnicity concept, may also be used, but are rare.

Mostly, surveillance systems have adopted racial and ethnic classifications that were developed for political or health policy purposes. The Office of Management Budget classification, first published in 1977, dominates in the USA. Some databases sometimes report an even cruder classification of White and non-White.

Hahn and Stroup (1994) recommend that a surveillance category should be conceptually valid, measurable accurately, exclusive and exhaustive, meaningful to respondents, reliable, consistent, and flexible. They and others have questioned the conceptual validity of categories such as Hispanic, Latino and Asian but they have not criticized the category White. Bhopal and Donaldson (1998) have pointed out the severe limitations of White as a valid category. While the USA census has 10 subcategories for Asian or Pacific Islanders, it has none for White, which accounts for most of the population. The focus of surveillance is therefore, necessarily, on non-White minority groups. This is not justifiable rationally even in an anti-discriminatory policy, as some White populations may be disadvantaged e.g. not only those coming as refugees, particularly from non-English-speaking countries, but also economically disadvantaged populations.

Surveillance has been constrained by the need to use classifications used in censuses to obtain the population size (denominator of the rate) data so essential for constructing the rates and summaries of rates (such as SMRs) which are the basis of surveillance. If changes are to be made to surveillance systems, whichever race and ethnicity categories are used need to be amenable to matching to census codes.

For reasons of cost, simplicity and stability over time the classifications used in surveillance divide populations in a fairly crude way and continue to be based on the relatively narrow factors underlying the race concept rather than on the broader concepts underlying ethnicity. That said, the weaknesses of racial classifications, even for surveillance, are clear—for example, as discussed in Chapters 1 and 2, there is no objective, valid measure of a person's race, self-reporting of race varies over time, and there is no classification which copes well with those of mixed race. It would be unfortunate if the uses of these categories in pragmatic surveillance systems imply that they were in any sense fixed, natural, or scientifically validated. Future surveillance systems are likely to change to more specific variables, and to self-reported ethnic group (albeit from a limited set of categories).

9.3.2 Health services research

Unlike surveillance, health services research is not easily defined and it takes many forms. Essentially, it is about the organization, costs, effectiveness, quantity and quality of health services. Where health services research is examining issues of equity of access, utilization of care or the evaluation of policy, the racial and ethnic concepts to be used and classifications needed are likely to be similar to those for surveillance and subject to the same limitations and criticisms. However, even more so than for surveillance, heterogeneity within an ethnic category is a major limitation.

Consider the uptake of breast cancer mammography. The health services research question 'Is the programme being accessed by all racial or ethnic groups?' is akin to surveillance. There is an important difference, however, and that is of heterogeneity. Categories used in surveillance—perhaps sufficient to detect change—such as South Asian, Hispanic, Black etc. are unreliably crude in this health care context. The programme may be accessed well by South Asians, overall, but not well by an important subgroup such as, say, Bangladeshi Muslims. Nonetheless, in terms of answering this question and tracing progress, a relatively simple racial or ethnic classification would suffice. The South Asian group might be subdivided into Indian, Pakistani and Bangladeshi and perhaps also (or alternatively) by religion and language. A mix of racial and ethnic labels could be derived, the relevant data could be collected quickly and this research question could be answered.

When the issue is research for the development of new policy or to effect change, or the evaluation of the quality or effectiveness of care, a deeper understanding is necessary. The question here might be 'Why is breast mammography less well taken up by some racial and ethnic groups?' To understand why, say, the uptake of breast cancer mammography was low in the South Asian community, is a question which focuses on causes. Here issues such as the group's religious views, language of communication and beliefs about the importance of prevention, cancer and on the service become important. This is also the case, of course, for all populations, including White ones.

In addition, the attitudes and behaviours of service providers are crucial too. In so far as racial discrimination may play a role both the ethnicity and race of a group will be important. In exploring this question, then, crude indicators such as religion, colour or place of birth are no more than a means of identifying a problem and a way of deriving a sample for more detailed work which will include measuring directly those population characteristics thought to be encapsulated by race and ethnicity. Here, race and ethnicity are variables which, in themselves, generate little or no understanding of the problem and hence do not serve the purpose on their own. The 'black box' that is race and ethnicity needs to be opened to answer the causal question. This theme is developed below.

9.3.3 Causes of disease

As stated, this issue was introduced in Chapter 3. For research on disease causation the principles are the same as in the kind of health services research which seeks to understand why something happens. Here the question is 'Why is there variation in disease pattern by ethnic group?' The explanation is that either the variation is chance, artefact or real. If it is real either exposure to the risk (causal) factors varies by ethnic group or the effects of the risk (causal factors) differ.

Ethnicity and race are, without question, good markers (or indicators) of variations which merit investigation, and are excellent for identifying relevant populations. They are also appropriate for sparking hypotheses but are rarely in themselves the source of causal knowledge. The contribution of population sciences to scientific understanding of causation is too complex to do justice to it here, but it has been discussed in my book *Concepts of Epidemiology* (2002, p316). The process is a long and difficult one, starting with associations—links between risk factors and the diseases (or other health outcomes)—of interest. Mostly, the associations arise by chance or from errors and biases in the research methods. Confounding is a huge problem in population sciences where experiments are not possible. It arises when there are differences between populations that have not been fully controlled. The classic example is the observation that those who drink alcohol are more likely to develop lung cancer. There is an association between alcohol consumption and the disease, but is it causal?

Assume that we have assembled a group of male 50-year-old alcohol drinkers and compared them with male non-alcohol drinkers of the same age, and that there are no errors and the results are unlikely to have arisen by chance. What explanation is there except that alcohol causes lung cancer? Is it possible that alcohol drinkers are either more likely to be smokers or to be exposed to tobacco smoke? Perhaps, therefore, alcohol is not itself a cause of lung cancer but tobacco use is? This phenomenon is known as confounding.

The best way of controlling confounding is experimentation. We can imagine animal experiments where the effects of alcohol on lung cancer are studied. We can with more difficulty imagine experiments on humans too, either where people are given alcohol, or perhaps more likely, stopped from drinking alcohol, to see the effects on disease outcome (here lung cancer or its precursors, e.g. malignant change in cells). The comparison in the population sciences such as epidemiology is, ideally, between the population with the risk factor and exactly the *same* (so-called counterfactual) population without the risk factor. This is obviously impossible. Changing the exposure of one randomly chosen subgroup of the population in an experiment and comparing with a similarly chosen control group, where exposure has not been altered, comes close to the ideal but impossible comparison described above. In epidemiology experimentation with randomization of populations is problematic and mostly we make do with a similar population (not randomly chosen) without the risk factor. The similar population is called the control, or reference, or comparison population. This thinking in epidemiology is based on the idea of counterfactuals and has been discussed in the context of ethnicity and health by Kaufman *et al.* (1997).

In causal epidemiology race and ethnicity are treated as risk factors and potential causal factors. These are, as discussed in Chapter 1, also known as exposure variables, as opposed to outcome variables. The focus here is on differences between ethnic groups. The ideal (counterfactual) population does not exist i.e. the same population but without the race or ethnicity it has, but a different one! The risk factor (or exposure) of race or ethnicity cannot be manipulated or changed by the investigator, so no experimentation is possible. This is similar to age, sex and adult height, to take some examples, but different from drug use, exercise habits and alcohol use. It follows that establishing causation is going to be difficult: the variable is not open to manipulation and change by investigators.

The specific components of ethnicity are, however, more amenable to change, e.g. the diet (rapidly), religion (rarely), language (between generations and slowly within one). The closest model we can find in terms of a natural experiment in race is studying mixed race or ethnic group populations (admixture studies). The admixture studies tend to be associated with genetics and put an emphasis on the genetic underpinning of racial and ethnic variations in disease. It is hard to predict where this kind of research will lead us, but hopefully it will not return us to the dark days of race as biology. One of the most influential ethnicity and health researchers in the UK, Paul McKeigue, is developing this field, and the quotations are illustrative of his thinking.

> When migrant groups living in the same environment have different disease rates that are not accounted for by adjusting for known environmental determinants of disease risk, genetic explanations should be considered. Genetic explanations are most likely where differences in disease rates persist even in migrants who have been settled outside the home country for several generations and where such differences are consistently found in all countries where the migrant group has settled. On these criteria, genetic factors are likely to underlie the high rates of coronary heart disease and non-insulin-dependent diabetes that have been reported in people of South Asian (Indian, Pakistani, Bangladeshi, and Sri Lankan) descent settled overseas.
>
> McKeigue (1997: 189)

If suitable markers can be identified, this analysis shows that linkage-disequilibrium mapping in recently admixed populations has much greater power than allele-sharing designs to detect loci contributing to ethnic differences in disease rates. With realistic sample sizes it is possible to detect loci that would account for one-third to one-half of the observed ethnic differences in prevalence of conditions such as hypertension, non-insulin-dependent diabetes, or obesity.

McKeigue (1997: 195)

Most ethnicity and health research is non-experimental, and is not using admixture type approaches. So, what is to be the control group? In practice, the control is another racial or ethnic group, but we already know that this does not come close to a true control, i.e. the counterfactual population. First, the control group cannot be without the risk factor (the particular ethnic or racial group), and second, the ethnic and racial group signals a multiplicity of differences. It is not possible to control confounding in these circumstances. This does not mean that race and ethnicity have no role to play in the causal endeavour of medical sciences, but it does mean that there are limitations that are both theoretically grounded and that create enormous practical problems.

Since all disease arises from the interaction of the genome, the human and the environment, in causal research both the concepts of race (as biology) and ethnicity are of interest. Historically, the role of biology has been invoked too readily as the prime explanation for racial differences. For example, as mentioned in Chapter 1 and earlier in this one, in the nineteenth century inherited biological susceptibility was wrongly assumed to be a prime explanation for syphilis, tuberculosis, conjunctivitis and nutritional disorders in African-Americans. Unfortunately, contemporary research also gives prominence to genetic explanations and downplays environmental (and especially economic) ones. To take one modern example, the high rates of hypertension in African-origin populations are widely attributed by medical scientists and clinicians to genetic and related biological factors with comparatively little attempt to test other explanations. The role of genetics in explaining hypertension in African-origin populations is slowly being clarified but nonetheless needs to be studied along with environmental and social factors, including the experience of racism. New studies across the globe, led by Richard Cooper (Cooper *et al.* 1997), are contradicting the emphasis on genetics by showing that there is a tremendous variation in blood pressure in African-origin populations across the world, and that their blood pressure is by no means uniquely high, being lower than some European populations.

To contribute usefully to hypothesis generation and testing requires measuring directly the components of the concepts which define a population group's race and ethnicity. The black box needs to be opened. This time, unlike in most health services research, this will include genetic studies. The approach to genetics that needs to be taken is exemplified in the quotation below, which is one of a number of recommendations made by the authors.

Race/ethnicity should not be used as a proxy for genetic variation. Statements about genetic differences should be supported by evidence from gene studies. Genetic hypotheses should be firmly grounded in existing evidence, clearly stated, and rigorously tested.

Kaplan and Bennett (2003: 2712)

Table 9.2 Categorizing and analysing the factors which may underlie an epidemiological variable: the example of ethnic differences in stroke disease

Category of potential explanatory underlying difference	Example of possible specific differences by ethnic group	Implications for data collections
Biological	Unique variants of human genes, or varying frequencies of such variants (polymorphisms) lead to different biochemistry of physiology	Collect biological data including DNA, blood and other tissues
Co-existing diseases	One ethnic group may have more or less of another disease which raises or reduces the risk of stroke disease e.g. diabetes	Collect clinical data, including appropriate diagnostic tests
Behavioural	An ethnic group may eat more fruits, vegetable and salads than another, and perhaps smoke less	Collect data on behaviours relating to health
Social	Members of an ethnic group may spend less time with friends and family, and other social networks, so increasing psychosocial strain	Collect psychosocial data as potential explanations
Occupational	The pattern of working, including likelihood of employment, the hours worked and the type of occupations is substantially different	Collect data on employment histories
Economic	Members of an ethnic group may earn less than the average	Collect data on differences in wealth and their effect on lifestyles and stress
Health care	Members of an ethnic group may be treated differently from the expected standard by health care professionals	Collect date on quality, quantity and timing of health care interventions

The first step in bioscience may indeed be work using racial and ethnic categories but it needs to move to the next step rapidly. The study of heart failure in African-American populations has caused huge controversy and this will need genetic studies to resolve, as the investigators have concluded.

> Our finding of the efficacy of isosorbide dinitrate plus hydralazine in black patients provides strong evidence that this therapy can slow the progression of heart failure. A future strategy would be to identify genotypic and phenotypic characteristics that would transcend racial or ethnic categories to identify a population with heart failure in which there is an increased likelihood of a favourable response to such therapy.
>
> Taylor *et al.* (2004: 2055)

Table 9.2 illustrates the approach I am recommending using the example of ethnic variations in stroke.

Overall mortality rates and life expectancy differ among racial and ethnic groups living in the USA and Britain. Far Eastern origin populations do well. Are these differences attributable to genetic or environmental factors? Until genetic studies of ageing demonstrate otherwise, the differences ought to be largely attributed to environmental and social factors. The mortality differences might be partly attributed to excesses of specific diseases, for which the biology and hence genetic basis is better understood than for ageing. To continue with the example of breast cancer, the mortality rate differs greatly by country of birth group in England and Wales as shown most recently by Wild and colleagues. The rate was comparatively low in South Asian, Chinese and East European-born, and high in North and West African-born groups. Since genetic factors are a demonstrated cause of breast cancer, it is important to ask whether such differences are attributable to genetic differences. It is imperative that the question is answered by direct measurement of the presence or absence of the relevant gene variants. The race and ethnicity of the population give no clue (at least to date) to their risk of possessing the causative genes linked to breast cancer, for the (few) genes which are responsible for the anatomic features which underlie the racial or ethnic classifications give no indirect clue as to the distribution of breast cancer-causing genes. In future, when a large number of specific disease genes are identified and the population distributions are more precisely known, this general principle may change.

The difference in breast cancer might arise from other factors which vary across the groups, e.g. diet, economic circumstances, environmental pollutants, contraception, and the age at first pregnancy. These are a few of the many social and environmental factors which have biological consequences. Again, the racial and ethnic group gives no direct information on these factors at the individual level though the population distribution is better known than for genetic variants. Information on such social factors needs to be collected directly and not assumed.

For causal analysis in this context biological, environmental and social factors need to be directly measured, both as potential contributors to the causal pathway and as confounding variables.

9.4 Undertaking research on the health of ethnic minorities: back to basics

Try Exercise 9.4 before reading on.

Exercise 9.4 Challenges for researchers and balancing ideals with practicalities

- What particular challenges do ethnicity and health researchers face when setting research questions, defining concepts, recruiting populations, asking questions, calculating rates, interpreting data, publishing and acting on the results?
- What can researchers do to overcome these challenges?
- What ideals may need to be sacrificed to make research practical and which ideals are sacrosanct?

The ideal research study in a multi-ethnic society would include all ethnic groups, have uniformly high response rates, provide data that are comparable across all groups, collect information on all facets of ethnicity, include data on all potential confounding variables and be analysed and interpreted in a way that both advances science and develops better health care. In practice many of these ideals are sacrificed to make the study feasible. In making pragmatic choices researchers should make themselves and their audience aware of the limitations of the work. Research on the health of ethnic minorities will not pay the dividend either in better services, or in yielding insights about the causes of disease, if the basic principles of research are breached. These basic principles are reviewed below although many of them have been covered already.

9.4.1 Define the question, aims, purpose and relevance of the research

Good research starts with clear-cut and unbiased research questions, explicit aims and specific, measurable, achievable, relevant and timely—SMART being the acronym—objectives. The way to formulate these is fundamental to guidance on how to do research but readers will need to access research textbooks (see references e.g. Bowling and Ebrahim 2006). The key point, from this book's perspective, is that the questions, aims and objectives must be designed to benefit and not harm ethnic minority groups. If there is to be a bias, then it should be anti-racist and anti-discriminatory to help balance past injustices. Neutrality, if it can be achieved at all (and most philosophers and researchers on the nature of science tend to the view it cannot be), is the ideal stance for good research.

The underlying purpose of the research— e.g. whether it is for health care planning or to enhance causal understanding of the causes of disease—guides the design and detail of the study, analysis of data, and the presentation and publication of the results. These twin objectives are rarely accomplished by one set of data analyses, or even by the one study, and then only if the investigator is equally interested in achieving both. For example, if the aim is to understand the causes of cancer then listing the standardized morbidity/mortality ratios or the incidence rates by ethnic group is of limited value. At best this would yield hypotheses for future study. Disease incidence lists are of value to the health planner, but only if the population studied is representative and the data are presented so as to highlight needs and priorities. Rankings of mortality and morbidity rates and years of life lost serve this purpose admirably but summary statistics of relative frequency (e.g. SMR) do not. The principles have been discussed in Chapters 6, 7 and 8 (readers can consult Bhopal, Concepts of Epidemiology, 2002—see p316).

Whatever the purpose, the research questions need to be credible to funders, study populations, journal editors and readers. Major research projects in the population sciences need to be on the important causes of death, disability or illness within ethnic minority communities, not on interesting cultural quirks, however tempting these are. It is easy to be sidetracked into the mode of thinking that all differences are interesting and that similarities are boring. My first proper research project in 1984 fell into this trap—I was misled into thinking that traditional medicines were very important in South Asian communities in Glasgow, Scotland. It was very interesting work for me and it led to publications (Bhopal 1986a and b) and useful experience. Only later did I realize that I was delving into a minor issue. In the small scale survey I did (100 people) the importance of diabetes was brought to my attention by several respondents but my mind was unprepared. At about the same time Mather (1985) and colleagues published their landmark paper showing diabetes in UK South Asians was about four times commoner than in the population as a whole. I had been sidetracked!

9.4.2 Definition of concepts and precision of terms is essential

Chapters 1 and 2 provide information relevant to this section.

Try Exercise 9.5 before reading on.

Exercise 9.5 The need to explain concepts and devise classifications

◆ Why do researchers need to specify and explain their use of the race and ethnicity concepts?

◆ Why should they devise their own classifications of race and ethnicity?

◆ In practice, why are they limited in their inventiveness in devising classifications?

Researchers need to make explicit how they are using the concepts of ethnicity and race, and should adapt classifications and methods of assessing ethnicity to the research questions under study. Researchers should not always be constrained by available classifications designed for administrative purposes. They need to explain in some detail what they are doing and why, and writing as if the text was for a reader in another country and time would help. The current terminology used to describe ethnic minority populations (Hispanics, Asians, Blacks, Whites, Chinese etc.) may suffice for everyday conversation or political exchange but is too crude for scientific studies. An internationally agreed vocabulary is the ideal. In its absence researchers should use either existing glossaries such as the one here—based on the one I published in the *Journal of Epidemiology and Community Health* (Bhopal 2004) or supply their own, if not in their publication then on a web site.

This encouragement to inventiveness in regard to classifications should not be seen as an invitation to violate common sense. Researchers should not invent ethnic groups or create irrational labels e.g. the use of the word Urdus to denote an ethnic group based on the language Urdu, or the phrase Chinese and Asian. Equally, it is not sensible to try to use the word Indian to include all South Asians for political and other reasons of great importance e.g. Bangladeshis, Pakistanis and Sri Lankans are not Indians (even although they have been at times in the past). Similarly, researchers have a misleading tendency to treat Africans from Africa and those from the Caribbean as one. They also have a tendency to treat all Africans as one, which they clearly are not. It is not sufficient for researchers to simply inform the readers that they are misusing concepts in these ways! It is disrespectful to the populations studied if terms used by researchers misrepresent them. The definition of terms aims to make the work of researchers and practitioners, as well as readers, easier and better. As such, definitions should be agreed in advance of the research, not in retrospect.

9.4.3 **Denominators and numerators need to match to calculate rates**

Issues relevant to this section were discussed in Chapters 2, 3 and 5. The census is the essential resource for denominators for most population-based research, and nearly all work that is based on vital statistics. The census also paints the backdrop for all forms of research that require an understanding of the size and composition of the population. However, for ethnic minority communities the accuracy of the denominator may be questioned for several reasons, including frequent travel abroad, difficulties in the completion of forms, non-completion, and errors in some details e.g. age. Further, the numerator for disease may also be inappropriate and, in particular, be inflated by the inclusion of visitors.

Name searching is currently a popular tool among researchers. This tool is usually applied only to derive the numerator from health status and disease outcome databases. The denominator usually remains that obtained from the census, thus creating a serious mismatch and source of error. The error is an elementary one, but presumably researchers cannot find another solution. Name searching the census would not be an easy task, but it is the logical action to derive a more valid denominator. These questions of the accuracy of denominators and numerators are fundamental but are rarely studied in the detail required. Researchers need awareness of these matters for they are of great importance to them and to health needs assessors.

9.4.4 **Ensure that there is comparability of populations: the confounding variable**

The concept of confounding was discussed above. To infer that a disease is commoner in one ethnic group as compared to another requires, at the very least, that the two groups are comparable in terms of age and sex. To go further and attempt to ascribe the differences to cultural or genetic factors requires that the explanation does not lie in other domains eg. socio-economic status. The onus is on the researcher to tease out the reasons for the differences observed. This is not easy, so as a minimum, the favoured explanation needs to be set in the context of alternatives.

If causal understanding is to result from studies, painstaking attention to the characteristics and comparability of the populations under study will be necessary; much more so than in studies comparing subgroups of one ethnic group, where it may sometimes be reasonable to accept broad comparability, say on religion or diet, although even then it is better to assume heterogeneity. As already discussed the problem of confounding is great in epidemiology, with the exception of large randomized trials. Researchers need a high degree of awareness that control of confounding will be incomplete (technically, that there will be residual confounding). Inferences can change radically once interacting and confounding factors are accounted for. Lillie-Blanton *et al.* (1993) challenged the observation that crack cocaine smoking was commoner in African-Americans and Hispanic Americans, showing that once social and cultural environmental factors were accounted for there were no differences.

9.4.5 Identification of representative populations

Researchers who are knowledgeable about the ethnic groups under study are more likely to be trusted and more likely to achieve the high response rates and informed consent that are essential to studying representative populations. Recruitment is achievable although it would be wrong to imply it is easy. A review of the evidence came to these conclusions.

> It is widely believed that racial and ethnic minorities are less willing to participate in health research. Such claims often focus on the US, where it is believed that minority groups' relative unwillingness to participate in health research traces to historic abuses, especially the notorious Tuskegee Syphilis Study. We found that racial and ethnic minorities in the US, particularly African-Americans and Hispanics, are as willing to participate, and in some instances more willing to participate, in health research than non-Hispanic whites, when eligible and invited to participate.
>
> Wendler *et al.* ((2006: 8)

> There are now sufficient examples of studies on marginalised communities that clearly show that it should really be possible to engage with people, irrespective of their ethnic background, and encourage them to participate in research that is ultimately in their and/or their community's best interests. What is now needed is less blame directed at already marginalised people. Instead, those with the power to change the way in which research is conducted should translate the important insights provided by Wendler and colleagues' study into significantly more invitations extended to minority ethnic and racial groups to participate in the research endeavour.
>
> Sheikh (2006: 1)

The truly representative ethnic minority population sample would be nigh impossible to obtain, unless the sampling was linked to the census, which in turn would need to be correct and up to date. The validity of the convenience samples we use in practice needs study, and the likely error measured. Ecob and Williams' (1991) work in the MRC Medical Sociology 'Asian' lifestyle and health study has shown that there are substantial differences between people who live in areas where the proportion of the ethnic minority population is high and those who live elsewhere. Such studies of methods are all important. Inner city populations are different from whole population samples, but ethnicity and health studies continue to focus on them for convenience. In the very important, and at the time ground-breaking, Health Education Authority survey the comparison population, unlike the ethnic minority populations, was not an inner city sample. Lessons have been learned and implemented in the Policy Studies Institute Study (Modood *et al.* 1997) and Health Survey for England (1999 and 2004 sweeps (see websites p348)) where time- and resource-consuming approaches to sampling from low ethnic minority concentration areas were used.

There are several ways of sampling (all with drawbacks) depending on the type of information that is required. One can take a random sample of people listed on a population register (e.g. electoral roll, municipal register, health service registration). Alternatively one can sample people who have used a service using admission, discharge or consultation registers. More informal networking can be used to find people. The populations assembled in the latter way may be culturally homogeneous, already know each other and therefore comfortable with the situation, and trust the researchers. The commonest method, particularly for small scale work, is to use the register of a community organization e.g. the Chinese/Bengali/Indian/Vietnamese Association.

Unless the study is set in a place where the ethnic minority group of interest is a substantial proportion of the population, a truly random sample might yield few people in that ethnic group. The answer here is a stratified sample i.e. the list of people potentially eligible for study (the sampling frame) is organized by the factor of interest (here ethnic group) and samples are taken from the relevant sections. Sampling frames that hold information by ethnicity are rare, so such reorganization of lists is problematic. Proxy indicators such as country of birth are more likely to be on sampling frames than ethnic group, and in many places using them is the easiest option.

Organizing the list by name is another partial solution—the limitations were discussed in Chapter 3. Sampling by name works for some groups. The South Asian and Chinese populations do have fairly distinctive names which are being retained across generations. Names have even been used to identify Irish people in Scotland. Analysis of names can help define, though far from perfectly, groupings based on religion and language. This technique relies on using the knowledge and skills of trained staff. The characteristic and distinctive nature of the surnames of Urdu, Punjabi, Hindi and Gujarati speakers permits this approach. Muslim names are similar across the world and names are common to Sikhs and Hindus. My name, Raj Bhopal, is recognizably Indian, but most knowledgeable observers would think it to be of a Hindu. My full name is, however, Rajinder Singh Bhopal. The first name identifies me clearly as Punjabi and probably a Sikh, as the ending 'inder' is adopted by Sikhs. The middle name Singh is adopted for Sikh men (women are Kaur), although it is not unique to Sikhs. Bhopal is a rare Indian surname but is immediately recognizable as Indian because there is a city called Bhopal (and formerly there was a State). The region of family origin for this name is, nonetheless, likely to be Punjab because of the first and second names and the language most likely to be associated with it is Punjabi. The religion is almost certainly Sikh. This example illustrates how much information there is in a name. The name Macdonald, alone, tells you the holder has Scottish origins, is likely to be a protestant Christian and speaks English. Of course, these guesses could well be wrong, but they are a fair starting point. Occasionally, South Asian names, particularly among Christian Indians, are similar (if not identical) to traditional names. Name analysis is not reliable as a tool for identifying people of African-Caribbean origin.

One major problem with sampling from population registers is that often the addresses (and sometimes names too) listed are incorrect. Accuracy of information for ethnic minority groups, who are relatively mobile, is usually worse than in the population as a whole. Addresses on such lists may need to be cross-checked against manual or computerized records e.g. in the telephone book or the electoral register, the list of people eligible to vote in local and national elections. Of course, these other sources of information may also be wrong.

Although health services may be required to collect ethnic status of users, many do not have accurate data.

Another approach is to ask people using a service to provide their ethnic group and use this newly collected information to select a sample. Although it is not currently judged as best practice the investigator can select people on the basis of observation—whether of physical features, clothing or other markers or ethnicity. It would be presumptuous for the investigator to assume ethnicity using these markers. As a first step, however, in identifying people who can then be asked about their ethnicity this may well be pragmatic and justified.

Where an ethnic minority group is hard to contact and recruit, and no reasonable lists of contact details exist, the so-called snowball technique can be used. The phrase is a metaphor based on the observation that rolling a snowball down a hill makes it bigger as it accumulates more snow around it.

In the *Bristol Black and Ethnic Minorities Health Survey Report* (Pilgrim and colleagues 1993) the Caribbean/African origin respondents were the most difficult to contact and the 'snowball' method of sampling was used, with some success. In this method an initial group of people already known to the researchers are asked to start a chain of contacts, i.e. each respondent is asked to give names and addresses of other potential participants. These people are then approached and invited to take part in the research. They in turn are asked to supply more names.

A mix of pragmatic approaches may be needed to recruit study participants in multi-ethnic studies, as illustrated below.

A needs assessment on the family planning and sexual health needs of the Chinese living in Kensington, Chelsea and Westminster was undertaken by the London Chinese Health Resource Centre with the aim of assessing the level of needs of the Chinese around the issues of sexual health and family planning. A quota sample size of 200 was established, representing 5 per cent of the total population of Chinese residents over the age of 16 years, in the boroughs of Kensington and Chelsea and the City of Westminster. Field interviewing was used to obtain as accurate and complete a response to the sensitive nature of the questionnaire as possible. Respondents were located and interviewed at Chinese community centres, libraries, student centres, tube stations, women's group sessions, and other locations.

London Chinese Health Resource Centre 2005

The possibility that there may be differential response rates to both self-report (and other forms of measurement) is an obvious consideration. The biases of non-response are difficult to judge but non-response makes representativeness of samples hugely difficult. There is evidence that those who participate are different from those who do not, although in some studies the differences have been modest. I am not aware of studies examining response biases by ethnic group. It is likely, though to be verified, that as in most studies, non-responders in minority ethnic groups are likely to have a different profile than responders.

Response to one aspect of a study may not lead to response to another component. This kind of bias is easier to examine. In the above-mentioned multi-ethnic Health Survey for England, 1999, for example, the response rate to the questionnaire, was in relation to other ethnic groups, higher in Bangladeshis but participation in the physical measures and blood sample components of the study was comparably lower. This also adds to the problem of non-representativeness.

9.4.6 Data collection methods should be valid and cross-culturally equivalent: questionnaires and focus groups

The art and science of data collection is well developed and interested readers should consult textbooks (see references (including Bowling and Ebrahim 2006)), as here we can only touch upon the issues that are particularly pertinent to ethnicity and health research. In Chapter 3 the principles for maximizing cross-cultural validity of questionnaires were considered. Here we consider some of the issues in a study setting.

Ethnicity and health researchers are challenged to fill huge gaps in knowledge rapidly, and their studies are sometimes highly ambitious. Box 9.1 summarizes the span of self-report data, and methods used, in a study in the late 1980s by Williams and colleagues in Glasgow (1993).

Box 9.1 The span of interview data collected by Williams *et al.* and methods

Information was collected by interview-administered questionnaire on current and past health, physical measures of health, perceived health, health beliefs, health care, medications, and health-related lifestyle issues including smoking, exercise, drinking and diet, stress and other aspects of mental health. Additionally, details of origins, education, occupation, housing, household organization, child rearing, family support and religion were collected.

Dietary questions were designed to reveal broad patterns of food choice and frequency of consumption. Stress measures reflected the common division of the field into: (1) structural inequalities, which may or may not give rise to 2; (2) stressors (usually negative events or chronic strains); (3) mediators (usually coping resources or social support); and (4) stress outcomes (usually perceived distress). The focus was on structural inequalities in work, finance and housing, on possible chronic strains arising, on events involving violence, damage or perceived racial discrimination, and on social support (as a mediator often compromised by migration). The questionnaires were pre-translated from English into Urdu, Hindi and Punjabi by an educational psychologist fluent in all four languages. The quality of the translation was tested by the translator and another polylingual interviewer piloting the schedules, and by further discussion with a bilingual doctor (i.e. me) and other bilingual interviewers who between them covered all the languages concerned. Interviewers for the South Asian sample were all literate in English and in at least one of the three South Asian languages concerned, and were given a week's interview training and a further week's close individual supervision.

This study was a cross-sectional survey of about 200 South Asians sampled from the publicly available electoral register and local tax payers register and identified by name. The comparison group was a sample of the general population (predominantly White). The challenges of the study and particularly of ensuring cross-cultural validity are self-evident. These challenges are not confined to self-report but also to other types of data, e.g. anthropometric measurements and laboratory tests, though the problems there are less acute. The challenges of preparing validated questions are well known but to ensure they retain their meaning on translation and are suitable for several ethnic groups is a formidable undertaking, particularly for lengthy questionnaires in several languages as used by Williams and colleagues (1993).

As language barriers are common, the self-completion questionnaire may be unsuitable in multi-ethnic studies. The face-to-face interview, using professional interviewers, is the main alternative but it leaves the problems of finding and training appropriately qualified staff, and of high cost. (Interviews are about 10 times more expensive than self-completion methods.) Other models, e.g. computer, video, and audiotape-based interviews have promise but have not been widely tested (they need to be).

To gather self-report information on populations two main methods can be used—questionnaires (self-completion or interview) and focus groups. Focus groups are an effective way of allowing themes to be explored in an interactive way that cannot be achieved using questionnaires alone. Indeed such discussions are often a prerequisite for developing the questionnaire. Hanna and colleagues (in press; report on ASH Scotland website—see p344) have demonstrated the value of group work, in addition to individual interviews, in developing a questionnaire in several languages.

Translation of questionnaires is crucial for the successful collection of information on the health of minority ethnic groups, particularly those whose primary language is not English. Issues such as using words, phrases and accents (whether in English or not) appropriate for the community under study also need to be taken account of, particularly for interviews.

Respondents may not share common assumptions about health and well-being which underlie survey questions. Ethnic minority population usually comprise a mix—some preferring English, others not; some holding health beliefs very different from the majority, others with identical ones. In most research on ethnicity and health we accept participants' preferences even though from a methodological perspective we know that this is not ideal. In practice many people will, given a choice, use a mix of English and non-English, even when their knowledge of one language is superior. For example, I am much more familiar with English than Punjabi. If, however, there was a question on the properties of food described in English as hot/cold (not referring to temperature but to intrinsic properties of the ingredients), I would prefer the Punjabi equivalent words 'garam' (warm/hot) and 'thandha' (cold) because they convey the non-thermal meaning more clearly to me, simply because this variance in meanings is ingrained in the language (Bhopal 1986b).

In devising questionnaires, researchers should beware of using jargon, colloquialisms and sayings that are idiosyncratic to the English language, and it may be more appropriate to adopt a simple and descriptive question in order to minimize misinterpretation.

It is important for translations to be consistent. Some pointers to translating questions can be found in the *Bristol Black and Ethnic Minorities Health Survey Report* (Pilgrim *et al.* 1993) and an extract is in Box 9.2.

Box 9.2 Translating the interview schedule—example taken from the *Bristol Black and Ethnic Minorities Health Survey Report*

A variety of difficulties were dealt with in translating the interview schedule into Urdu/Punjabi, including:

♦ There is no equivalent word but the concept is clear, e.g. 'inpatient' is replaced by the Urdu phrase 'a stay in hospital';

♦ An equivalent word exists but is obscure or not easily understood by respondents (technical jargon etc.), e.g. 'cervical smear test': interviewers were told to ask initially using the English phrase. Many respondents replied by saying they did not understand. Therefore an explanation was given. 'The passage whereby you have a child, the doctor takes a sample from there to analyse for cancer.'

♦ There is no equivalent concept in Urdu/Punjabi-speaking culture e.g. 'social life' is replaced by the Urdu phrase 'meeting and interacting with people'.

♦ The concept is clear but the expression is culturally inappropriate, e.g. 'female doctor' is translated as 'lady doctor'.

♦ Both Urdu and English terms are commonly used, e.g. 'dentist', 'optician': here both the English and Urdu terms were used to ensure that there was no misunderstanding.

♦ The concept is difficult to convey in both English and Urdu, e.g. the concept of 'ethnic identity' is difficult in any language. For the Urdu version it was necessary to be specific and to ask directly if people saw themselves as Pakistani, Asian, Black etc.

Pilgrim *et al.* (1993)
(Adapted by author)

In devising and translating questions researchers need to be conscious that they may be interpreted quite differently by different ethnic groups, either because of subtle problems with translation or underlying concepts. Hanna and colleagues (in press) have explored this in a detailed study of a questionnaire focusing on tobacco related behaviours. The difficulties were numerous, and ranged from technical—the written and spoken language is different as in Cantonese, or there is no written language as in the Sylheti dialect of Bangla, itself the Bangali version of the language of Bangladesh—to conceptual—conveying the idea of a pipe or cigar in languages where there is no culture of using tobacco in these forms—to practical—gaining the involvement of lay members of the community in the process of establishing face validity of questions. The questionnaires were created in English, Punjabi, Urdu, Sylheti (written in English alphabet with Sylheti words), and Cantonese (written in the Chinese spoken form). These questionnaires are for use at interview.

The questionnaires used in ethnicity and health research tend to contain a mix of question types. There are three main types of questions—structured, semi-structured and open-ended, all of which can be asked by self-completion or at interview. The advantage of self-completed questionnaires is that people can consider questions carefully in their own time. They may also be less embarrassed about including details around personal issues. However, these require both familiarity with this format and good reading skills. Interview-based questionnaires allow the interviewer to ask the questions and convey the meanings of questions if they are not fully understood (possibly in an alternative language). The interview has great advantages when the study subjects do not read and write the language well. The interviewer must be trained rigorously or major biases can occur. Such biases will be easier to detect if the interview is tape recorded and not simply summarized by the interviewers, but that adds very considerable cost and complexity to an already difficult research task, particularly in large studies.

These methods also have fundamental drawbacks, e.g. both interviews and question-naires are subject to the problem of discrepancy between public and private accounts in that the respondent gives the answer that is perceived as acceptable, possibly desirable, in the circumstances. The more honest, but less acceptable, answer may be reserved for private discussions. These private accounts can sometimes be accessed by skilled interviewers over a series of interviews. The answers will also depend on how the respondent interprets the question. For this reason, questions should be kept simple whenever possible.

The researchers must also remember the social aspects of the interview situation, e.g. people from some cultures may find it rude not to be engaged in some polite formalities or to have their own questions, whether about the research or personal ones about the researchers and their families, ignored.

In focus groups people are gathered together (perhaps grouped according to sex, ethnic background etc.) and questions are put to them, e.g. what do you think of local hospital services? The people are then encouraged to talk in their own language if desired, to discuss issues and exchange experiences. Through these discussions, themes emerge and often rich and vivid stories of how people have interacted with health services are drawn out. A facilitator is present to keep the discussions relevant to the topic and the group views are collected through open-ended questions. The facilitator uses a topic guide. A questioning route is prepared which will allow for flexibility within the research. Box 9.3 is an example of a questioning route which was used in five focus group meetings held to assess the impact of cardiovascular disease and diabetes in the Chinese and South Asian communities in Newcastle (Elliot 1997).

The focus group gives insight into the attitudes, beliefs and behaviours of a group. The group is 'focused' in the sense that it involves a collective activity, such as discussing health beliefs. One of the advantages of focus groups is the capacity to exploit group dynamics. By encouraging the group participants to interact with one another, the researcher can gain insight into group/social processes. Focus groups and individual interviews elicit different material. Two major problems with focus groups are those of the emergence

Box 9.3 Example of a focus group questioning route

Questioning route for focus group on cardiovascular disease and diabetes in minority ethnic groups

1. Tell us about your diabetes.

   Prompts: Previous family history
   Tests and investigations
   Hospital admissions
   Emergencies
   Treatments
   Health problems
   Problems with family diet/cooking arrangements

2. Tell us about how diabetes has affected your life.

   Prompts: As a mother
   As the breadwinner
   As a religious person
   As a social person

3. Research shows that the best preventive and rehabilitative care for people with diabetes and heart disease is to lose weight and take more exercise. Tell us about this aspect of your lifestyle.

   Prompts: Do you want to lose weight?
   Have you tried to lose weight?
   What makes you put weight on?
   What makes it difficult to watch your weight?
   Do you exercise?
   Do you want to exercise?

Adapted from Elliot *et al.* 1997

of group ideology and an opinion leader, both constraining the range and value of opinion.

If the language of the researcher is different to that of the participants, trained interpreters will be needed so that participants may speak in their chosen language and the main issues can then be transmitted back to the facilitator. Facilitators and interpreters then need to agree on the main issues to have emerged. Analysis of data can use theoretically established approaches, and custom designed computer software. Box 9.4 is an example of how focus group data can be applied to bring about change, based on the work by Elliot and colleagues (1997).

Box 9.4 CHD/Diabetes focus group methods and use of data

Focus groups were used in Newcastle to explore CHD and diabetes services for the ethnic minorities. Four focus groups were set up; separate male and female South Asian groups, a mixed sex Chinese group and an ethnic minority professionals group. The facilitator asked the questions which were interpreted by the community workers and the answers were fed back via the community workers to the facilitator. Immediately after the meeting, there was a group discussion between the facilitator and the community workers (the research group) to go over and clarify the main points raised. This discussion was recorded and the results transcribed. The salient points made were placed under theme headings and discussed and changed until the research group was happy that what was emerging was a true record of what had occurred. Conclusions were that the minorities knew little about their conditions (as well as preventative strategies) but wanted to know more. All participants had or knew of people who had received inadequate health services. The professionals complained that they often did not have the resources to educate the community properly, e.g. materials were not translated and of those that were most were not easily understandable by the community. The professionals were often inundated with calls from people who wanted help with other matters, e.g. filling out social security forms. Some of the health workers had had to change their telephone numbers two or three times. The results were used in the ethnic health strategy of the local health authority and were influential in gaining funding for a primary care based service for ethnic minority groups with a special focus on diabetes.

Adapted from Elliott *et al.* 1997

9.4.7 Validity of physical and other measures needs to be assured

Cross-cultural validity is obviously important in relation to self-report data, but it also matters in other forms of information. Here the difficulty is less with the measurement tool (as for questions) but with the meaning of the result.

The problems with physical measures are far from negligible. The same value of a physical measure may have differential significance across ethnic groups, as illustrated by body mass index (BMI) and waist measurement. BMI is the person's height in metres squared divided by the weight in kilogrammes, and it has been the major method of studying overweight and obesity for several decades (although it is increasingly under attack in this regard and is likely to be discarded in favour of waist measures). Based on research linking BMI to adverse health outcomes the WHO set a value for adults of BMI at 25 or more as overweight, with a value of 30 or more as obesity. These cut-offs work well except for sports people and particularly bodybuilders, where a high BMI could reflect a large muscle mass. For most people a high BMI reflects excess body fat. The main reason why a high BMI is undesirable is because it is an indicator of a high proportion of body fat, a risk factor for many diseases including heart attack, stroke, diabetes and breast cancer. The studies that generated these WHO cut-off points were mostly in White populations.

Do these general observations and cut-off points apply across all ethnic groups? We would expect they would if the BMI accurately reflected fat composition. It turns out that at any BMI, on average, most Asian populations including the Chinese, Malays and South Asians, have more fat than White populations. The association between BMI and disease holds but the cut-points for overweight and obesity need to be lower. The exact cut-points are under intense discussion with most observers recommending a value of 23 for overweight in most Asian ethnic groups. (In my view this is too high.) The difference between a BMI of 23 and 25 for a man of about 5ft 9 inches (1.75m) weighing 70 kg is about 6 kg or 13 lbs. For decades Asian people have been badly misinformed about their ideal body weight because the interpretation of the key measure was not valid across ethnic groups. (There are echoes here of the use of IQ scales designed for European population but used across the world leading to the stigmatizing view that many other populations had a low IQ.)

Currently there is an emerging view that waist to hip ratio (WHR) or simply waist would be a better indictor of excess body fat than BMI. Several studies suggest this is so for many Asian populations. WHR requires that a tape measure is passed around the preferably bare or very lightly clad waist and hip. This may not be easy to do in some populations that put a premium on modesty. In any case a high WHR may reflect small hips rather than a large waist. The waist size may not reflect the same amount of body fat across ethnic groups. Pending further research the International Diabetes Federation has recommended that in the context of defining a condition characterized by a set of cardiovascular risk factors and called metabolic syndrome, in Asian populations the waist size be less than 90 cm in men (80 cm in women) compared to the recommendation of 94 cm in White men (80 cm in women). Thus cross-cultural validity in relation to physical measures requires adjustment of methods and normal values. The underlying principles are similar to those discussed in relation to self-report data. These arguments are relevant to laboratory measures too, e.g. the effect of a value of 6 mmol/L of LDL cholesterol may not be the same in one ethnic group as in another. The reason would relate to the presence and the biological interaction of other risk factors (arguments that are beyond the scope of this introductory book, but are covered in most intermediate level textbooks of epidemiology).

9.4.8 Choose the right control/standard/reference population

One central principle that arises from these considerations concerns the paradigm of the comparison or standard population, and specifically whether this can or ought to be the White population. We have seen how misleading this approach can be. The idea that one small but extremely rich and powerful segment of the global population—White people of European ancestry—can supply the norms against which other ethnic groups are to be judged has been unquestioningly applied for too long. It is impeding progress and misleading us on numerous fronts. For example, many ethnic groups are currently judged to have an abnormally high prevalence of type 2 diabetes mellitus, as judged by the norms of White populations. A better perspective would be to consider the White population to have an abnormally low prevalence. This population (and a few others) can be thought of as unusual or deviant. The question—What protects this population from diabetes even amidst plentiful nutrition?—may provide a greater return than why nearly all other human populations have a great tendency to diabetes amidst over nutrition. The relatively high BMI of European origin populations with comparatively low body fat may be one of the explanations.

In multi-ethnic studies there will be a need to develop normal values for physiological measures in different ethnic groups. On a general note there is a case for the group with the most favourable health status or risk factor profile providing the standard population, against which others are compared. This would potentially transform public health, with new and challenging targets.

9.4.9 Interpret data and use the findings to benefit the population studied

Try Exercise 9.6 before reading on.

Exercise 9.6 Publication, dissemination and impact of research

- What problems must researchers foresee and plan for in relation to interpretation of data, drawing conclusions and the publication and dissemination of research?
- How can such research stimulate change to improve the health of ethnic minority groups?

Research data do not provide answers. Only researchers and readers of research can do this through the advanced skill of data interpretation. Researchers who know the communities they work with are also more likely to interpret data with minimal error and bias. The researcher and ideally the reader of research needs insight into the history, culture and living conditions of the people studied, particularly to assess the plausibility of the hypothesis developed and the acceptability of any recommendations. Such insight, which may be taken for granted, perhaps wrongly so, when the researcher comes from the same ethnic group as the subjects, is not easily acquired. Furthermore, there is very limited guidance, support, training, and peer support to assist with interpretation of research on ethnic minorities.

Even with insights into analysis and interpretation, the researcher is often left with insufficient and inappropriate data to analyse, because of problems of small sample size, non-response bias, improper ethnic coding etc. The practical experience of reporting large multi-ethnic studies is very limited worldwide. Normally, such research reports on one ethnic group contrasted with another—usually the White majority. Reporting and interpreting data on three or more ethnic groups is unusual, and using a non-White reference population still more so. Such analysis and reporting is demanding both of intellect and publication space. We need to test its value and generate examples. The translation of research into policy and practice is a complex area in any field, including ethnicity and health. Such translational research is under active investigation and ethnicity and health researchers need to make contributions to it.

Presently, in the UK we are witnessing a rapid rise in the number of funded studies on South Asian populations. It is likely that this is in part because South Asians are firmly established in the health care professions, particularly medicine, and in the academic sector. The same is not true of most other ethnic minority groups e.g. gypsy travellers, East Europeans, Africans. While I would not wish to argue that only people from a particular ethnic group can do research on that group, for it is manifestly untrue, I do, however, argue that a multi-ethnic research workforce is needed to generate good research in multi-ethnic societies. The most important of all the tasks in research is to pose the important questions and to generate imaginative ideas and solutions. These tasks, surely, need deep insight into the nature of the populations to be studied, and one route to this insight comes from membership of the population, or from diligent study over many years.

9.4.10 Publishing the research and seeking the generalizations that avoid stereotypes

Try Exercise 9.8 before reading on.

Exercise 9.8 Using research

◆ What problems must researchers foresee and plan for in relation to funding, publication and dissemination of research?
◆ How can such research stimulate change to improve the health of ethnic minority groups?

Not all data gathering exercises are research. Research is characterized by the objective of extending the boundaries of known knowledge. How do we know this has been achieved? Researchers may need to go through a rigorous process of review and approval to gain resources and permission to do the work. Many funding sources demand external peer review before awarding funding. Peer reviewers are required to assess whether the proposed research will add to known work and whether the extra knowledge is worth the resources. The system is far from perfect, but it is the one that has been widely adopted internationally.

Once the work is done the ethics and conventions of research require that it is summarized as a research paper or monograph and submitted for potential publication as a journal article or book. The purpose of this is twofold. First, so the work can be subjected to peer and editorial scrutiny. Second, assuming it is found worthy of publication (usually after much painstaking revision), so that it can be made widely available and placed on the research record for posterity. Many research papers are now available throughout the world via the Internet on the day that the final editing takes place and before official publication. Research that is published in this way becomes highly influential. Other scholars, researchers, professionals and policy-makers will take such published findings much more seriously than those in in-house documents or verbal presentations. The published works have a stamp of quality and authority. These papers are often given media attention and brought to the attention of the public and their elected representatives. If such papers are to have a lasting impact beyond the place and time of their publication they need to emphasize generalizable findings and draw generalizable conclusions. It is also true that work that draws attention to problems is more likely to be published than work that shows there is no problem. Work that is novel is more publishable than work that confirms what is already known. Work that has a positive result, i.e. it demonstrates an association or that an intervention works, is more likely to be published than other works (the outcome is so called publication bias).

These issues pose great challenges to ethnicity and health researchers. The kind of knowledge they seek may already be published—though usually only for the White population. It will be hard to win scarce, competitively granted resources, and to win highly competitive publication space in top journals, for such necessary but not necessarily ground-breaking work. Researchers will need to make the work sound exciting—and that usually requires highlighting problems and giving attention to the positive findings.

In winning grants, writing up and publishing the work, however, researchers should have systems to minimize the danger of harm to the ethnic group studied, particularly the stigma associated with demonstration of problems, stereotyping and a fuelling of racism. This is a delicate path to tread. My major area of research at present is cardiovascular disease in South Asians. The problem is vast. Lest the population is seen in a negative light I remind audiences that overall mortality rates in South Asians are similar to those of the population as a whole, despite an excess of these diseases. The excess is balanced by a deficit of other causes of death, e.g. cancer. The South Asian population is not crumbling.

9.5 Conclusions—the challenge of studying minority ethnic groups

The challenge of ethnicity and health research includes demonstrating tangible health benefits in addition to satisfying curiosity. Ethnicity and health is a beguiling research theme, for: it is worthy as it often focuses on underprivileged groups; is interesting and unearths unusual and sometimes exotic results; differences between ethnic groups can be demonstrated with ease; and small studies can yield statistically significant and relevant results. The full range of public health science research methods—qualitative, case-histories, case series, analysis of routine statistics, case control studies, cohort studies, trials—and medical sciences, are potentially applicable to ethnicity and health (see Table 9.1). However, as the research literature has grown, so has criticism about its value.

Try Exercise 9.7 before reading on.

Exercise 9.7 Future research and challenges

+ What challenges will researchers need to overcome in the future?
+ What, in your opinion, is the future of ethnicity and health research?

There are numerous challenges in research. Some of these in relation to epidemiology are listed in Box 9.5. There are others relating to other social, population and medical sciences. One of the greatest overall challenges is doing good work in the light of complexity and amidst criticism. Who are we to believe—those who extol the concepts of race and ethnicity or those who condemn them? We are in the midst of a change of paradigm in the use of the race and ethnicity concepts (see Chapter 10). Meantime, researchers are left with the decision to either avoid the controversy and difficulty associated with race and ethnicity variables (an action which may be socially, politically, legally and scientifically unacceptable) or to do their best, with the express intention of continually improving their work. In this book I have demonstrated that even when operationalized with crude classifications, race and ethnicity have value in health politics, policy, planning, surveillance, health services and epidemiological research and occasionally in clinical care.

Box 9.5 Some challenges for epidemiological research on ethnicity, race and health

- Inclusion of minorities in research
- Clarification of the purpose of the research
- Definitions of concepts relating to ethnicity and race
- Definition and precision of terms, and ethnic/racial classifications
- Recognition of heterogeneity within ethnic minority groups
- Identification of representative populations
- Ensuring comparability of populations that are to be compared, requiring socio-economic data over the life-course
- Accurate measurement of the denominators and numerators, in calculating rates
- Ensuring the quality of data, particularly in cross-cultural comparability
- Maximizing completeness of data collection
- Avoiding misinterpretation of differences that are due to confounding variables
- Pinpointing genetic bases of genetic hypotheses
- Proper interpretations of associations as causal or non-causal
- Maximizing validity and generalizability of the research
- Presentation of research to achieve benefits for the population studied, and avoid stigmatization and racism
- Appropriate action to follow the research

Bhopal (2004: 444)

Reproduced from Bhopal R. Glossary of terms relating to ethnicity and race for reflection and debate. *Journal of Epidemiological Community Health* 2003; 58: 441–45

Both purpose and context are the prime determinants of the way that race and ethnicity concepts are applied, classifications are devised and employed, and data are analysed and presented. Researchers must overcome the many conceptual and technical problems of race, ethnicity and health research. One huge task is to achieve a shared understanding. In working with the tarnished race concept based on biology and the power of the idea of ethnicity we must avoid the mistakes of the past. In Chapter 1 I gave guidelines on how to do this and Box 9.6 offers some others.

Box 9.6 Recommendations on the use of ethnicity and race in health (a) generally (b) with refugees (see page 282)

(a) Generally

1. Scientific criteria, based on knowledge from the social, behavioural and biological sciences, should be used to define the concepts and measurement procedures for categories such as race and ethnicity.

2. Valid and reliable concepts of race, ethnicity, and related notions, such as ancestry or national origin, need to be explored.

3. The concepts of, and language used for, race, ancestry, ethnicity, and related notions need to be assessed among diverse segments of the USA population to ensure valid and reliable responses to survey questions.

4. Social, economic, and political forces underlying differences in health status among ethnic and racial populations should be investigated and reported in population studies of health status.

5. When researchers describe differing health status among racial and ethnic populations they should explain (a) why they collected the information, (b) how the information was collected, and (c) what the information means.

6. Active participation of racial and ethnic communities in survey design, application and dissemination should be used to avoid misunderstanding and promote goodwill amongst groups whose health is being assessed.

Warren *et al.* (1994)

Unfortunately, investigators are not putting them into practice, as the following euphemistically phrased quote indicates.

> Although previous authors who have questioned the value of using race and ethnicity as scientific variables have proposed methodological guidelines aimed at increasing the integrity of these variables, it is clear from our study that researchers have not yet come to a consensus concerning their use.

Comstock (2004: 619)

Migrant populations have provided a rich source of striking disease variations which have intrigued the epidemiological imagination. There is still massive potential for causal understanding through the in-depth investigation and explanation of such variations. Cohort and intergenerational effects could sharpen our understanding and prediction of disease frequency, disease causation and the control of risk factors. Unfortunately, as yet we have hardly begun to deploy these powerful designs.

The huge potential of research on ethnic minorities for service planning and delivery also needs good design and a clear focus, better data and experience of putting research to use. For future progress we need to recognize that such research should focus on high priority problems and that the planning of health services needs simple but validated data, different from the understanding of disease causes. Improvements will come from conceptual openness and explicit and defined terminology; and imaginative solutions to the fundamental problems of research on ethnic minorities, such as matching denominators and numerators, representativeness of the population, comparability of subgroups, and validity of the measurement tools.

The health of ethnic minorities would be served by:

- international conferences with the sole purpose of discussing terminology and other methodological issues;
- more fora (and perhaps journals) for discussion of the specific problems posed by research on ethnic minority groups;
- greater emphasis on research on methodological issues;
- a focus on the causes and prevention of the major causes of ill-health;
- a greater readiness to research the quality of health care offered to ethnic minority groups; and
- more research input from ethnic minority populations, as investigators, advisers and participants.

Most research on ethnic minority health has been by researchers whose interest is in one (or a group of) disorder(s). They seek a new perspective on that interest and are using the ethnic variations model for that primary goal; the ethnic minority population's health and well-being may well be peripheral. More research needs to be done by researchers whose main interest is in ethnic minorities and their health, with the disorder, methods and disciplines being peripheral. This requires, among other solutions, a stronger cadre of researchers from ethnic minority populations.

Participation by ethnic minorities in research, policy-making and the development of services might be one safeguard against repeating the mistakes of the past. The American College of Epidemiology has called for a greater contribution to epidemiology by researchers from ethnic minority groups, who are under-represented. The minorities' views may be interpreted as representing special interests so a partnership between scientists from a multiplicity of ethnic groups is needed.

Wider, constructive debate on the mounting criticisms of race and ethnicity research is essential as a step towards agreement on the way forward. This debate is more advanced in the USA than in Europe but on both sides of the Atlantic, papers intended to stimulate change have had surprisingly little impact. Even scientific journals are ignoring their own guidelines on reporting of race and ethnicity research.

The perception that the health of ethnic minority groups is poor can augment the belief that immigrants and ethnic minorities are a burden. The perception of poorer health arises from a focus on differences, where the excess of disease is in the ethnic minority population. It is naïve to believe that the demonstration of inequalities by race will narrow them and it is plausible that such studies can perpetuate and even augment inequalities. It is noteworthy that the concept of race is scarcely ever used to study racism, at least in medicine, but is still frequently applied to infer biological differences between populations. The quotation from Hilda Parker summarizes this mismatch, although it would be wrong to infer from the quotation that the USA has made great strides (through more than most countries) in studying racism in health care.

Recent British publications assessing the methods used in studies of ethnicity primarily considered the status of the variables 'ethnicity' and 'race' and advised on the use of appropriate categories. Such scrutiny of ethnicity research is welcomed, yet authors rarely emphasise the importance of racism as a variable. This paper discusses why racism matters as a variable and poses suggestions for its absence from British health services research. Reference is made to USA research to demonstrate that this focus is important and feasible. Health services research that considers ethnicity and excludes the effect of racism may result, at best in an incomplete understanding. At worst, this omission could itself be perceived as a racist practice.

Parker (1997: 256)

For many causes, morbidity and mortality rates are lower but these gain little attention. The promise of aetiological understanding has meant a focus on variation in diseases, as opposed to the quality of services. So there is a huge gap in the research record on the quality of care received by ethnic minority groups, to the detriment of the services and populations served. Ethnic minority populations are seriously under-represented in major studies, especially cohort studies and trials. The view that much research is institutionally racist is extant but suppressed. There is, at the least, a case to answer as Ranganathan and I have discussed (2006). It would be better that action were taken before the world of research, at least in Europe, is asked to account for itself, either by government, funders or the law. Europe has something to learn from the United States, although policy on the inclusion of racial and ethnic minorities in research has raised difficult questions that need to be resolved. Box 9.7 cites some material that poses the questions.

We should step forward but tread warily, for if we do not, the twenty-second century will look no more favourably upon present day research on race, ethnicity and health than we do upon the work of talented but, in today's light, misguided scientists of the nineteenth century.

Box 9.6b Proposed guidelines for research in refugee and internally displaced populations

(b) Refugees

- ◆ Undertake only those studies that are urgent and vital to the health and welfare of the study population
- ◆ Restrict studies to those questions that cannot be addressed in any other context
- ◆ Restrict studies to those that would provide important direct benefit to the individuals recruited to the study or to the population from which the individuals come
- ◆ Ensure the study design imposes the absolute minimum of additional risk
- ◆ Select study participants on the basis of scientific principles without bias introduced by issues of accessibility, cost, or malleability
- ◆ Establish highest standards for obtaining informed consent from all individual study participants and where necessary and culturally appropriate from heads of household and community leaders (but this consent cannot substitute for individual consent)
- ◆ Institute procedures to assess for, minimize, and monitor the risks to safety and confidentiality for individual subjects, their community, and for their future security
- ◆ Promote the well-being, dignity, and autonomy of all study participants in all phases of the research study.

Leaning (2001: 1432)

Box 9.7 Appropriate representation

The range of possible interpretations of the phrase 'appropriate representation' has left investigators struggling with the practical application of the National Institutes of Health guidelines on the inclusion of minorities in research. At least three goals might be reached by including minorities in clinical research; to test specific hypotheses about differences by race and ethnicity; to generate hypotheses about possible differences by race and ethnicity; and to ensure the just distribution of the benefits and burdens of participation in research, regardless of whether there are expected differences in outcome by race or ethnicity. In this paper, we describe possible interpretations of 'appropriate representation' as well as provide a general approach that investigators might use to address this issue. To expand scientific knowledge about the health of minority populations, investigators should be expected to state which goal they have selected and why that goal is appropriate as compared with other possible goals.

Corbie-Smith *et al.* (2004: 249)

Summary

Research is not a value-free activity, particularly when it is on living human beings. Race and ethnicity are important to the structure and function of human populations, and it is inevitable that research utilizing these concepts is of interest to, and has influence upon, society and will be interpreted to meet social goals. Just as modern day work is mostly used to further current goals of social equality and justice, so it was that much research in the past was used to further previous goals such as the continuation of slavery, the justification of Empire, the maintenance of social and material inequality (including Apartheid), anti-immigration policies focused on those who where not Northern Europeans, eugenics and the Nazi Final Solution. The most important lesson from this history is that research on race and health needs to be done within an ethical framework emphasizing benefit to the population studied, primarily, and to wider society secondarily.

The full range of public health sciences and their methodological approaches— literature review, qualitative studies, case-histories, case series, analysis of routine statistics, case control studies, cohort studies, trials—and medical sciences, are potentially applicable to ethnicity and health. It is likely that an explosion of research on the genetic basis of ethnic/racial variations will occur as all societies become multi-ethnic ones. More cooperation with social scientists is needed to help resolve the issues that will arise.

Researchers need to make explicit how they are using the concepts of ethnicity and race, and to adapt classifications and methods of assessing ethnicity to the research questions under study. Researchers should not be constrained by available classifications designed for administrative purposes. Researchers who are knowledgeable about the ethnic groups under study are more likely to be trusted and more likely to achieve the high response rates and informed consent that are essential, and to interpret data with minimal error and bias. In writing up and publishing their work, researchers should minimize the danger of harm to the ethnic group studied, particularly the stigma which can ensue from associating them with problems for health care systems, the propensity for stereotyping and a fuelling of racism.

The ideal research study in multi-ethnic societies would be inclusive of all ethnic groups, have uniformly high response rates, provide data that are comparable across all groups, collect information on all facets of ethnicity, include data on all potential confounding variables and be analysed and interpreted in a way that both advances science, improves health status and develops better health care. In practice, many of these ideals are sacrificed to make the study feasible. In making pragmatic choices researchers should make themselves and others aware of the limitations of the work. The excitement of this research theme means we can expect a rapid increase of research in this field. The challenge includes demonstrating tangible health benefits in addition to satisfying curiosity.

Chapter 10

Theoretical, ethical and future-orientated perspectives

Many epidemiologists continue to use the variable race uncritically and with little attention to theory. That is, they fail to consider possible social determinants of racial inequalities in health, including mechanisms originating from exposure to multiple forms of racial discrimination.

Muntaner *et al.* (1996: 535)

In generally trying to explain why some people are more susceptible to disease, health researchers propose that one clear, essential set of characteristics is shared by everyone in a category. This essentialism assumes we each have a 'true' identity inherent in us, and that we carry it from the moment of conception, or at least from the cradle to the grave.
    Essentialism can be social as well as biological.

Pfeffer (1998: 1382)

Contents

Objectives

On completion of this chapter you should be able to:

◆ consider the theories and principles learnt earlier, in an ethical, enquiring and future-orientated way, to improve the health of ethnic minority groups

◆ analyse and articulate the future potential of the concepts of race and ethnicity in a number of health settings—clinical care to individuals, public health initiatives, health care planning, research and policy-making

10.1 Introduction: theory

Before reading on try Exercise 10.1.

Exercise 10.1 Theories

◆ What theories, if any, can you discern as underlying the concepts of race and ethnicity?

◆ What theories have lost favour?

◆ What theoretical ideas about health and disease in epidemiology do the concepts of race and ethnicity uphold?

◆ Why are these concepts growing in importance?

A scientific theory is a rational exposition, based on general principles, that explains disparate observations, ideas and mechanisms about the natural world and allows predictions to be tested. Although many theories about race and ethnicity have been developed, both in the biological and social sciences, presently none command wide acceptance. We need more and better theories, and much more time spent on discussing these, as the quotations opening this chapter testify.

Biological theories based on species and subspecies and on gene variants have almost certainly had their 'moment of glory'. This is another reminder that widespread acceptance of a theory does not make it right—race as biology was deemed self-evident and even now commands attention despite its flaws.

Hopefully, we will never return to the kind of thinking of Gilbert Murray considered by Michael Banton in the quotation below.

> Consider the remarks of Gilbert Murray (1900: 156) the classical scholar, humanitarian and devoted supporter of the League of Nations:
>
> 'There is a world a hierarchy of races...those nations which eat more, claim more, and get higher wages, will direct and rule the others, and the lower work of the world will tend in the long-run to be done by the lower breeds of men. This much we of the ruling colour will no doubt accept as obvious.'
>
> In these remarks nations, as political units, are equated with race, as biological units. The position of white people as the top of the hierarchy is attributed to their racial character and the future division of labour throughout the world is represented as an expression of this hierarchy. So the statements reflect a theory that is simultaneously biological and sociological.
>
> Michael Banton (1987; vii)

Although genetic research continues to examine the global distribution of genetic variants, and to match the findings to racial and ethic groupings, a renaissance of biology in the race and ethnicity fields seems improbable. The theory that all humans evolved in one place—probably Africa—and migrated from there fairly recently in evolutionary terms is the key to understanding this viewpoint. While it stands—and at present it is rooted firmly despite continuing scientific scrutiny—it is hard to envisage how the concept of race as clearly separable subspecies can work. The idea that the human species *Homo sapiens* evolved in several places has been relegated to the fringes of scientific study. Should it ever return to centre stage then the concept of races as ancient and separate species/subspecies that have converged over long time periods might return. Presently, the continuum of genetic variation across the globe, and hence among human populations internationally, means that a genetically based classification of races is not feasible. This does not mean that genetically based factors cannot contribute to race (or ethnicity), but, that they cannot hold centre stage in the great drama of ethnic variations in human health.

Population sciences such as demography and epidemiology have made only modest contributions to theoretical debates on concepts of race and ethnicity (in contrast to general theories about health and disease where the contributions have been considerable). Rather, they have used theories and concepts primarily from biology, anthropology and sociology. Their contribution has been more at practical levels e.g. the development of classifications and comparison of the value of different means of assessing race and ethnicity.

Population sciences and the professions and disciplines that use them have, however, stimulated theoretical work by continuing to demonstrate the importance of ethnic variations in health and disease, and hence to public health. The concepts of race and ethnicity fit very well into the general theories of health and disease developed by the population sciences. This type of pragmatic and, at least ostensibly, atheoretical approach is common in these disciplines, for example, in the lack of well-developed theories on sex, gender, age, education and class-based variations in health and disease. While the approach may, ostensibly, be pragmatic as James Nazroo has correctly stated, it is underpinned, nonetheless, by theories.

> ... it is a mistake to assume that the process of identifying 'ethnic' groups is theoretically neutral (hence my use of the term 'un-theorised' rather than atheoretical).
>
> Theory is brought in surreptitiously—ethnicity, however measured, equals genetic or cultural heritage. This then leads to a form of victim blaming where the *inherent* characteristics of the ethnic (minority) group are seen to be at fault and in need to rectifying.
>
> Nazroo (715–716)

In all these areas—and more—population scientists and practitioners look to biological or social sciences for theories. Collaborations between social, population and biological scientists in theoretical work are needed as already happens so successfully in empirical research. Users of concepts in empirical and applied research have a role and responsibility to help develop theory too.

Since the Second World War the social sciences have dominated theoretical discussions on race and ethnicity. Clearly, this is wholly appropriate as these concepts shape societies and social interactions between populations, population subgroups and individuals. The contribution of social sciences, however, goes much deeper than merely describing how race and ethnicity impact on society, and two profound insights have emerged that seem all too evident once articulated.

First, the theory that societies have created race and ethnicity to meet their own social purposes i.e. the concepts are socially constructed. If so, racial and ethnic groups do not actually exist in any biological or natural way. (According to social constructivism all labels and values are also social constructs—a perspective that I largely accept.) Leaving aside philosophical debates on existence of objects and ideas (outside one's mind), this is a powerful and provocative idea. If it is correct then we could also envisage societies that have no concepts of this kind. We could envisage societies that socially construct in radically different ways, for example thinking of African-origin and European-origin populations as one race or ethnic group and Indians and Pacific Islanders as another. Many medical scientists concur, generally, with this view as the following quotation shows.

> National, religious, geographic, linguistic and cultural groups do not necessarily coincide with racial groups: and the cultural traits of such groups have no demonstrated genetic connection with racial traits.
>
> UNESCO statement on race, 1950 in Kuper *et al.* (1975: 344)

This view implies that our current concepts and classifications have no secure foundation in nature. It is a much needed correction to the biological ideas that preceded it but in my view it goes a little too far. The social construction of races and ethnic groups, whatever groupings are chosen, needs to be based on information to permit such social construction. What is this information? Is it not the biological and cultural factors that underpin the concepts of race (colour, hair texture, physiognomy etc.) and ethnicity (language, ancestral origins, clothing, traditions and so on)? Is this information not processed by humans to make important social decisions? The neurological research studying humans' responses to faces indicates that it is so (Golby *et al.* 2001). No doubt, some of this processing is innate and some of it is socially conditioned. As is so often the case a clean separation of the social and the biological is impossible in the human species, which is characterized by its socialization.

The second huge contribution from the social sciences is encapsulated by the terms racialization and reification. Racialization is the process whereby for individuals, groups and institutions perceiving the social world in terms of racial and ethnic groups becomes an ingrained habit, one that seems normal and necessary. Epidemiological research in the USA is racialized to see health problems in terms of Black and White populations.

Once this happens it is a small step to perceiving these racial and ethnic divisions as real, perhaps even inviolable. This latter step is called reification—making real something that does not deserve that status. A complex and somewhat nebulous concept, here race and a

Black/White division, becomes over time a natural way of thinking and in due course the classification arising becomes rigid and unchanging.

Habits and routines are an ingredient of our social worlds, and sometimes they can be helpful. Eating is natural but eating three meals a day is not. Other routines are possible. To achieve the objectives of this book other approaches, and other words, are not only possible, but probably desirable. In the same way, I believe, perceiving humans as different using the cues underlying race and ethnicity is natural but the divisions we create are not. Other divisions are possible. It is even possible to have no divisions at all. Difference does not necessarily need to be enshrined in divisions. The choice is ours and we should do what is best for human society, and this is a task for all of us, led by our politicians. It is far from easy to work out what is the best way forward. It depends on viewpoint and goals. Here are two world viewpoints, one from Carl Coon, who published an extensive classification of the races of humanity in 1953, perhaps the last work of its kind. The other is from the Bikhu Parekh, one of the leading UK academics in race relations.

> If the races of man stay where they are best adapted, it creates much less trouble than when they move into each other's territories.
>
> Do the minds of all races work in the same fashion, do not their emotions differ with differences in their hormonal peculiarities, and is it not possible that cultures vary to a certain extent in terms of these variations? These questions require research, and the results may mar the vision of a single world culture.
>
> If the world is to become united, the union must be a loose confederation of very different units, or it will not long endure.
>
> Coon (1963: 130–1)

> A multicultural society should be based on equal citizenship, and five areas have been identified for consideration, and commitment for change:
>
> 1. elimination of discrimination
> 2. equality of opportunity
> 3. equal respect
> 4. acceptance of immigrants as a legitimate and valued part of society
> 5. the opportunity to preserve and transmit their cultural identities including their languages, cultures, religions, histories and ethnic affiliations.
>
> Parekh, ix in Modood et al. (1997)

Theoretical work is needed to both understand and to reconcile such different view-points. It is time for a new and hopefully more integrated theory. When scientists in a field of endeavour cannot agree on basic concepts, according to Thomas Kuhn, a major shift in thinking is underway, and if it is not, it is overdue. In his words, it is time for a paradigm shift (Kuhn 1996). Pending developments of new paradigms people using race and ethnicity need to be thoughtful and aware, and be ready to contribute their own views to ongoing and forthcoming debates.

10.2 **Ethics of ethnicity and race**

Before reading on try Exercise 10.2.

Exercise 10.2 Ethics

◆ Why is an ethical code so important in the ethnicity and health arena?
◆ Reflect on the codes that require professionals to:
  (i) do no harm
  (ii) do good
  (iii) offer autonomy
  (iv) be just
◆ How can these codes prevent the return of misuses of race?

Ethics is a code of right behaviour. Such codes must, necessarily, change with time and differ to some extent from place to place. Ethical codes are not rigid and incontestable, even although they may be given stability by fundamental principles (sometimes enshrined in religions). Furthermore, they are different for different disciplines. Ethical codes are highly developed in medicine, and these codes have deeply influenced public health—not least because public health is often dominated or strongly influenced by medicine. Adaptations of these codes for epidemiology and for medical and public health are available (see websites for International Epidemiological Association—p 345). As discussed in Chapter 8, there are ethical codes for undertaking research with ethnic minorities that are based on general ones. Ethical codes are vital to the ethnicity and health field. While it would be wasteful and possibly even harmful to create separate and new ethical codes for ethnicity and race research, we do need to consider the potential influences that might require a change of emphasis or application of such codes.

10.2.1 **Do no harm (non-maleficence)**

In my view this is the most important ethical pillar in the ethnicity and health field. The mere act of articulating the concept of race or ethnicity draws attention to differences, potentially magnifying their importance. These differences can be used in damaging ways, as emphasized throughout this book. The way that data are put to use depends on the social milieu.

Researchers and practitioners need to be sensitive to wider events. At the time of writing, the suicide missions that destroyed the twin towers in New York, the war against Iraq, the furore over the proposal by Iran to develop nuclear energy, the Islamic world's revulsion at the cartoons of the Prophet Muhammad published in Denmark and carried by other European newspapers, and the backlash as others defend their right to freedom of speech, are a few of the background issues that matter. It is a difficult time, even with the best of intentions, to release research or make proposals relating to improving the health of Muslims or even to publish this book. These proposals, and particularly research data, could be used to drive wedges between Islam and other religions. This is not to advocate self-censorship or to suggest that no change should be proposed—but that researchers should have awareness of the primary goal of health improvement in relation to potential adverse outcomes that could take them further from it. The health researcher has a secondary duty that is a companion to the primary one of gaining and using knowledge—to foster a milieu of equality, justice, tolerance and sensitivity. Only then, I propose, can benefits occur, as discussed next.

10.2.2 Beneficence—doing good

Doing good—beneficence—lies at the heart of public health, medicine and all health professions. Unfortunately, the intention to do good often, and perhaps even mostly, does not lead to good. As so often is the case, a historical analysis gives clarity. It is worth reflecting upon the harm done by the extensive use in medicine of enemas, blood letting, heavy toxic metals, electroconvulsive treatment (ECT), thalidomide, hormone replacement therapy (for heart disease prevention) and a multiplicity of drug and other interventions. Health and health care interventions are not usually implemented in a climate of undiluted beneficence and there are additional social, political, commercial and other motives. As discussed in some detail in this book beneficence towards minority ethnic groups is by no means universal, either across time or place.

Doing good in this context requires a special effort of will, and a struggle against lack of knowledge, information, expertise, leaders, finances and against competing priorities. Nonetheless, the general imperative of medical ethics to do good also provides the specific imperative to ensure that some populations, ethnic minorities being an example, are not excluded. This general ethic is, in the long term, more powerful than even legislation and policy, for it is an ingrained part of every health professional's training and mental make-up. Doing good is also the governing value of health institutions including those responsible for training and education. Without the ethic of beneficence in place it is possibly better not to draw attention to ethnic differences. With it the daunting challenges we have explored in this book are worth tackling.

To do good in professional settings needs competency in a variety of attitudes and skills. Competency is moving to the core of clinical education. It is achieved through education, training, research and an understanding and respect for both the individuals and groups that comprise the population to be served. Respect is a key word and it may develop in a variety of ways. Education, research or training does not always engender respect for others, perhaps the opposite. It is proving rather difficult to integrate ethnicity and race into medical curricula in a rigorous and solid way, but we must keep trying, as Joe Kai attests.

> As learning to value ethnic diversity begins to feature more consistently in medical training it will inevitably include 'token' approaches that lack coherence. However, even imperfect first steps can provide useful lessons and create momentum for change. In an increasingly diverse society, which serves to enrich our lives and experiences, doctors must learn to value ethnic diversity to deliver effective health care. In doing so, they will bring mutual benefits for their patients and themselves.
>
> Kai *et al.* (1999: 622)

While one can respect the autonomy and differences of others without understanding them, the current view is that increasing the knowledge base of professionals is a necessary prerequisite. A professional culture that requires respect for everyone, irrespective of ethnic group, is the goal. Admittedly, it seems sad that such a goal needs to be set.

10.2.3 Respect and autonomy

Respecting and understanding others is not easy for anyone. At the minimum it requires a tolerance of others, but it also needs an interest in others, a wish to learn about them, and an active effort to perceive their world view in a positive light. Clearly, minority ethnic groups need to do this also, if only to adjust to living in multi-ethnic societies: the majority populations have no such immediate need, but in a healthy society they should reciprocate. The idea that the process of learning should be two-way lies at the heart of multiculturalism. Multiculturalism seems to me to be the only possible direction for the modern world, and hence for modern health-care systems, yet it is coming under attack (see Chapter 4, particularly the section on the Netherlands). The alternative, that the dominant culture remains wholly or largely unchanged while the minority ones integrate, assimilate and conform to the norms of the majority is, in my view, both impossible and undesirable.

Just as with the force of gravity, where each object in the universe exerts a force on surrounding objects, so it is with individuals and social subgroups. (Unlike gravity and inanimate objects the mutual social influence is not subject to formulaic assessment.) The correct response, I propose, is for active but sensitive debate to seek changes that benefit society. By respecting and understanding minority populations we might learn of the cultural and other forces that are leading in the UK, for example, to superb educational achievements among Chinese and Japanese children, the low levels of psychological stress in Bangladeshis in East London despite economic deprivation, the continuing low prevalence of smoking amongst Sikhs and South Asian women, and the low levels of coronary heart disease in African-origin men. There are also other values that may exist in ethnic minority communities but which are not so valued although they may bring many health benefits e.g. practising religion on a daily basis, close-knit families, traditional health care, herbal remedies and systems of health such as yoga. There may be much to be learned from practices that are portrayed negatively by the media, for example, arranged marriages. These are only a small sample of the potential benefits of multiculturalism in public health.

Respect is the pre-condition for autonomy. In medical ethics the competent patient (hence excluding young children and the mentally impaired, for example) must give informed consent for all procedures and for research. Autonomy is a pre-eminent medical ethic in current times. It overrides beneficence, as the classic example of the Jehovah's Witness patient right in refusing a life-saving blood transfusion against medical advice illustrates. The competent person even has the right to end their life, with medical help, in some societies.

Autonomy of ethnic minority populations to live in their own traditional way is not easy to achieve in multi-ethnic societies. Compromises are essential. Tensions have arisen on matters such as Sikhs refusing to wear helmets while motorcycling, the lack of organ donations from some ethnic minority populations, the larger family sizes of some ethnic minority groups because of positive attitudes to children and negative ones to contraception, female circumcision (usually called genital mutilation), pressure exerted on young people by the family in favour of arranged marriages, and so-called honour killings where people going against the tradition are murdered. These are a few examples of issues that relate to culture, health care and public health. These are very difficult issues that require very sensitive consideration to create a sense of fairness and can be handled justly. Justice requires that such issues are properly considered and appropriate laws and policies are framed that balance the needs of the individual, the group and society as a whole.

10.2.4 Justice, fairness and equality

Justice is the core value that underpins equity. Justice is fairness—fairness that is built into social structures. Justice also underpins law. The importance of justice to the equity, ethnicity and health agenda is great.

Justice changes when human values on right and wrong change, and therefore it varies in time and place, for change does not occur at a constant rate everywhere. In the modern era in many countries justice requires that individual people are treated equally. Moreover, justice also requires that social groups are also treated equally. Perhaps most remarkably of all, justice may include compensation for historical injustices. In this special circumstance, everyone may not be treated equally, and there may be positive action in favour of some individuals and groups. Remarkably, such affirmative action can create great tensions around ethnic and racial identities, and the use of genetics to resolve these, as indicated in the quotations below.

> Genetics can affect questions of ethnic identity (such as who counts as Cherokee or Maori), religious identity (who counts as Parsee or Jewish), family identity (who counts as a descendant of Thomas Jefferson), or caste (who counts as Brahman or Dalit). These identities overlap in various ways, and genetic evidence will not affect them all equally. But clearly confusion looms when genetic markers conflict with other kinds of markers of group membership, such as a shared culture or historical narrative. Does it make you any more English, or Sioux, or Jefferson if your identity has been corroborated by a genetic marker?
>
> Two years ago, after a bitter monetary dispute, the Seminole Nation of Oklahoma passed a resolution that will effectively expel most black Seminoles, or Seminole Freedmen. The Freedmen are the descendants of former slaves who fought alongside the Seminoles in the Seminole Wars and who have been officially recognised as members of the Seminole Nation of Oklahoma since 1966. The new constitution says that to be part of the tribe, a person must show that he or she has one eighth Seminole blood.
>
> Elliot and Brodwin (2002: 1469–70)

This viewpoint that equality and equity is social justice is now enshrined in constitutions, treaties, international conventions and laws (whether local, national or international).

The full consequences of a social justice stance are never easy to grasp or implement, and this applies in the ethnicity and health arena. It is, in most modern societies, unfair, unjust and in some places illegal to deliver a service, knowingly or unknowingly, to one racial or ethnic group that is either superior or inferior to that delivered to another group.

It is acceptable, and perhaps even mandatory, to target resources and expertise to redress historical wrongs so creating temporary conditions that favour the previously discriminated against population. There are many examples, including the Indian Health Service in the USA that was set up to meet the specific needs of Native Americans, the reservation of jobs and university places for scheduled castes in India, and the reservation of lands for Aborigines in Australia. This is a deep paradox—to promote equality, we may need to treat people and groups unequally, a point captured by the phrase 'fair discrimination'.

The Scottish Executive's strategy for ethnic minority health is aptly called Fair for All, a title that is to be used for the wider diversity agenda to include inequalities in sex, sexual orientation, disability and other grounds for potential discrimination (see Chapter 8). Fairness is something that is intuitively right and something virtually all agree with, at least in theory.

Justice is important not only to the allocation of resources and setting of priorities, but also to autonomy, and human rights. Competition between varying ethical principles, or even within a principle, is inevitable. For example, justice requires proper and effective use of resources—it is not fair on those paying the money to waste resources when there are unmet needs. It would be fair and just, arguably, at least in an ideal world where all needs could be met, to translate hospital information in the hundred or so languages read in a typical metropolitan area such as London, Amsterdam, New York or Sydney. Then the public could exercise its choice and equity would be achieved. The cost of simply developing (and not even distributing) would, however, be very high—at present perhaps £100,000 for a typical 2–4 page pamphlet translated in 100 languages. If there were 500 such pamphlets, a reasonable estimate considering the complexity of health care, that would be £50 million. The materials would need updating every couple of years. The printing, storage and distribution costs would be additional. The materials in many languages would probably not be read for lack of demand, interest, illiteracy and the fact that people are often able to read several languages including English. This apparent ideal of meeting every group's needs for information conflicts with the inherent injustice in wasting scarce resources, an act that deprives people with other equally or more pressing needs. The need for delicate judgements cannot be escaped and a balance needs to be found. Some principles for finding such a balance were discussed in Chapter 7 on priority-setting.

On a larger scale than the delivery of health care, laws against racism and for equality may infringe other deeply held values, ethics and laws, for example, those promoting freedom of speech and action. These clashes usually require resolution on a grand scale— by parliamentarians or the law courts, not only nationally but internationally. The ethics of medical research are, indeed, governed by international codes.

10.2.5 Research ethics

This is a topic too big to be addressed fully in this book, but I touched on it in Chapters 8 and 9. As is often the case, it is safe to conclude that the ethics of research generally are applicable to ethnic minority groups. The principles enshrined in the Nuremberg

Code, for example, those emphasizing informed consent, are excellent as a starting point for use with ethnic minority populations. Indeed, such codes are usually written following the abuse of minorities—and this one was designed to prevent a repetition of the abuses of Nazi scientists (see Chapter 6).

Yet some modifications may be necessary. Ethical codes may need to be modified to emphasize the importance of including ethnic minority populations in research and not bypassing them on non-scientific grounds such as researchers' unfamiliarity with them, heterogeneity of populations, real or perceived communication barriers and extra costs. This may require purposive strategies, policies and even laws, as has already happened in the USA (see Chapter 8). Above all, it will require that researchers have the necessary awareness, expertise and resources to achieve inclusivity.

Ethical codes on confidentiality and informed consent may also need modifications. It is absolutely correct that potential research participants' personal details are guarded as far as possible. If such a person, however, does not read it is unethical on the grounds of waste of resources to send written information about a project. It may even alienate such persons by pointing to their illiteracy, and hence belittling them. It may be ethical to tele-phone or even call at the doorstep of such a person, a behaviour that ethical committees may frown upon, because it is considered a greater infringement of privacy than a letter. The right to be invited in an appropriate manner needs to be balanced against the right to privacy of personal data such as a telephone number. To take another example, informed consent may not be easy to gain or to record in writing. Some small leap of imagination may be needed such as recording of the consent on a video or audio recorder. Where this is not possible, a witness may need to confirm oral consent. A thumbprint should be considered as a time-honoured alternative to a signature. Ethical codes should also consider research in cultures where it is most common for the head of the household or the whole family to decide on participation. Thus individual informed consent is not always the only or best way forward.

The point of research is to learn and apply that knowledge. It is important that we can see the effects—and that requires research on outcomes, i.e. evaluation. In Chapter 8 I discussed evaluation of policies, with a focus on checking they were being implemented, and in Chapter 9, I discussed briefly some research methods including trials (the gold standard for evaluation).

10.3 **Evaluating interventions in ethnicity and health**

Before reading on try Exercise 10.3.

Exercise 10.3 Evaluation

- How can we demonstrate the benefits of working with race and ethnicity?
- Why is our endeavour in the ethnicity and health field difficult to evaluate?
- Why is it necessary to evaluate it?

Evaluation is difficult, even for specific effects of circumscribed actions such as giving a drug to treat pneumonia or such easily definable conditions. Even this type of intervention usually requires the complexities and expense of a randomized, double-blind, placebo controlled trial so that biases and confounding factors can be taken into account. Evaluation of the combined effects of laws, policies, strategies and interventions on ethnic minority health poses challenges of a higher order. Nonetheless, it is important for us to ask the question, 'Is this activity benefiting our society, and the ethnic minority populations within it, and are the costs in line with the benefits?' Posing the question is valuable, even although it may be almost impossible to answer it in a definitive way. The question needs to be tackled by a mix of approaches including political, historical and social policy analysis; monitoring of health and related states; and both observational and experimental research on specific interventions. Societies need to be ready to change direction if necessary.

The underlying premise of this book is that ethnic variations in health care, health and disease are too large to be ignored and that acknowledging and acting upon them is better than ignoring them. I have acknowledged one of the prices to be paid—highlighting differences may widen ethnic divisions in society. If the discovery and study of ethnic variations does no good, or does harm, then it would be better to retrace our steps, dismantling research policies, ethnic monitoring programmes and research projects. It is largely a matter of faith, and inference from general observations, that currently the benefits exceed the harms. (This is not to deny the sheer intrinsic interest of the topic from a scholarly, research point of view.)

International comparisons hold one, admittedly difficult, approach to analysis and evaluation. The period 2005–2006 has been fraught with racial tensions, as witnessed by such examples as riots across France, in Sydney in Australia, and great unhappiness at the possible role of racism in the weak response of USA authorities to the flooding of New Orleans. There has been disorder in England, the Netherlands and Denmark over a number of matters that have been linked to socio-economic deprivation and social segregation. Across the world, surveys report a negative attitude to immigration.

It is not apparent that racial disharmony is less in multi-ethnic countries which proclaim themselves as single identity nations that have no place for race-based policies or data. France is such a country. For many years France either was, or was perceived to be, a haven for people suffering from racism. Now, problems have come to the fore. It is likely, in my view, that these problems have existed for a long time and have not been tackled openly, because of ostensibly race-free policies. Since 1999, by contrast, Scotland has openly declared a social justice agenda with equality in race and ethnicity as one of several core components. To date we have seen no social backlash, and the accrual of small but noticeable benefits to the health care of ethnic minority and majority populations alike (for example, areas for prayer and meditation in hospitals that are suitable for people of any religion, or no religion, alike; more choice in the type of food in hospitals; and more choice in the gender of the health professional treating you).

On the smaller scale, beneficial impacts of interventions to better manage and control numerous health problems in ethnic minority groups including diabetes, heart disease and tuberculosis, have been demonstrable. The methodology of controlled trials is increasingly being applied to evaluate specific interventions targeted at ethnic minority populations in relation to their costs. The most important principle is that the benefits, harms and costs of working with race and ethnicity need to be kept under close scrutiny. The scrutiny should be international and continuing.

10.4 Continuing education in ethnicity, race and health

The study of race as, primarily, a biological indicator is outdated and no longer trusted. The modern approach whereby race is perceived as a socially constructed concept encapsulating the social history of a group, and ethnicity is seen as a complex variable that combines cultural, social and biological features, are still under development.

The perspective that these variables are of greatest value for pinpointing and tackling inequalities, rather than exploring causes (aetiology) of disease, is newer still. The number of people trained formally in ethnicity and health, either for research or health care practice, is small, and opportunities for attending courses are limited. Textbooks designed to teach the concepts and principles of the subject in the health context in a comprehensive way are few. There are, however, numerous textbooks on specific topics as listed in the references (p316–319). There are also excellent online overviews of the subject (see p344–350).

It is hard to predict how history will judge current efforts to make use of race and ethnicity. As a minimum we should show our successors that we were conscious of our need to probe and question our subject matter, to learn, and to do better.

Learning in this field will come largely from peers, who are grappling with problems that have no easy answers. How are we to move from theory and concepts to classifications, to data systems, to information, to policy, to plans, to projects, to routine health care, and to show such actions are effective and even better cost-effective? The concrete answers to this question do not exist, and may never exist because the world is rapidly changing. Perhaps all we can hope for are general principles and experiences that we can apply to specific circumstances using our judgement.

We are seeing a rapid rise in the number of web sites, academic journals, e-mail lists, conferences, research projects, newspaper and newsletter articles and student and research staff projects on ethnicity. Networking to a regional, national and even international community offers a route to more efficient management of tough challenges. Some of the numerous portals to web-based knowledge, books and articles are given at the end of this book.

Ultimately, in multi-ethnic nations and continents virtually everyone will need to know more, and that requires foundational education in schools, colleges and universities. For health professionals and health researchers—at least those in population sciences—a solid and comprehensive knowledge base will be necessary. The current largely ad-hoc approach to ethnicity and health education, sometimes based on a few introductory lectures or seminars, will need to be substituted with both core and integrated teaching spanning the subject.

In this field the exemplars (classic works illustrating success) are relatively few, but as a compensation, we have the excitement of now developing them and creating a better future.

10.5 **Predicting a future for race, ethnicity and health: a peek into the crystal ball**

Try Exercise 10.4 before reading on.

Exercise 10.4 Future

- ◆ What would an ideal (but realistic) future for ethnic health be like?
- ◆ Imagine this from the point of view of a hospital practitioner, public health practitioner, a health planner, a policy-maker and a researcher

---

Gazing into the crystal ball is a hazardous action for a writer—it is far safer to pontificate in the impermanent form of a lecture, seminar and discussion over coffee. The written word can be held to account, with no chance of obfuscation, and rare opportunities for retraction or modification.

Some predictions, however, seem absolutely safe. Unless a global catastrophe occurs that leads to retrenchment and mass repatriation probably leading to world war, there will be an inexorable mixing of nations and their peoples that has already been accelerated by migration, international trading, exploration, colonization and the rise of tourism in the last 600 years. In a hundred years from now the idea of a nation founded on a single (or a few) ethnic groups bound by one language or religion will seem quaint. Rather, the global problems of climate change, energy needs and shortages of essentials such as water will bring people in close contact to generate solutions or share in tragedies (as tens, perhaps hundreds, of millions of people are probably going to be displaced by rising sea levels and other natural disasters). The multi-ethnic nation will be the normal one. The creative power of such societies, already so obvious in places such as London, New York, Sydney and Vancouver, will be unquestioned.

What is less easy to predict is the effect of these changes on ethnic and race relations. If solutions to cultural clashes are not found we could find ourselves in a world at war, whether between or within countries. Given solutions we could be immensely enriched by sharing cultures. To continue with this particular point, the teachings of a Prophet who can win the hearts and minds of hundreds of millions of Muslim people across the globe and unite them so strongly to a common purpose—here the defence of his respect— surely deserve a worldwide audience. Perhaps in these teachings there are solutions to the myriad of problems we face, the greatest of these being poverty. The Prophet requested all his followers to give 10 per cent of their earnings as charity. Perhaps this teaching holds the solution to poverty. Equally, perhaps Muslims can also find the solution to the problems that trouble them through peaceful means that would have won the approval of the Prophet and will win widespread respect. How do we move from the clashing of cultures to their cross-pollination and mutual enrichment?

In a world of clashes, the content of this book and its focus on health and health care will become irrelevant and even derisory. In a world of cross-pollination, the approaches discussed here may offer great opportunities to entire populations, minorities and majorities alike, by applying the best in health that each culture has to offer. Let us strive for the better future, illustrated by the health setting scenarios below.

10.5.1 Clinical care scenario: a look into the crystal ball

The health professional of 2017 has the concepts of race and ethnicity ingrained in her through direct exposure to multi-ethnic societies. While at school she learned about the unity yet diversity of humanity. This foundation was essential to her medical studies where the importance of race, ethnicity and related concepts such as religion and language were emphasized not only in the formal curriculum, but also at the bedside by the teaching staff, who themselves typified a multi-ethnic society. Her class comprised of students from 20 countries, and six ethnic groups from her own country. Curricular activities fostered opportunities for learning about all the ethnic diversity represented in the class, with a strong focus on how people maintain their heath in different cultures.

She did a project in one of the local ethnic minority community organizations, both learning about, and earning the respect of, the people she served. Her elective was in a village overseas, where she enjoyed her immersion in a foreign setting. Her postgraduate studies and work encouraged her to apply and extend her learning. She took a special interest in the health beliefs and attitudes of the Chinese population (the longest-lived population in her country), and took a lot of pride in integrating their good ideas into the advice on healthy living she gave to all her patients. She made a special study of traditional Chinese medicine, which she found to be effective for several difficult to manage conditions.

By the end of her training she was comfortable with her own ethnicity, that of her patients, and ready to teach the next generation of health professionals. She always made a point of emphasizing the criticisms about the routine and simplistic use of race labels in Caldwell and Popenhoe's paper, and set an example by making sure that there was a very good clinical reason for mentioning her patient's ethnic group, and if there was, explaining it. She made sure the ethnic group was never the fourth routinely spoken word in her case presentations.

> In regions of the United States such as ours, where the population is predominantly of European-American or African-American descent, the description of race is often distilled down to 'black' or 'white'. Thus, in our institution and in those with similar demographics, the fourth spoken word of many case presentations broadly describes the patient as black or white.
>
> Caldwell and Popenhoe (1995: 614)

She took special pride in her work in helping to train interpreters on medical matters, and the fact that the health service's policy-makers and her peers turned to her for advice on improving services for ethnic minorities in her locality. Her roles and skills were amply and appropriately recognized in the awards and promotions committees.

10.5.2 Public health scenario: 2017

The public health practitioner of 2017 knew, as his predecessors did, that information is the key to success in health improvement. The difference is that he has it at his fingertips. In 2012 the WHO convened an International Working Group that prepared a handbook defining and operationalizing the concepts of ethnicity and health. The handbook was revised every two years with an ongoing online commentary on potential improvements. The handbook, despite controversy, led to sharing of ideas and information, particularly on terminology and classifications, such that everyone can now access these, together with an interpretation, online. Moreover, the accompanying active electronic discussion allows global sharing of ideas and practice.

The public health practitioner works with the national ethnic coding system that ensures every existing and all new databases have a common approach and one that itself maps onto the census classification. Commonality in numerators and denominators, and opportunity for international comparison, means that he can produce data and a cogent commentary including international, national, regional and local comparisons. All the problems of small numbers are still present but the ability to aggregate data for 5, 10 and even 15 years is a boon. Primary research also now pays attention to meticulous description of the ethnic composition of study populations so that aggregation of data by systematic review and meta-analysis is possible.

The health authority, hospitals and primary care services and individual health professionals are very interested in these data and as a result work hard to ensure the information they supply is accurate. The most satisfying aspect of the work is that the data are used to help both modify and evaluate the local ethnic health strategy. For several years, no one has questioned the worth of these data and it seems amazing that there was a time when strategy and plans on ethnicity and health were made by guesswork.

The public health practitioner took special pride when Waqar Ahmad (see the quotation) spoke to him at a conference and said that his reports were not racialized, but helpful to ethnic minority populations. Rather, his reports pinpointed both similarities and differences and extracted the key messages for health improvement, paying particular attention to those conditions where ethnic minority populations were doing well.

> 'For black people this focus (racialization) is almost exclusively on cultures and ethnicities, genetics and metabolisms, being different and therefore inferior'.
>
> Ahmad (1993: 22)

10.5.3 Health care planning: 2017

The Director of Health Care Planning, responsible for implementing policy for six million people, had found it very hard to meet competing demands, and in particular to persuade the Director of Finance to set aside extra funds to develop the service to meet the needs of ethnic minority populations. One particular problem was that short term funding increases from the period 2003–2008 led to developments that could not be sustained when funding was tight (most of the time since 2008). There have been some improvements recently, resulting from the implementation of important policy and strategic principles in the last ten years.

First, the policy and strategic documents on ethnicity and health were firmly integrated into the region's overall strategy on health and health care improvement and linked to the challenge of reducing inequalities, the top political priority for the last 15 years. Second, the emphasis on quality and effectiveness of services, and particularly the resources saved by getting the services right first time for ethnic minority populations, has resulted in huge satisfaction among patients, staff and managers.

The merging of the business case with the ethical one, only achieved once funding became tight in 2008, has been powerful. Third, the funding formula for our population's share of health care resources has been changed to make explicit, and take into account, two important points that generally hold:

1. that most of the ethnic minority groups are younger so they use fewer resources for diseases of old age e.g. dementia, and cancers
2. they do use more resources in relation to time spent in consultations, services for children and women, and diabetes and one or more cardiovascular diseases.

Readjustment of the overall formulae for each component of health care has made it possible to meet demands within specific services without altering the overall budget. Even the finance director was happy with these changes. Finally, we have solved the problem of mainstreaming. No project is funded for less than three years, rules for what will happen after this time are established at the outset and an evaluation is done before decisions are taken to mainstream and these are based on demonstrable success. The decision to mainstream is heavily influenced by our Ethnic Health Forum, a committee comprised of professionals and members of ethnic minority communities. Then, we have a three-year timeframe for mainstreaming of successful projects i.e. a time-frame of at least 6 years in total.

The Director of Planning's satisfaction has been in having made some inroads into a really tough assignment. She can hold her head high and say her department has conformed to the spirit of national policy and, of course, the law. Not surprisingly, as some people knew even in the twentieth century, many of the changes have benefited everyone. For example, the Caribbean-style menus are very popular, cheap and healthy, and the signs around the hospital based on symbols are really appreciated by all our older patients, not just the ethnic minority patients.

10.5.4 **Policy-making: 2017**

The policy-maker of 2017 frames her ideas in the light of widespread experience of what does and does not work. Of course, politics isn't primarily about evidence, but ideas and visions can be moulded, shaped and improved by experience and evidence. So when the Minister for Health asked for a speech on where the nation was going in relation to the health of ethnic minority groups her office was able to summarize the successes and failures of the last ten years and compare approaches with other nations. Then, working quickly with the National Diversity and Health Forum's ideas that had themselves been shaped in debates over the preceding few years she was able to come up with realistic proposals that would gain wide support, help the country stay in the vanguard and not exceed available budgets.

Policy-making became easier because of cross-party political consensus that ethnic diversity is essential to our nation; increase in participation in the political processes by ethnic minority groups that resulted in sharing of responsibility in decision-making and implementation; national information systems that produced data by ethnic group; and, sad to say, since a health authority was taken to court under the race relations laws. Thankfully, the case was withdrawn by mutual consent when her department agreed to review all policies once again and set up systems to do a diversity check on all relevant policies. On this occasion the health authorities implemented their race equality policies fully. The policy makers greatest satisfaction is from the observation that the policy-making is generic—the principles that work for one disadvantaged group seem to work for others too and what works for one ethnic group helps others, even new groups arriving as refugees. Finally, the policies are getting the best out of people, by creating a healthy and participating population and environment.

10.5.5 Research: 2017

The researcher of 2017 takes it for granted that ethnicity is a core if not essential feature of population-based research, but also that ethnic minority groups are both invited and expected to participate in other kinds of research based on tissues and organs and done mainly in the laboratory. The research community does not simply do this from a sense of what is right, or even because of the intrinsic interest of ethnic variations, but to maintain the long-term health of the research infrastructure. If researchers did not do this, in some parts of the country there would be insufficient people to participate in research.

The turning point was a statement, to a large extent inspired by the leadership of the National Institute of Health in the USA, on required good practice in research issued jointly by the research councils, the Department of Health, the major research charities, and some key leaders of ethnic minority organizations. This stated that research funding was contingent upon, and would be inclusive of associated costs of, attention to issues of population diversity. The aim was to both fill a deep hole in the research database relating to the health and health care of ethnic minorities, and create an extensive infrastructure that would make the research possible. One big job was education about the limits and potential of this kind of research. Ethnic minority communities themselves participated.

Everyone was pleasantly surprised how much cooperation and interest there was. The recruitment and training of a cadre of researchers from a wide range of ethnic minority populations was also pivotal. A strategic and proactive approach was taken to finding, training and retaining in long-term careers people from previously under-represented ethnic groups. We now have people from most ethnic groups and a network that allows sharing of expertise. Ethical committees have been instrumental in monitoring how well the research policy has been implemented, and to be frank, forcing the recalcitrant to comply. We have more equity in research. The academic journals are brimming with good quality ethnicity and health research. The press, and particularly the sector catering to ethnic minority populations, has shown a real appetite for this work. Research has helped to identify and reduce racism. Luckily, the emergent opinion in the early twenty-first century that the research establishment itself was institutionally racist was quickly deflected by decisive action. Finally, the controversy about the relative value of race and ethnicity died down when most researchers switched to the latter. Effectively, Oppen-heimer's view (see quotation) prevails now and Huxley and Haddon's recommendation of 1935 is implemented. Raj Bhopal's book in its second edition in 2012 had one single paragraph on race!

> Unlike race, 'ethnic group' is more obviously a social construct. Its weakness is also a strength. It shifts the researcher's focus away from race, which carries the taint of its biological heritage and offers a powerful alternative approach ... to seek explanations for the distribution and determinants of disease. As a social construct, each ethnic group contains a history ... and alters over time; the use of ethnic group should make the researcher sensitive to the effects of generation, changing economic status, social class, relations with other groups, discrimination, and relative political power.
>
> Oppenheimer (2001: 1053)

10.6 Conclusions

The concepts of race and ethnicity are constructed on factors that are pivotal in the lives of humans, and to the way humans organize their societies. As societies have become more complex, and the typical size of human settlements has risen, these concepts have become more important. Fundamentally, race and ethnicity are among the factors, or strictly conglomerates of factors, that allow humans to differentiate themselves, and their social groups, from others and others' social groups. This is not to deny that similarities far outweigh differences. Equally this does not imply that race or ethnicity are features of nature. They are not. They are created from fundamental factors, some of which are natural and some social. The composite of factors that are considered to comprise race and ethnicity is subject to change over time and may vary by place. Of course, the choice of the underlying factors of interest is also dependent on the purposes and contexts of the work.

The theoretical basis of these concepts is not easy to define. This does not make them atheoretical just, to echo Nazroo, untheorized. It is difficult, if not impossible, to think about complex matters without a theory, even although the theory cannot be articulated easily, at least in a way that commands respect and consensus. Achieving a stronger and more explicit theoretical base is a continuing challenge. This book has pointed to some of the theories that have informed discussion of race and ethnicity. This book has also focused on how race and ethnicity are relevant to epidemiology, public health and

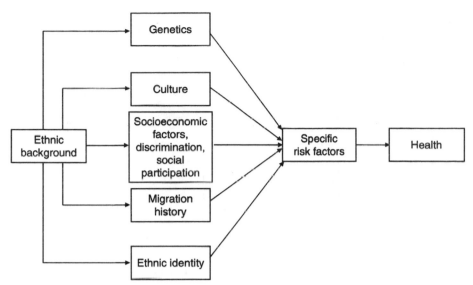

Fig. 10.1 Characteristics of ethnic groups that play a role in the interpretation of ethnic inequalities in health.
Reproduced with permission from Stronks K, Uniken Venema P, Dallan N, Gunning-Schepers LJ, T Soc Gezondneidsz 1999; 77: 33–40.

health care, with somewhat less emphasis on their role in individual health care, and in the wider spheres of health, science and society. This emphasis reflects not only the disciplinary background of the author but the historical and contemporary importance of these concepts in these disciplines.

Epidemology is based on finding and explaining population differences, and the race and ethnicity concepts are among the most powerful tools available though they are better at finding than explaining. Race, ethnicity and health scholars have created a number of models that explore how the associations between these concepts and health appear. Naturally, such models are based upon underlying theories, and they can also be used to contribute to them. Four such models are given in Figures 10.1–10.4, with no comment from me, but with encouragement to readers to study the original publications. (See references.) Figure 10.1 shows how ethnicity fits an epidemiological model showing the genesis of variations in health status.

Public health and medical care are humanitarian disciplines that are focused on the most needy (the sick) who are so often also the most disadvantaged. Race and ethnicity are good at pinpointing need and economic disadvantage. For these and other reasons the relationships between these disciplines and concepts will not be severed, notwithstanding the potential to harm that is inherent in the work. It is imperative for us to improve our work so that the benefits substantially outweigh the harm at.

I have argued that the key to doing good in this field is a social and cultural milieu of equality, and freedom from racism. Given this, the thoughtful application of the approaches of the social and population sciences should yield workable classifications and data that can be interpreted using epidemiological frameworks for analysis including

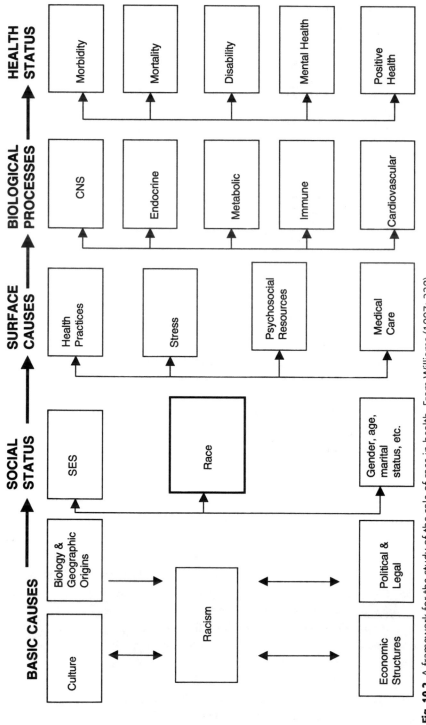

Fig. 10.2 A framework for the study of the role of race in health. From Williams (1997: 328).

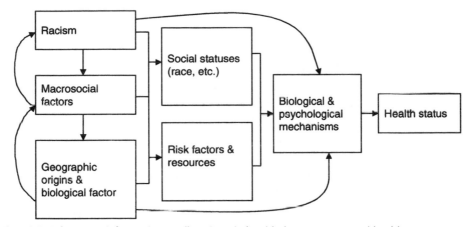

Fig. 10.3 A framework for understanding the relationship between race and health.

Reprinted with permission from Williams DR, Lavizzo-Mourey R, Warren RC, The concepts of race and health status in America. *Public Health Reports* 1994; 109: 26–41.

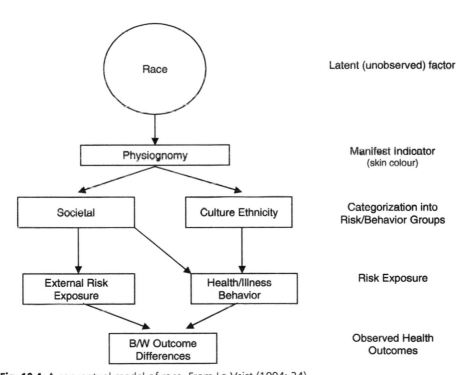

Fig. 10.4 A conceptual model of race. From La Veist (1994: 24).

Reproduced from La Veist TA, 'Why we should continue to study race . . . but do a better job: An essay on race, racism and health.' *Ethnicity and Disease* 1996; 6: 21–29. Permission requested from International Society on Hypertension in Blacks (ISHIB).

those for assessing error and bias (misclassification, mismeasurement, information, selection, confounding); and cause and effect (see Chapter 9). The analysis arising can feed into needs assessment (Chapter 5), priority-setting (Chapter 7), the inequalities debate (Chapter 6), policy- and strategy-making (Chapter 8), and scholarship and research (Ch 9). There is a virtuous cycle around data—the more it is used the more the enthusiasm for its collection and for improvement in data systems (Chapters 2, 3 and 5). Data also improves services both directly (through better decisions) and through the Hawthorne Effect, whereby awareness of being monitored is a motivator for better performance.

This age of equality of humans, enshrined in international legislation, has coincided with, or perhaps has been caused by, the intermingling of the inhabitants of the globe. The mixing of the world's ethnic groups is not without its problems, but the benefits probably outweigh these. The response of the health care system in each country is shaped by local circumstances, and yet, in broad historical terms there are many features in common (Chapter 4). The intermingling through migration has brought, in the wake of slavery, colonialism and scientific racism, a freer exchange than ever before of ideas, labour, art, culture, business, science and technologies. Who can deny that, notwithstanding tensions and setbacks, increasing mutual respect and opportunity has accompanied this intermingling? I was born in 1953 in India six years after the end of the British Raj, to parents who were governed by the British. My parents had, in this 'jewel of the British Empire', three years of schooling between them, before they emigrated to Glasgow, one of the great cities of the motherland. I was raised by them in Scotland from the age of two. That I have penned this book while holding the Chair of Public Heath at the University of Edinburgh testifies to the power of such intermingling. I have benefited hugely from this cross-cultural opportunity, but so has society at large, locally, nationally and internationally.

The combination of cultural perspectives is an advantage. This is shown par excellence in the world of literature. Travel has been extolled, since time immemorial, as a core component of the experience of life. The benefits, and the costs, are shared by the minorities and majority alike. It behoves us all to maximize the benefits. There is no greater goal for any society than that its citizens should be long-lived, free of disease and disability, brimming with energy, creative and full of ideas. In other words, that they are healthy. In so far as the concepts of race and ethnicity can contribute to the creation of a healthier society they should be coveted. As with children, so it is with ideas such as race and ethnicity. How they develop and mature depends on us. Race has been a disappointment. Ethnicity has a future.

Summary

There is no single theory (or group of theories) on race and ethnicity that is widely accepted. Biological theories based on species and subspecies have not withstood testing and social theories have not as yet made a major impact in medical sciences. Advances in the science of genetics are reopening old debates on the biological underpinnings of racial and ethnic differences. Articulating coherent theories on race and ethnicity in the health domain is a continuing challenge. Race and ethnicity concepts conform, and contribute, to the general epidemiological theories on the forces that shape population differences in health status and hence they are important in public health.

International migration and greater international exchange through tourism and communication media are creating a multi-racial, multi-ethnic global society, demanding clarity of understanding around both similarities of, and differences between, subgroups of populations. Used wisely the concepts of race and ethnicity have the potential to improve public health, health care, clinical care and medical science, but used unwisely they can do immense damage. Stringent attention to ethics and justice is essential.

A rational, analytic approach to the interpretation of data, set within broader epidemiological theories of health, is needed. Interventions utilizing the concept of race and ethnicity need to be carefully evaluated to judge the balance of benefits to costs, and to counteract the weaknesses of the concepts. There is an imperative to achieve benefits in terms of health improvement and to demonstrate this unequivocally. This imperative mandates that we continue to learn. A vision for better clinical practice, health care planning, health policy and research is in place and is realistic. Scholarship to advance theoretical understanding, as well as underpin practical advances, has been done, and continues. In the future, historians and health scholars and researchers will subject our work to scrutiny. We should ensure that they conclude that we not only did our best with our limited knowledge, but that we built well on our legacy, and learned the painful lessons of the past.

A brief glossary

Absolute risk The actual rate of a disease/illness event occurring in a population under study i.e. without comparison with another population.

Acute An adjective commonly applied to diseases that have a short time course, as opposed to a long one (see chronic).

African A person with African ancestral origins who self-identifies, or is identified, as African, but excluding those of other ancestry e.g. European and South Asian. This term is the currently preferred description for more specific categories, as in African-American, for example. (In terms of racial classifications, this population approximates to the group historically known as Negroid or similar terms.) In practice, Northern Africans from Algeria, Morocco and such countries are excluded from this category. (See also Black.)

Afro-Caribbean/African-Caribbean A person of African ancestral origins whose family settled in the Caribbean before emigrating and who self-identifies, or is identified, as Afro-Caribbean (in terms of racial classifications, this population approximates to the group known as Negroid or similar terms). (See also Black.)

Allele See gene.

Asian Indian A term currently used synonymously with South Asian (see below), but with the important limitation that major South Asian populations such as Pakistani and Bangladeshi may not identify with it. This term is being used in North America to distinguish this population from Native Americans, previously known as American Indians.

Asian Strictly, this label applies to anyone originating from the Asian continent. In practice, this term is used in the UK to mean people with ancestry in the Indian subcontinent. In the USA, the term has broader meaning, but is mostly used to denote people of Far Eastern origins, e.g Chinese, Japanese and Philipinos. More specific terms should be used whenever possible.

Bangladeshi A person whose ancestry lies in the Indian subcontinent who self-identifies, or is identified, as Bangladeshi. (See also South Asian.) Between 1947 and 1971 the land known as Bangladesh was East Pakistan and before that India. There is no clear-cut equivalent in terms of racial classifications, though historically northern Indians have been classified as Caucasian, and some Indian tribes as aboriginal. (The racial term Malayan, coined by Blumenbach, is forgotten as purposeless.)

Black A person with African ancestral origins, who self identifies, or is identified, as Black, African or Afro-Caribbean (see African and Afro-Caribbean). The word is capitalized to signify its specific use in this way. In some circumstances the word Black signifies all non-White minority populations, and in this usage serves political purposes. While this term was widely supported in the late twentieth century there are signs that such support is diminishing.

Blood pressure Usually refers to the pressure in the arteries supplying the body except for the lungs (i.e. not veins and pulmonary arteries) as measured by sphygmomanometer (see below).

Case control study A study where cases are compared with controls (see below), people who usually do not have the disease or problem under investigation. These comparisons help to test hypotheses about the causes of disease.

Case A person with the disease or problem under investigation.

Caucasian An Indo-European. This is Blumenbach's eighteenth-century term for the White race of mankind, which he derived from the people who lived in the Caucasus. This term is usually used synonymously with Caucasoid European or White. Alone amongst terms derived from traditional racial classification, Caucasian remains popular in both science and everyday language.

Cause Something which has an effect, in the case of epidemiology, this effect being (primarily) a change in the frequency of risk factors or adverse health outcomes.

Chinese A person with ancestral origins in China, who self-identifies, or is identified, as Chinese. (In terms of historical racial classifications, Chinese approximate to the group known as Mongolian or Mongoloid.)

Cholesterol A lipid (fatty substance) that is essential to many bodily functions that is transported in the blood via lipoproteins. Cholesterol and other lipids carried by low density lipoproteins (LDL/VLDL) are a risk factor for coronary heart disease (and like vascular diseases), while those carried by high density lipoproteins (HDL) seem to be protective.

Chromosome See gene.

Chronic An adjective commonly applied to diseases that have a long-lasting time course, and usually applied to non-toxic and non-infectious diseases.

Cohort study A study where people with a risk factor or health problem of interest are followed up to observe the outcomes, e.g. new cases of disease. It is also known as a longitudinal study.

Competing causes A concept where alternative causes of disease, usually as causes of death, are in competition with each other, e.g. in Afro-Caribbean population one explanation of the comparatively low CHD rates is that the atherosclerotic process kills people from stroke. If this were to be controlled, it may be that CHD would become commoner.

Confounding The distortion of an association by other (confounding) factors that influence both the outcome and risk factor under study.

Congenital A health problem present at birth.

Control/control group A comparison population that is used in a number of study designs so as to permit inferences about the pattern of risk factors, health outcomes, or treatment effects in the study population of interest.

Coronary heart disease A group of diseases resulting from reduced blood supply to the heart, most often caused by narrowing or blockage of the coronary arteries that provide the blood supply to the heart.

Cot death A synonym for the sudden infant death syndrome, which is unexplained death in infancy.

Creole An uncommon word used to describe people of mixed European and African ancestry living or originating from the West Indies and parts of South America. The main use of this term in ethnicity and health research is in Dutch studies of the Surinamese, who are divided mainly into Creole and Hindu (see also Hindu).

Dementia See senile dementia.

Demography The scientific study of population, particularly the factors that determine its size and shape. A cousin of epidemiology.

Diabetes (mellitus) A disease characterized by high levels of glucose in the blood caused by either lack or ineffectiveness of the hormone insulin.

Disease A bodily dysfunction, usually one that can be described by a diagnostic label. (For simplicity, this book concentrates on discussing diseases and uses this word when describing other health problems, e.g. death, disability, illness, etc.).

Distribution The frequency with which each value (or category) occurs in the study population. The distribution of many variables take on a characteristic shape. (See normal distribution).

Down's Syndrome A congenital, genetic disorder, leading to mental retardation and a characteristic face caused by the presence of three chromosomes instead of two at the site of the 21st chromosome.

Environment A broad conception, sometimes to mean everything except genetic and biological factors, and sometimes qualified and narrowed, e.g. physical environment.

Epidemiology The science and craft that studies the pattern of diseases (and health, though usually indirectly) in populations to help understand both their causes and the burden they impose. This information is applied to prevent, control or manage the problems under study.

Ethnic minority group Usually, but not always, this phrase is used to refer to a non-White population. Alternatively, it may be used to describe a specific identifiable group e.g gypsy travellers, and less commonly, Irish in the UK. Some people consider the phrase inaccurate and prefer minority ethnic group, but the two phrases are used synonymously.

Ethnicity The social group a person belongs to, and either identifies with or is identified with by others, as a result of a mix of cultural and other factors including one or more of language, diet, religion, ancestry, and physical textures traditionally associated with race (see race). Increasingly, the concept is being used synonymously with race but the trend is pragmatic rather than scientific.

Ethnocentrism The tendency to perceive and interpret the world from the standpoint of one's own culture. In epidemiology the tendency is reflected in the practice of using the White population as the norm or standard (see White).

European European primarily means an inhabitant of Europe, or one with ancestral origins in Europe. Effectively this is used in epidemiology and public health as a synonym for White (see below). Europeans are placed in the racial classification Caucasian, more recently known as Europid (the latter has not proven popular).

Exposure A general term to indicate contact with the postulated causal fctors (or agents of diseasese) used in a way similar to risk factor.

Fetal origins of disease hypothesis The phrase encapsulating the idea that early life circumstances, particularly *in utero*, have an important and lasting effect in determining health and disease in later life.

Gene The discrete basic unit (made of DNA or deoxyribonucleic acid) of the chromosome, which itself consists of numerous genes and other DNA material. Genes carry information coding for specific functions, e.g. making proteins. There are two genes at a particular location on a chromosome—both for the same function. Variants of the same gene on a particular location are called alleles. There are 23 pairs of chromosomes in each cell in human beings (46 in total), and the number of genes is variously estimated as 25–35,000.

General population Everyone in the population being studied, irrespective of race or ethnicity.

Genetic drift Genetic evolution, characteristically observable in small populations, arising from random variations in gene frequency.

HDL See cholesterol.

Health care needs Effective preventative or medical interventions which improve health in its broadest sense.

Health needs Factors needed to improve the health of individuals and populations.

Health A desired ideal, that includes being free of disease, disability and infirmity, that is characterized by well-being and functioning in society.

Hindu An old, now seldom used, term for Indians. A term occasionally used more or less synonymously with South Asian. In some countries such as the Netherlands the term is used to describe the ethnicity of Surinamese of Indian subcontinent ancestry.

Hispanic A person of Latin American descent (with some degree of Spanish or Portuguese ancestral origins), who self-identifies, or is identified, as Hispanic irrespective of other racial or ethnic considerations. In the USA this term, often used interchangeably with Latino, is considered (wrongly) an indicator of ethnic origin

Hypertension A condition of having blood pressure above an arbitrarily defined level (presently usually set at 140/90). Hypertension is associated with many adverse outcomes, particularly atherosclerotic diseases

Hypothesis A proposition that is amenable to test by scientific methods. (See null hypotheses).

Illness The state of being unwell, often due to disease.

Incidence/incidence rate The number of new cases of a disease or other condition in a defined population within a specified period of time. When this number is divided by the numbers of people in the relevant population we have the incidence rate.

Indian A person whose ancestry lies in the Indian subcontinent who identifies, or is identified, as Indian (see South Asian). (There were major changes to India's geographical boundaries in 1947 when Pakistan was created.)

Indigenous This term is usually used to mean a person who belongs naturally to a place in the sense of long-term family origins (see Native). This term is sometimes used to identify the majority population, for example, in the UK as an alternative to the word White. In some parts of the world e.g. Australia, the word indigenous is used specifically to refer to aboriginal populations (e.g. Aborigine).

Institutional racism See racism

Irish A person whose ancestry lies in Ireland who self-identifies as Irish but generally restricted to the White population (see White).

LDL/VLDL See cholesterol

Longitudinal study See cohort

Majority population When used in race/ethnicity studies this phrase is usually used as a synonym for White or European.

Minority ethnic group See ethnic minority group. Increasingly used as the preferred phrase and replacing ethnic minority group

Mixed and other race or ethnic group This glossary omits a clear exposition on these terms, which require fresh thought. The increasing importance of the category mixed (ethnicity or race) is self-evident. The increasing acceptance of sexual unions that cross ethnic and racial boundaries is adding both richness and complexity to most societies. The way to categorize people born of such unions is unclear and the current approaches are inadequate, partly because the number of potential categories is huge. Another category seen in racial classifications is 'other', this permitting those not included to identify themselves, or be identified by the observer. In both instances the solution is, most probably, to offer space for free-text responses for individuals to identify themselves. These responses, however, need to be coded, analysed, summarized, quantified and published. Without this, individually small but collectively large populations remain hidden when policy on ethnic diversity is made.

Native Sometimes this word is used to refer to populations born, or with family origins, in a place (see indigenous). This was also a pejorative term meaning populations belonging to a non-European and imperfectly civilized or savage race, so writers need to take care.

Non-Asian/Non-Chinese etc. This type of term is rarely defined but self-evidently implies those not belonging to the group under study. This degree of non-specificity is not usually recommended, but is used where there is little or no alternative.

Normal distribution A distribution that describes well a great many biological variables. The mean, median and mode values are identical, the distribution is symmetrical around this value, and one standard deviation encapsulates 68 per cent of the population.

Occidental This is a very rarely used term meaning a native or inhabitant of the Occident (West), and effectively a synonym for European, but readers need to be aware of it as the antonym of Oriental.

Oriental A term meaning a native or inhabitant of the Orient (East). This term is in occasional use in epidemiology, usually referring to Far Eastern populations. It is too general to be useful.

Pakistani A person whose ancestry lies in the Indian subcontinent who identifies, or is identified, as Pakistani (see South Asian). Some Pakistanis may have birth or ancestral roots in the current territory of India but identify with Pakistan, a country created in 1947.

Participant The word that is replacing subject, as in study participant.

Placebo An inactive substance or procedure used as a medicine for psychological effect; and commonly used in the control group in a trial.

Population A complex concept with a multitude of meanings in epidemiology, but crucially, the people in whom the problem under study occurs, and in whom the results of the research are to be applied.

Prevalence/prevalence rate The number of cases of a given disease or other condition in a given population at a designated time. When this number is divided by the number of people in the relevant population we have the prevalence rate.

Proportional mortality (or morbidity) ratio (PMR) A summary measure of the proportion of deaths/disease due to a specific cause in the study population compared to either all causes or another cause.

Public health An activity to which many contribute, most usually defined as the science and art of prolonging life, preventing disease and promoting health through the organized efforts of society.

Race By historical and common usage the group (subspecies in traditional scientific usage) a person belongs to as a result of a mix of physical features such as skin colour and hair texture, which reflect ancestry and geographical origins, as identified by others or, increasingly, as self-identified. The importance of social factors in the creation and perpetuation of racial categories has led to the concept broadening to include a common social and political heritage, making its usage similar to ethnicity. Race and ethnicity are increasingly used as synonyms causing some confusion and leading to the hybrid terms race/ethnicity (see Ethnicity).

Racial prejudice Negative beliefs, perceptions or attitudes towards one or more ethnic or racial groups.

Racism/institutional racism A belief that some races are superior to others, used to devise and justify individual and collective actions which create and sustain inequality among racial and ethnic groups. Individual racism is usually manifested in decisions and behaviours that disadvantage small numbers of people. Institutional racism, whereby policies and traditions, sometimes unwittingly, favour a particular racial or ethnic group, may be less obvious but may disadvantage large populations.

Reference/control/comparison This refers to the standard against which a population that is being studied can be compared to permit an analysis of similarities and differences. The concept is fundamental to epidemiology, and this terminology is preferable to non-specific ethnic or racial terms such as non-Asian, or general or even White population.

Relative risk The ratio of the incidence of disease in one population (the study population) compared to another (the control population).

Risk Factor A factor associated with an increased probability of an adverse outcome, but not necessarily a causal factor.

Senile dementia Brain disease characterized by loss of intellect, usually irreversible and caused by degenerative processes associated with old age.

Sexually transmitted diseases (STD) The group of diseases mainly transmitted during sexual behaviour, e.g. syphilis. Some STDs may be transmitted in other ways too, e.g. AIDS.

Sickle cell disease/anaemia A genetic disorder, whereby the haemoglobin, the oxygen carrying molecule in red blood cells, crystallizes and distorts the blood cell into a sickle shape when oxygen in the cell is low. The result is anaemia.

Sickness The state of being unwell or dysfunctional, often as a result of disease.

SMR (Standardized Mortality/Morbidity Ratio) The ratio of the number of events observed in the study population to the number that would be expected if it had the same specific rates as the standard population (usually the fraction is multiplied by 100). A figure of more than 100 reflects an excess of disease, less than 100 a deficit. The SMR takes into account age differences between populations.

South Asian A person whose ancestry is in the countries of the Indian sub-continent, including India, Pakistan, Bangladesh and Sri Lanka (in terms of racial classifications, most people in this group probably fit best into Caucasian or Caucasoid but this is confusing and is not recommended). This label is usually assigned, for individuals rarely identify with it. (See also Indian, Indian Asian, Asian, Pakistani, Bangladeshi).

Standardized mortality (or morbidity) ratio (SMR) See SMR.

Stratified sample The people selected for (or participating in) a study where the sampling frame is organized by subgroups, e.g. men and women, or age groups. Then random samples are chosen within each subgroup

Subject A person who is studied, i.e. a member of the population under study (see participant).

Theory A system of ideas offered to explain and connect observed factors or conjectures. A statement of general principles or laws underlying a subject.

Trisomy 21 See Down's Syndrome.

Tuberculosis A multisystem infection caused by the bacteria Mycobacterium tuberculosis.

Western A person or populations with ancestry in a region conventionally known as the west, effectively European countries, as distinguished from Eastern or Oriental populations. This loose term is not recommended.

White The term usually used to describe people with European ancestral origins who identify, or are identified, as White (sometimes called European, or in terms of racial classifications, the group usually known as Caucasian or Caucasoid). The word is capitalized to highlight its specific use. The term has served to distinguish these groups from those groups with skin of other colours (black, yellow etc.), and hence derives from the concept of race but is used as an indicator of ethnicity. There are problems of poverty and excess disease in subgroups of the White population, which cannot be unearthed and tackled by solely using the label White.

From Bhopal R, Glossary of terms relating to ethnicity and race: for reflection and debate. *Journal of Epidemiological Community Health* 2003; 58: 441–45.

Bibliography

This is a small selection, and much of it is for general reading.

Publications that have been reworked (invariably in part) for the purposes of this book are marked with the symbol *

Publications that have been cited in the text are marked with the symbol †

Publications that are sources of quotations are marked with the symbol ‡

Publications that provided the four models of race or ethnicity are marked with the symbol §

Glossary

The major sources for the glossary were:

* Bhopal RS (2002) *Concepts of Epidemiology*. Oxford: Oxford University Press.
* Bhopal R (2003) Glossary of terms relating to ethnicity and race: for reflection and debate. *Journal of Epidemiology and Community Health* 58: 441–5.

Books

Several thousand books are listed on Amazon.com under key words race, ethnicity and health. Here is a small selection. A selected bibliography on ethnicity and health.

Ahmad WIU (ed.) (1992) *The Politics of Race and Health*. Bradford: University of Bradford and Bradford and Ilkley Community College, Race Relations Research Unit.

‡ Ahmad WIU (ed.) (1993) *Race and Health in Contemporary Britain*. Milton Keynes: Open University Press.

Ahmad WIU and Atkin K (1996) *Race and Community Care*. Buckingham: Open University Press.

Arora S, Coker N, Gillam S and Ismail H (2000) *Improving the Health of Black and Minority Ethnic Groups: a guide for primary care organisations*. London: King's Fund.

† Bahl V and Hopkins A (1993) *Access to Health Care for People from Black and Ethnic Minorities*. London: The Royal College of Physicians of London.

Barkan E (1992) *The Retreat of Scientific Racism*. London: Cambridge University Press.

Bernal M (1987) Black Athena. London: Free Association Books.

Bhugra D, Bahl V (eds.) (1999) *Ethnicity: An agenda for mental health*. London: Gaskell.

Biddiss MD (ed.) (1970) *Gobineau Selected Political Writings*. London: Johnathan Cape.

Blakemore K and Boneham M (1994) *Age, Race and Ethnicity. A comparative approach*. Philadelphia, PA: Open University Press, 1994.

† Blumenbach JF (1865) *The anthropological treatises of Johann Friedrich Blumenbach*. London: Anthropological Society.

British Medical Association (1995) *Multicultural Health Care. Current practice and future policy in medical education*. London: BMA.

Cashmore E. (1996) *Dictionary of Race and Ethnic Relations*, 4th edn. London: Routledge.

† Coker NE (2001) *Racism in Britain. An agenda for change*. London: King's Fund.

† College M, van Geuns HA, Svensson PG (1986) *Migration and Health: towards an understanding of the health care needs of ethnic minorities*. Proceedings of the Consultative Group on Ethnic Minorities, The Hague, Netherlands, 28–30 November. Copenhagen: World Health Organization, Regional Office for Europe.

Cruickshank JK and Beevers G (1990) *Ethnic Factors in Health and Disease*. MA: Butterworth.

Diamond J (1998) *Guns, Germs and Steel*. London: Vintage.

Ebling FJ (ed.) (1974) *Racial Variation in Man*. London: Institute of Biology.

† Erens B, Primatesta P, Prior G. (2001) *Health Survey for England: the health of minority ethnic groups '99*. London: Stationery Office.

Fernando S (1991) *Mental Health, Race and Culture*. Basingstoke: Macmillan in association with MIND (National Association for Mental Health).

Gerrish K and Husband C (1996) *Nursing for a Multiethnic Society*. Buckingham, Philadelphia, PA: Open University Press.

† Gould SJ (1984) *The Mismeasure of Man*. London: Pelican Books Ltd.

† Gunaratnam Y (1994) *Checklist. Health and Race: a starting point for managers on improving services for black populations*. London: King's Fund.

Helman CG (2000) *Culture, Health and Illness: an introduction for health professionals* Oxford: Butterworth Heinemann.

Henley, A (1987) *Caring in a Multiracial Society*. London: Bloomsbury Health Authority.

* Institute of Medicine Committee on Understanding and Eliminating Racial and Ethnic Disparities in Health Care. *Unequal Treatment: confronting racial and ethnic disparities in health care*. Washington, DC: National Academy Press.

† Johnson MRD, Owen D, Blackburn C (2000) *Black and Minority Ethnic Groups in England: the second health and lifestyle survey*. London: Health Education Authority.

Jones JH (1993) *Bad Blood. The Tuskegee Syphilis Experiment, 2nd edn*. New York: Free Press.

Kai J (ed.) (1998) *Valuing Diversity—an Educational Resource for Effective Health Care*. London: Royal College of General Practitioners.

Kai J (2003) *Ethnicity, Health and Primary Care*. Oxford: Oxford University Press.

‡ Karmi G (1996) *The Ethnic Health Handbook: a factfile for health care professionals*. Oxford: Blackwell Science.

Karmi G and McKeigue P (1993) *The Ethnic Health Bibliography*. London: NE and NW Thames RHA.

Kelleher D and Hillier SM (1996) *Researching Cultural Differences in Health*. London, New York: Routledge.

‡ Kiple KF and King V (1981) *Another Dimension to the Black Diaspora: diet, disease, and racism*. Cambridge: Cambridge University Press.

Kumar D (ed.) (2004) *Genetic Disorders of the Indian Subcontinent*. Dordrecht: Kluwer Academic Publishers.

Kuper L (ed.) (1975) *Race, Science and Society*. London: Allen and Unwin.

LaVeist T (2002) *Race, Ethnicity and Health: a public health reader*. San Francisco, CA: Jossey Bass.

Loue S (1998) *Handbook of Immigrant Health*. New York: Plenum Press.

* Macbeth H and Shetty P (eds.) (2000) *Ethnicity and Health*. London: Taylor and Francis.

* Mackintosh J, Bhopal RS, Unwin N, Ahmad N (1998) *Step-by-step Guide to Epidemiological Health Needs Assessment for Ethnic Minority Groups*. Newcastle upon Tyne: Department of Epidemiology and Public Health, University of Newcastle upon Tyne.

Mares P, Henley A, Baxter C (1985) *Health Care in Multiracial Britain*. Cambridge: Health Education Council and the National Extension College.

McAvoy BR and Donaldson LJ (eds) (1990) *Health Care for Asians*. Oxford: Oxford University Press.

McNaught A (1985) *Race and Health Care in the United Kingdom*. London: Health Education Council.

McNaught A (1988) *Race and Health Policy*. London, New York: Croom Helm.

† Modood T, Berthoud R, Lakey J, Nazroo J, Smith P, Virdee SBS (1997) *Ethnic Minorities in Britain: diversity and disadvantage*. London: Policy Studies Institute.

† Nazroo JY (1997) *The Health of Britain's Ethnic Minorities: findings from a national survey*. London: Policy Studies Institute.

Nazroo JY (2001) *Ethnicity, Class and Health. PSI research report 880*. London: Policy Studies Institute.

† Patel KC, Bhopal RS (eds.) (2004) *The Epidemic of Coronary Heart Disease in South Asian Populations: causes and consequences*. Birmingham: South Asian Health Foundation.

† Polednak AP (1989) *Racial and Ethnic Differences in Disease*. Oxford: Oxford University Press.

Qureshi B (1994) *Transcultural Medicine: dealing with patients from different cultures. Including 35 articles published in the British medical press, 1981–1988*. Dordrecht: Kluwer Academic.

Rack P (1982) *Race, Culture, and Mental Disorder*. London: Routledge.

Rathwell T and Phillips DR (1986) *Health, Race and Ethnicity*. London, Dover, NH: Croom Helm.

† Rawaf S and Bahl V (eds) (1998) *Assessing Health Needs of People from Minority Ethnic Groups*. London: Royal Colleges of Physicians of the United Kingdom, Faculty of Public Health Medicine.

Robinson M (2002) *Communication and Health in a Multiethnic Society*. Bristol: The Policy Press.

Sana L (1999) *Gender, Ethnicity, and Health Research*. New York, London: Kluwer Academic/Plenum Publishers.

† Smaje C (1995) *Race and Ethnicity: making sense of the evidence*, London: King's Fund.

Smith DB (1999) *Health Care Divided: race and healing a nation*. Ann Arbor, MI: University of Michigan Press.

Stepan N (1982) *The Idea of Race in Science*. London: Macmillan.

Suman F and Campling J (2002) *Mental Health, Race, and Culture*, 2nd edn. Houndmills, Hampshire: Palgrave.

World Health Organization (1983) *Migration and Health*. Netherlands: World Health Organization.

Preface

‡ Azuonye IO (1996) Who is black in medical research? *BMJ* 313: 760.

Chapter 1

† Afshari R, Bhopal RS (2002) Changing pattern of use of 'ethnicity' and 'race' in scientific literature. *International Journal of Epidemiology* 31: 1074–76.

Alper JS and Natowicz MR (1992) The allure of genetic explanations. *BMJ* 305: 666.

Balarajan R, Bulusu L (1990) Mortality among immigrants in England and Wales, 1979–83. In Britton M (ed.) *Mortality and Geography*, pp. 103–121. London: HMSO.

Bhatnagar D, Anand IS, Durrington PN, Patel DJ, Wander GS, Mackness MI *et al.* (1995) Coronary risk factors in people from the Indian subcontinent living in West London and their siblings in India. *The Lancet* 345: 405–9.

* Bhopal RS (1997a) Ethnicity. In Boyd KM *et al.* (eds) *The New Dictionary of Medical Ethics*, pp. 89–90. London: BMJ Books.

* Bhopal RS (1997b) Is research into ethnicity and health racist, unsound, or important science? *BMJ* 314: 1751–6.

* Bhopal RS (2001) Race and ethnicity as epidemiological variables: centrality of purpose and context. In Macbeth H (ed.) *Ethnicity and Health*, pp. 21–40. London: Taylor and Francis.

* Bhopal RS (2002) *Concepts of Epidemiology*, pp. 317. Oxford: Oxford University Press.

* Bhopal R (2003) Glossary of terms relating to ethnicity and race: for reflection and debate. *Journal Epidemiology and Community Health* 58: 441–5.

Bhopal R, Rahemtulla T, Sheikh A (2005). Persistent high stroke mortality in Bangladeshi populations. *BMJ*, 331: 1096–97.

Byrd WM and Clayton LA (2002) An American health dilemma, vol. 1. A medical history of African Americans and the problem of race: beginnings to 1900. *New England Journal of Medicine* 346: 458.

† Chadwick J and Mann WN (1950) *The Medical Works of Hippocrates.* London: Blackwell Scientific Publications Ltd.

‡ Clinton WJ (1997) Remarks by the President in apology for study done in Tuskegee. Washington, DC: Office of the Press Secretary, The White House.

† Coon CS (1939) *The races of Europe.* New York: Alfred A. Knopf.

‡ Cooper R (1984) A note on the biological concept of race and its application in epidemiological research. *Am Heart J* 108: 715–23.

Cooper RS, Kaufman JS, Ward R (2003) Race and genomics. *New England Journal of Medicine* 348: 1166–70.

† Cooper R. Rotimi C, Ataman S, McGee D, Osotimehin B, Kadiri S *et al.* (1997) The prevalence of hypertension in seven populations of West African origin. *Am J Public Health* 87: 160–8.

‡ Down JLH (1867) *Observations on an Ethnic Classification of Idiots.* Reprinted in: Mental Retardation, 1995, 54–57.

† Ellison GTH, de Wet T, Ijsselmuiden CB, Richter LM (1996) Desegregating health statistics and health research in South Africa. *SAMJ* 86: 1257–62.

Ellison GTH and de Wet T (1997) *Re-examining the content of the South African Medical Journal during the formalisation of 'racial' discrimination under apartheid. Health and Human Rights Project. In: The Final Submission of the HHRP to the Truth and Reconciliation Commission*: 112–131. Cape Town: Health and Human Rights Project.

Ellison GTH (1998) Contemporary medical definitions of 'race' and 'ethnicity'. *Annals of Human Biology* 1998; 25: 555.

Ellison GTH and de Wet T (1998) *The South African Medical Journal, the medical profession and 'racial' categories in the era of apartheid.* 1–31. Brighton, Centre for Sourthern African Studies, University of Sussex.

Ellison GT (2005) Population profiling and public health risk: When and how should we use race/ethnicity? *Critical Public Health* 1: 65–74.

Farrar FW (1867) Aptitudes of races. *Transactions of the Ethnological Society* 5: 115–26.

Fullilove MT (1998) Comment: Abandoning 'Race' as a variable in public health research—an idea whose time has come. *Am J Public Health* 88: 1297–98.

* Gill PS, Kai J, Bhopal RS, Wild S (2006) Health care needs assessment: black and minority ethnic groups. In Raftery J (ed.) *Health Care Needs Assessment. The epidemiologically based needs assessment reviews, 3rd series,* pp. 000–000. Abingdon: Radcliffe Medical Press Ltd. (in press, expected in print 2006). Available at http://www.hcna.radcliffe-oxford.com/bemgframe.htm.

† Golby AJ, Gabrieli JDE, Chiao JY, Eberhardt JL (2001) Differential responses in the fusiform region to same-race and other-race faces. *Nature Neuroscience* 4: 845–50.

Hinds DA, Stuve LL, Nilsen GB, Halperin E, Eskin E, Ballinger DG, *et al.* (2005) Whole-genome patterns of common DNA variation in three human populations. *Science* 18: 1072–9.

Huth EJ (1995) Identifying ethnicity in medical papers. *Ann Intern Med* 122: 619–21.

† Huxley JS, Haddon AC (1936) *We Europeans: a survey of 'Racial' problems.* New York: Harper.

‡ Jackson FL (1992) Race and Ethnicity as Biological Constructs. *Ethnicity and Disease,* 2: 120–25.

† Jones JH (1993) *Bad Blood. The Tuskegee Syphilis Experiment,* 2nd edn. New York: Free Press.

Jones S (1991). We are all cousins under the skin. *The Independent.* 14. London. 12-12-1991.

‡ Kaplan JB, Bennett T (2003) Use of race and ethnicity in biomedical publication. *JAMA* 289: 2709–16.

† Kiple KF and King VH (1981) *Another Dimension to the Black Diaspora.* London: Cambridge University Press.

† La Veist TA (1994) Beyond dummy variables and sample selection: what health services researchers ought to know about race as a variable. *Health Services Research* 29: 1–16.

† Linnaeus C (1806) *A general system of nature through the three grand kingdoms of animals, vegetables, and minerals.* Systema Naturae: London: Lackington Allen & Co.

* Mackintosh J, Bhopal RS, Unwin N, Ahmad N (1998) *Step-by-step Guide to Epidemiological Health Needs Assessment for Ethnic Minority Groups*. Newcastle upon Tyne, Department of Epidemiology and Public Health, University of Newcastle upon Tyne.

Marmot MG (1989) General approaches to migrant studies: the relation between disease, social class and ethnic origin. In Cruickshank JK, Beevers DG (eds) *Ethnic Factors in Health and Disease*. London: Wright.

† Marmot MG, Adelstein AM, Bulusu L (1984) *Immigrant mortality in England and Wales 1970–78*. London: HMSO.

Miller EM (1994) Tracing the genetic history of modern man. *Mankind Quarterly* 35: 71–108.

‡ Morrison T (1993) *Beloved*. London: Chatto and Windus.

Mountain JL, Risch N (2004) Assessing genetic contributions to phenotypic differences among 'racial' and 'ethnic' groups. *Nat Genet* 36: S48–S53.

‡ Olumide J (2002) *Raiding the Gene Pool: the social construction of mixed race*. London: Pluto Press.

† Osborne NG and Feit MD (1992) The use of race in medical research. *JMA* 267: 275–9.

† Pinker S (2002) *The Black Slate: the modern denial of human nature*. London: Penguin Press.

† Ramaiya KL, Swai ABM, McLarty DG, Bhopal RS, Alberti KGMM (1991) Prevalence of diabetes and cardiovascular risk factors in Hindu Indian sub-communities in Tanzania. *BMJ* 303: 271–6.

† Rankin J and Bhopal RS (1999) Current census categories are not a good match for identity. *BMJ* 318: 1696.

‡ Reynolds G (1993) Foreword. *Ann Epidemiol* 3: 119.

* Senior P and Bhopal RS (1994) Ethnicity as a variable in epidemiological research. *BMJ* 309: 327–9.

Sheldon TA and Parker H (1992) Race and ethnicity in health research. *J Public Health Med* 14: 104–10.

Special section: papers from the CDC-ATSDR Workshop on the Use of Race and Ethnicity in Public Health Surveillance. *Public Health Rep* 1994 109: 4–45.

Temple B & Moran R (2006) *Doing Research with Refugees—Issues and Guidelines*. Bristol: Policy Press, University of Bristol.

Turshen M (1996) Unhealthy paradox: a nation of immigrants debates harsh immigration controls. *Current Issues in Public Health* 2: 61–7.

Varma JK (1996) Eugenics and immigration restriction: lessons for tomorrow. *JAMA* 275: 734.

‡ Walker APR (1997) Data are not now collected by ethnic group in South Africa. *BMJ* 314: 220.

† Wild S and McKeigue P (1997) Cross-sectional analysis of mortality by country of birth in England and Wales, 1970–1992. *BMJ* 314: 705–10.

Wilkinson DY (1987) Conceptual and methodological issues in the use of race as a variable: policy implications. *The Milbank Quarterly* 65(Suppl. 1): 56–71.

Williams DR (1994) The concept of race in health services research 1966–1990. *Health Services Research* 29: 261–74.

Williams R (1996) The health legacy of the emigration: the Irish in Britain and elsewhere, 1845–1995. *Irish Journal of Sociology* 6: 56–78.

Williams, DR (1997) Race and health: basic questions, emerging directions. *Ann. Epidemiol.* 7: 322–333.

Winker MA (2004) Measuring race and ethnicity: why and how? *JAMA* 292: 1612–14.

Witzig R (1996) The medicalization of race: scientific legitimization of flawed social construction. *Annals of Internal Medicine* 125: 675–9.

Wolffers I, Verghis S, Marin M (2003) Migration, human rights, and health. *The Lancet* 362: 2019–20.

Yoon E (1996) Asian American and Pacific Islander Health: a paradigm for minority health. *JAMA* 275: 736.

Chapter 2

† Agyemang C, Bhopal RS, Bruijnzeels M (2005) Negro, Black, Black African, African Caribbean, African American or what? Labelling African origin populations in the health arena in the 21st century. *Journal of Epidemiology and Community Health* 59: 1014–18.

Ahdieh L and Hahn RA (1996) Use of the terms 'race', 'ethnicity', and 'national origins': a review of articles in the American Journal of Public Health, 1980–1989. *Ethnicity and Health* 1: 95–8.

Anderson M and Fienberg SE (1995) Black, white, and shades of gray (and brown and yellow). *Chance* 8: 15–18.

Albin B, Hjelm K, Ekberg J, Elmstahl S (2005) Mortality among 723,948 foreign- and native-born Swedes 1970–1999. *Eur J Public Health* 15: 511–17.

‡ Aspinall PJ (1995) Department of Health's requirement for mandatory collection of data on ethnic group of inpatients. BMJ 311: 1006–9.

Aspinall PJ (1998) Describing the 'white' ethnic group and its composition in medical research. *Social Science and Medicine* 47: 1797–808.

Aspinall PJ (2002) Collective terminology to describe the minority ethnic population: the persistence of confusion and ambiguity in usage. *Sociology* 36: 803–16.

Aspinall PJ (2003) Who is Asian? A category that remains contested in population and health research. *Journal of Public Health Medicine* 25: 91–7.

Barton Laws M, Rachel A, Heckscher MPH (2002) Racial and ethnic identification practices in public health data systems in New England. *Public Health Reports* 117: 50–61.

Bennett T (1997) 'Racial' and ethnic classification: two steps forward and one step back? *Public Health Reports* 1122: 477–80.

Bennett T, Bhopal RS (1998) US health journal editors' opinions and policies on research in race, ethnicity and health. *Journal of the National Medical Association* 90: 401–8.

Bhopal RS (1988) Respiratory illness and home environment of ethnic groups. BMJ 297: 69.

Bhopal RS, Phillimore P, Kohli HS (1991) Inappropriate use of the term 'Asian': an obstacle to ethnicity and health research. *J Public Health Med* 13: 44–6.

* Bhopal RS and Donaldson LJ (1998) White, European, Western, Caucasian or what? Inappropriate labelling in research on race, ethnicity and health. *Am J Pub Health* 88: 1303–7.

Bhopal RS, Rankin J, Bennet T (2000) Editorial role in promoting valid use of concepts and terminology in race and ethnicity research. *Science Editor* 23: 75–80.

* Bhopal R (2004) Glossary of terms relating to ethnicity and race: for reflection and debate. *Journal of Epidemiology and Community Health* 58: 441–5.

‡ Bogin B (1998) Letter to the Editor. *American Journal of Human Biology* 3: 279.

‡ *British Medical Journal* (1996) Ethnicity, race and culture: guidelines for research, audit and publication. BMJ 312: 1094.

Bouwhuis CB and Moll HA (2003) Determination of ethnicity in children in The Netherlands: two methods compared. *Eur J Epidemiol* 18: 385–8.

‡ Campbell C & McLean C (2002) Representations of ethnicity in people's accounts of local community participation in a multi-ethnic community in England. *Journal Community Appl. Soc. Psychol* 12: 13–29.

Cashmore E (1996) *Dictionary of Race and Ethnic Relations*, 4th edn. London: Routledge.

† Ellison George TH, Mikey Rosato, and Simon Outram. The Impact of Editorial Guidelines on the Classification of Race/Ethnicity in the *BMJ* The Fifth International Congress on Peer Review and Biomedical Publication was held September 16–18, 2005, in Chicago, Illinois. http://www.ama-assn.org/public/peer/abstracts.html

Evinger S (1995) How shall we measure our nation's diversity? *Chance* 8: 7–14.

Freedman BJ (1994) Caucasian. BMJ 288: 696–8.

* Gill PS, Kai J, Bhopal RS, Wild S (2006) Health care needs assessment: black and minority ethnic groups. In Raftery J (ed.) *Health Care Needs Assessment. The epidemiologically based needs assessment reviews. Third Series*, pp. 000–000. Abingdon: Radcliffe Medical Press Ltd. (Book in press, expected 2006). At http://www.hcna.radcliffe-oxford.com/bemgframe.htm.

‡ Gimenez ME (1989) Latino/Hispanic—who needs a name? The case against a standardized terminology. *International Journal of Health Services* 19: 557–71.

Gomez S, Kelsey JL, Glaser SL, Lee MM, Sidney S (2005) Inconsistencies between self-reported ethnicity and ethnicity recorded in a health maintenance organisation. *Annals of Epidemiology* 15: 71–9.

Hahn RA (1992) The state of federal health statistics on racial and ethnic groups. *JAMA* 267: 268–71.

Hahn RA (1996) Identifying ancestry: the reliability of ancestral identification in the United States by self, proxy, interviewer, and funeral director. *Epidemiology* 7: 75–80.

Harwell TS, Hansen D, Kelly R, Moore MD, Jeanotte D, Gohdes D *et al.* (2002) Accuracy of race coding on American Indian death certificates, Montana 1996–1998. *Public Health Reports* 117: 44–9.

Hayes-Bautista DE, Chapa J (1987) Latino terminology: conceptual bases for standardised terminology. *Am J Public Health* 77: 61–8.

Jones CP, LaVeist TA, Lillie-Blanton M (1991) 'Race' in the epidemiologic literature: an examination of the *American Journal of Epidemiology*, 1921–1990. *Am J Epidemiol* 134: 1079–84.

‡ Lawrence E (1982) Just plain commonsense: the 'ropes' of racism. In Centre for Contemporary Cultural Studies, *The Empire Strikes Back: Race and Racism in 70s Britain*. London: Hutchinson and Co (Publishers) Ltd.

Lee SS, Mountain J, Koenig BA (2001) The Meanings of 'race' in the new genomics: implications for health disparities research. *Yale Journal of Health Policy, Law and Ethics* 1: 33–75.

Lillquist E, Sullivan CA (2004) The law and genetics of racial profiling in medicine. *Harvard Civil Rights—Civil Liberties Law Review* 39: 391–483.

* Mackintosh J, Bhopal RS, Unwin N, Ahmad N (1998) *Step-by-step guide to Epidemiological Health Needs Assessment for Ethnic Minority Groups*. Newcastle upon Tyne: Department of Epidemiology and Public Health, University of Newcastle upon Tyne.

McKenzie K (1995) Accuracy of variables describing ethnic minority groups is important. *BMJ* 310: 333.

‡ McKenzie K and Crowcroft NS (1996) Describing race, ethnicity and culture in medical research. *BMJ* 312: 1054.

Mays VM, Ponce NA, Washington DL, Cochran SD (2003) Classification of race and ethnicity: implications for public health. *Annu Rev Public Health* 24: 83–110.

Nazroo JY (1997) *The Health of Britain's Ethnic Minorities: findings from a national survey*. London: Policy Studies Institute.

Office of Management and Budget (1997) *Revisions to the Standards for the Classification of Federal Data on Race and Ethnicity*. Washington, DC: OMB.

Oppenheimer GM (2001) Paradigm lost: race, ethnicity, and the search for a new population taxonomy. *American Journal of Public Health* 91: 1049–55.

* Rankin J & Bhopal RS (1996) Current census categories are not a good match for identity. *British Medical Journal*, 318: 1696.

Rankin J, Bhopal R, Wallace B (1997) *Factors Influencing Heart Disease and Diabetes in South Asians: the South Tyneside Heart Study*. University of Newcastle upon Tyne: Department of Epidemiology and Public Health.

† Sangowawa O and Bhopal, R (2000) Can we implement ethnic monitoring in primary health care and use the data? A feasibility study and staff attitudes in North East England. *Public Health Medicine* 2: 106–8.

Schoendorf KC (1993) Comparability of the birth certificate and 1988 maternal and infant health survey. *Vital and Health Statistics* 2: 19.

‡ Schwartz RS (2001) Racial profiling in medical research. *New England Journal of Medicine* 344: 1392–3.

SHARE (1995) A note on views and terminology from Share. *Share Newsletter* 10: 16.

Shaunak S, Lakhani SR, Abraham R, Maxwell JD (1986) *Differences among Asian patients*. (letter). Br. Med. J., 293: 1169.

Stillitoe K (1978) Ethnic origin: the search for a question. *Population Trends* 13: 25–30.

Williams HC (2002) Have you ever seen an Asian/Pacific Islander? *Archives of Dermatology* 138: 673–4.

Chapter 3

Albin B, Hjelm K, Ekberg J, Elmstahl S (2005) Mortality among 723,948 foreign- and native-born Swedes 1970–1999. *Eur J Public Health* 15: 511–17.

Aspinall PJ (1995) Department of Health's requirement for mandatory collection of data on ethnic group of inpatients. *BMJ* 311: 1006–9.

Beckles GLA, Kirkwood BR, Carson DC, Miller GJ, Alexis SD, Byam NTA (1986) High total and cardio-vascular mortality in adults of Indian descent in Trinidad, unexplained by major coronary risk factors. *The Lancet* 1: 1298–1300.

† Bhopal RS, Unwin N, White M *et al.* (1999) heterogeneity of coronary heart disease risk factors in Indian, Pakistani, Bangladeshi and European origin populations: cross-sectional study. *BMJ* 319: 215–20.

* Bhopal RS (2000) Race and ethnicity as epidemiological variables. In Macbeth H (ed.) *Ethnicity and Health*, pp. 21–40. London: Taylor and Francis.

* Bhopal RS (2002) *Concepts of Epidemiology.* Oxford, Oxford University Press.

* Bhopal R, Fischbacher CM, Steiner M, Chalmers J, Povey C, Jamieson J, Knowles D (2005) *Ethnicity and health in Scotland: can we fill the information gap? A demonstration project focusing on coronary heart disease and linkage of census and health records.* Edinburgh, Edinburgh University 1–94.

† Bhopal R (2006) Race and Ethnicity: Responsible Use from Epidemiological and Public Health Perspectives. *Journal of Law, Medicine and Ethics* 500–507.

Blakely T and Salamond C (2002) Probabilistic record linkage and a method to calculate the positive predicitve value. *International Journal of Epidemiology Association* 31: 1246–52.

‡ Booth H (1984) *Identifying Ethnic Origin: the Past, Present and Future of Official Data Production.* 1–26. Sheffield.

Bos V, Kunst AF, Keij-Deerenberg IM, Mackenbach JM (2002) Mortality amongst immigrants in the Netherlands. *European Journal of Public Health* 12: S41.

† Bos V, Kunst AE, Deerenberg IMK, Garseen J, Mackenbach JP (2004) Ethnic inequalities in age- and cause-specific mortality in the Netherlands. *International Journal of Epidemiology Association* 33: 1112–19.

† Bos V (2005) *Ethnic Inequalities in Mortality in the Netherlands And the Role of Socioeconomic Status.* Rotterdam: University Medical Center.

Bos V, Kunst AE, Garseen J, Mackenbach JP (2005) Socioeconomic inequalities in mortality within ethinic groups in the Netherlands, 1995–2000. *J Epidemiol Community Health* 59: 329–35.

† Cabinet Office (2000) Minority ethnic issues in social exclusion and neighbourhood renewal. London, Cabinet Office.

† Caldwell SH and Popenhoe R (1995) Perception and misperceptions of skin colour. *Annals of Internal Medicine* 122: 614–17.

Chaturvedi N and McKeigue PM (1994) Methods for epidemiologic surveys of ethnic-minority groups. *J Epidemiol Community Health* 48: 107–11.

Coldman A, Braun T, Gallagher R (1988) The classification of ethnic status using name information. *J Epidemiol Community Health* 42: 390–5.

† Cooper RS, Rotimi CN, Kaufman JS, Owoaje EE (1997) Prevalence of NIDDM among populations of the African Diaspora. *Diabetes Care* 20: 343–8.

Cummins C, Winter H, Cheng KK, Maric R, Silcocks P, Varghese C (1999) An assessment of the Nam Pehchan computer program for the identification of names of South Asian ethnic origin. *Journal of Public Health Medicine* 21: 401–6.

† Ecob R and Williams R (1991) Sampling Asian minorities to assess health and welfare. *J Epidemiol Commun Health* 45: 93–101.

† Erens B, Primatesta P, Prior G (eds) (2001) *Health Survey for England: the health of minority ethnic groups '99* vols 1 and 2. London: The Stationery Office.

Faculty of Community Medicine and WHO (1988) Proceedings of the 1987 Summer Scientific Conference of the Faculty of Community Medicine of the Royal Colleges of Physicians of the United Kingdom in Collaboration with the World Health Organization 1987. *Equity A Prerequisite for Health Intersectoral Challenges For Health For All 2000.* 1–62.

Gill PS & Johnson M (1995) Ethnic monitoring and equity: Collecting data is just the beginning. *BMJ*, 310: 890.

* Gill PS, Kai J, Bhopal RS, Wild S (2006) Health care needs assessment: black and minority ethnic groups. In Raftery J (ed.) *Health Care Needs Assessment. The epidemiologically based needs assessment reviews, 3rd series*, pp. 000–000. Abingdon: Radcliffe Medical Press Ltd. (in press, expected in print 2006). Available at http://www.hcna.radcliffe-oxford.com/bemgframe.htm.

‡ Gomez S, Kelsey JL, Glaser SL, Lee MM, Sidney S (2005) Inconsistencies between self-reported ethnicity and ethnicity recorded in a health maintenance organisation. *Annals of Epidemiology* 15: 71–9.

Hahn RA, Mulinare J, Teutsch SM (1992) Inconsistencies in coding of race and ethnicity between birth and death in US infants. *JAMA* 267: 259–63.

Hammar N, Kaprio J, Hagstrom U, Alfredsson L, Koskenvuo M, Hammar T (2001) Migration and mortality: a 20 year follow up of Finnish twin pairs with migrant co-twins in Sweden. *Journal of Epidemiology and Community Health* 56: 362–6.

* Harland J, Unwin N, Bhopal RS, White M, Watson B, Laker M, Alberti KGMM (1997) Low levels of cardiovascular risk factors and coronary heart disease in a UK Chinese population. *J Epidemiol Community Health* 51: 636–42.

Harland J, White M, Bhopal R, Raybould S, Unwin NC, Alberti KGMM (1997) Identifying Chinese populations in the UK for epidemiological research: experience of a name analysis of the FHSA register. *Public Health* 111: 331–7.

† Hazuda HP, Haffner SM, Stern MP, Eifler CW (1988) Effects of acculturation and socioeconomic status on obesity and diabetes in Mexican Americans: the San Antonio heart study. *Am J Epidemiol* 128: 1289–301.

Health Education Authority (2000) *Black and Minority Ethnic Groups in England: the second health and lifestyles survey*. London: HEA.

Heath I (1991) The role of ethnic monitoring in general practice. *Br J Gen Pract* 41: 310–11.

† Home Office (2001) Race Relations (Amendment) Act 2000. New laws for a successful multi-racial Britain. London: Home Office Communication Directorate.

Jeffreys M, Stevanovic V, Tobias M, Lewis C, Ellison-Loschmann L, Pearce N *et al.* (2005) Ethnic inequalities in cancer survival in New Zealand: Linkage study. *Research and Practice* 95: 834–7.

Kai J and Bhopal R (2003) Ethnic diversity in health and disease. In Kai J *Ethnicity, health and primary care*, pp. 15–25. Oxford: Oxford University Press.

Kljakovic M (1993) Is it easy collecting ethnicity data in general practice? *N Z Med J*, 106: 103–4.

† La Veist TA (1996) Why we should continue to study race ... but do a better job: an essay on race, racism and health. *Ethnicity and Disease* 6: 21–9.

London Health Observatory (2003) *The Case for Recording Ethnicity at Birth and Death Registration*. London, London Health Observatory.

* Mackintosh J, Bhopal RS, Unwin N, Ahmad N (1998) *Step-by-step Guide to Epidemiological Health Needs Assessment for Ethnic Minority Groups*. Newcastle upon Tyne: Department of Epidemiology and Public Health, University of Newcastle upon Tyne.

Marmot MG, Adelstein AM, Bulusu L (1984) Lessons from the study of immigrant mortality. *The Lancet* i: 1455–8.

† Miller GJ, Beckles GL, Maude GH, Carson DC, Alexis SD, Price SG *et al.* (1989) Ethnicity and other characteristics predictive of coronary heart disease in a developing community: principal results of the St James Survey, Trinidad. *Int J Epidemiol* 18: 808–17.

Nanchahal K, Mangtani P, Alston M, dos Santos Silva I (2001) Development and validation of a computerized South Asian names and group recognition algorithm (SANGRA) for use in British health-related studies. *Journal of Public Health Medicine* 23: 278–85.

Newcombe H (1988) *Handbook of Record Linkage: methods for health and statistical studies, administration and business.* Oxford: Oxford University Press.

Nicoll A, Bassett K, Ulijaszek S (1986) What's in a name? Accuracy of using surnames and forenames in ascribing Asian ethnic identity in English populations. *J Epidemiol Community Health* 40: 364–8.

‡ Office for National Statistics: *Ethnicity, Identity, Language and Religion Census Topic Group; working paper no. 1.* (unpublished draft, 2005).

Patel KV, Eschbach K, Ray LA, Markides KS (2004) Evaluation of mortality data for older Mexican Americans: implications for the Hispanic paradox. *American Journal of Epidemiology* 159: 707–15.

Pringle M (1996) Practicality of recording patient ethnicity in general practice: descriptive intervention study and attitude survey. *BMJ* 312: 1080–1.

Public Health Reports (1994) Special Section. Papers from the CDC-ATSDPR workshop on the use of race and ethnicity in public health surveillance. *Public Health Reports* 109: 4–45.

Razum O, Zeeb H, Akgun S (2001) How useful is a name-based algorithm in health research among Turkish migrants in Germany? *Tropical Medicine and International Health* 6: 654–61.

* Sangowawa O and Bhopal R (2000) Can we implement ethnic monitoring in primary health care and use the data? A feasibility study and staff attitudes in North East England. *Public Health Medicine* 22: 124–5.

* Senior P and Bhopal RS (1994) Ethnicity as a variable in epidemiological research. *BMJ* 309: 327–9.

† Shaw J (1994) *Collection of Ethnic Group Data for Admitted Patients (EL(94)77).* Leeds: NHS Executive.

† Sheth T, Nair C, Nargundkar M, Anand S, Yusuf S (1999) Cardiovascular and cancer mortality among Canadians of European, south Asian and Chinese origin from 1979 to 1993: an analysis of 1.2 million deaths. *Canadian Medical Association Journal* 161: 132–8.

‡ Sheth T, Nargundkar M, Chagani K, Anand S, Nair S, Yusuf S (1997) Classifying ethnicity utilizing the Canadian Mortality Data Base. *Ethnicity and Health* 2: 287–95.

Sprotson K, Pitson, Whitfield, Walker (1999) *Health and Lifestyles of the Chinese Population in England.* London: Health Education Authority.

Stenhouse NS and McCall MG (1970) Differential mortality from cardiovascular disease in migrants from England and Wales, Scotland and Italy, and native-born Australians. *Journal of Chronic Disease* 23: 423–31.

‡ Stoep AV (1998) Public health then and now. *American Journal of Public Health* 88. 1390–402.

† Terris M (1973) Desegregating health statistics. *American Journal of Public Health* 63: 477–80.

* Unwin N, Harland J, White M, Bhopal R, Winocour P, Stephenson P, Watson W, Turner C, Alberti KGMM (1997) Body mass index, waist circumference, waist-hip ratio, and glucose intolerance in Chinese and Europid adults in Newcastle, UK. *J Epidemiol Comm Health* 51: 160–6.

Weitoft GR, Gullberg A, Hjern A, Rosen M (1999) Mortality statistics in immigrant research: method for adjusting underestimation of mortality. *International Journal of Epidemiology* 28: 756–63.

† Wild S and McKeigue P (1997) Cross sectional analysis of mortality by country of birth in England and Wales, 1970–92. *BMJ* 314: 705–10.

Wild SH, Laws A, Fortmann SP, Varady AN, Byrne CD (1995) Mortality from coronary heart disease and stroke for six ethnic groups in California, 1985 to 1990. *Annals of Epidemiology* 5: 432–9.

Chapter 4

† Agyemang C, Bindraban N, Gideon M, Gert van M, Koopmans R, Stronks K (2005) Prevalance, awareness, treatment, and control of hypertension among Black Surinamese, South Asian Surinamese and White Dutch in Amsterdam, The Netherlands: the SUNSET study. *Journal of Hypertension* 23: 1971–7.

Ahmad WIU (ed.) (1993) *'Race' and Health in Contemporary Britain*. Milton Keynes: Open University Press.

Anonymous (1981) X-rays, age, and immigration. *Lancet*, 1:1301.

Beecham L (1983) Health problems of ethnic minorities—call for Board of Science Study. *BMJ* 286: 1226–7.

* Bhopal R (1997) Is research into ethnicity and health racist, unsound, or important science? *BMJ* 314: 1751–6.

* Bhopal RS (1998) The spectre of racism in health and health care: lessons from history and the USA. *BMJ* 316: 1970–3.

* Bhopal RS (2002) *Concepts of Epidemiology*. Oxford: Oxford University Press.

Black JA (1984) NHS thik hai. *BMJ* 289: 1558–9.

† Bos V, Kunst AE, Keij-Deerenberg IM, Mackenbach JM (2002) Mortality amongst immigrants in the Netherlands. *European Journal of Public Health* 12: S41.

† Browne A (2005) Dutch unveil the toughest face in Europe with a ban on the burka. *The Times* 13 October, 35.

Cameron WI, Moffitt PS, Williams DRR (1986) Diabetes mellitus in the Australian Aborigines of Bourke, New South Wales. *Diabetes Research and Clinical Practice* 2: 307–14.

‡ Clyne MB (1964) Indian patients (General Practitioners' Forum). *Practioner* 193: 195–9.

Clyne MB, Hasmi F, Nandy D (1976) Racial and cultural factors of relevance for the General Practioner. *Proc Roy Soc Med* 69: 635–7.

† Coker N (ed.) (2001) *Racism in Medicine: an agenda for change*. London: King's Fund.

† Cooper R, Rotimi C, Ataman S, McGee D, Osotimehin B, Kadiri S *et al.* (1997) The prevalence of hypertension in seven populations of West African origin. *Am J Public Health* 87: 160–8.

Dowse G, Gareeboo H, Zimmet P, Alberti KGMM, Tuomilheto J (1990) High prevalence of NIDDM and impaired glucose tolerance in Indian, Creole and Chinese Mauritians. *Diabetes* 39: 390–6.

† Esmail A and Everington S (1993) Racial discrimination against doctors from ethnic minorities. *BMJ* 306: 691–2.

† Gamble VN (1993) A legacy of distrust: African Americans and medical research. *American Journal of Preventive Medicine* 9: 35–8.

Geiger H (1996) Race and health care—an American dilemma? *New England Journal of Medicine* 335: 815–16.

‡ Geronimus AT, Bound J, Waidmann TA, Hillemeier MM, Burns PB (1996) Excess mortality among blacks and whites in the United States. *The New England Journal of Medicine* 21: 1552–8.

Gillum RF (1999) The epidemiology of cardiovascular disease in black Americans. *New England Journal of Medicine* 335: 1597–9.

‡ Hausfeld RG (1977) Social, ethnic and cultural aspects of Aboriginal health. *Aust. Fam. Physician* 6: 1301–7.

Hawthorne K (1994) Accessibility and Use of Health Care Services in the British Asian Community. *Family Practice* 11: 453–9.

Health Education Authority (1999) *Black and Minority Ethnic Groups and Tobacco Use in England; a practical resource for health professionals*. London: Health Education Authority.

† Johnson M (1984) Ethnic minorities and health. *J Roy Coll Physicians London* 18: 228–23.

King TE Jr (2002) Racial disparities in clinical trials. *New England Journal of Medicine* 346: 1400–2.

† Kiple KF and King VH (1981) *Another Dimension to the Black Diaspora*. London: Cambridge University Press.

† Krieger N (1992) The making of public health data: paradigms, politics, and policy. *J Public Health Policy* 65: 412–27.

‡ Kreiger N (2000) Counting accountability: Implications of the new approaches to classifying race/ethnicity in the 2000 census. *American Journal of Public Health* 90: 1687–9.

† Kreiger N, Rowley D, Herman A (1993) Racism, sexism and social class: implications for studies of health, disease and wellbeing. *American Journal of Preventive Medicine* 9: 82–122.

Kushnick L (1988) Racism, the National Health Service and the health of black people. *Int J Health Services* 18: 457–70.

† La Veist TA, Wallace JM, and Howard DL (1995) The color line and the health of African Americans. *Humboldt Journal of Social Relations* 21: 119–37.

Loue S (1998) *Handbook of Immigrant Health*. New York: Plenum Press.

* Mackintosh J, Bhopal R and Ahmad N (undated). *Step by Step Guide to Epidemiological Health Needs Assessment for Ethnic Minority Groups.* 1–99. Newcastle Upon Tyne, University of Newcastle.

McBride G (2005) The coming of age of multicultural medicine. *PLoS Med* 2: e62.

McLeod H. (2002) Pharmacokinetic differences between ethnic groups. *The Lancet* 359: 78.

NAHA (1988) *Action not Words*. Birmingham: NAHA.

Oberman A & Cutter G (1984) Issues in the natural history and treatment of coronary heart disease in African American populations: surgical treatment. *American Heart Journal* 108: 688–94.

† Patel KC, Bhopal RS (eds.) (2004) *The Epidemic of Coronary Heart Disease in South Asian Populations: causes and consequences.* Birmingham: South Asian Health Foundation.

Pineda MD, White E, Kristal AR, Taylor V (2000) Asian breast cancer survival in the US: a comparison between Asian immigrants, US-born Asian Americans and Caucasians. *International Journal of Epidemiology* 30: 959–82.

Pockley P (1991) Increase in death rate among Aborigines. *BMJ* 302: 551–2.

† Porter R (1997) *The Greatest Benefit to Mankind—A medical history of humanity from antiquity to the present.* London: Harper Collins.

Reijneveld SA, Westhoff MH, Hopman-Rock M (2003) Promotion of health and physical activity improves the mental health of elderly immigrants: results of a group randomised controlled trial amoung Turkish immigrants in the Netherlands aged 45 and over. *Journal Epidemiol Community Health* 57: 405–11.

Royal College of General Practitioners (North London Faculty) (1967) *A Symposium on the Medical and Social Problems of an Immigrant Population in Britain.* London: Royal College of General Practitioners.

Scottish Executive Health Department (2002) *Fair for All: working together towards culturally competent services*, NHS HDL 51. Edinburgh: Scottish Executive.

† Tesh SN (1988) *Hidden Arguments*. New Brunswick: Rutgers University Press.

Thomas HE (1968) Tuberculosis in immigrants. *Proc Roy Soc Med* 611: 21–3.

Uitewaal PJM, Bruijnzeels M, Bernsen RMD, Voorham AJJ, Hoes AW, Thomas S (2004) Diabetes care in Dutch general practice. *European Journal of Public Health* 14: 15–18.

† Ward L (1993) *Race equality and employment in the National Health Service*. In Ahmad WIU (Ed.), 'Race' and Health in Contemporary Britain: 167–182. Buckingham: Open University Press.

Welshman J, Bashford A (2006) Tuberculosis, migration, and medical examination: lessons from history. *J Epidemiol Community Health* 60: 282–4.

‡ Whittle J, Conigliaro J, Good CB, Lofgren RP (1993) Racial differences in the use of invasive cardiovascular procedures in the Department of Veterans Affairs medical system. *New England Journal of Medicine* 329: 621–627.

† Wild S and McKeigue P (1997) Cross-sectional analysis of mortality by country of birth in England and Wales, 1970–92. *BMJ* 314: 705–10.

World Health Organization (1983) *Migration and Health*. Netherlands: World Health Organization.

Chapter 5

Aspinall PJ (2005) Why the next census needs to ask about language. *BMJ* 331: 363–4.

* Bhopal RS (1988) Health Care for Asians: conflict in need, demand and provision. In *Equity. A prerequisite for health. The proceedings of the 1987 Summer Scientific Conference of the Faculty of Community Medicine.* Faculty of Community Medicine and the World Health Organisation.

* Bhopal RS and Donaldson LJ (1988) Health education for ethnic minorities: current provision and future directions. *Health Ed J* 47: 137–40.

Bhopal R, Vettini A, Hunt S, Wiebe S, Hanna L, Amos A (2004) Review of prevalence data in, and evaluation of methods for cross-cultural adaptation of, UK surveys on tobacco and alcohol in ethnic minority groups. *BMJ* 328: 76–80.

† Bowling A (1997) *Measuring Health: a review of quality of life measurement scales.* Buckingham: Open University Press.

† Bowling A and Ebrahim S (2006) *Handbook of Health Research Methods: investigation, measurement and analysis.* Maidenhead: Open University Press.

† Crosthwaite L (1994) *Equal Access Survey. Asian and African Working Group.* Walsall, Walsall Health Authority.

‡ Elliott B for the Newcastle Strategy Group (including RSB) (1997) *Taking Heart. Reducing diabetes and cardiovascular disease among Newcastle's South Asian and Chinese communities.* Newcastle upon Tyne: University of Newcastle upon Tyne.

* Gill PS, Kai J, Bhopal RS, Wild S (2006) Health care needs assessment: black and minority ethnic groups. In: Raftery J (ed.) *Health Care Needs Assessment. The epidemiologically based needs assessment reviews. Third Series,* pp. 000–000. Abingdon: Radcliffe Medical Press Ltd. (in press, expected 2006). Available in full at: http://www.hcna.radcliffe-oxford.com/bemgframe.htm.

‡ Hawthorne K (1994) *Accessibility and Use of Health Care Services in the British Asian Community.* Family Practice, 11: 453–459.

Hopkins A and Bahl V (eds) (1993) *Access to Health Care for People from Black and Ethnic Minorities.* London: Royal College of Physicians.

* Hunt S, Bhopal R (2004) Self-report in clinical and epidemiological studies with non-English speakers: the challenge of language and culture. *Journal Epidemiology and Community Health* 58: 618–22.

* Mackintosh J, Bhopal R, Unwin N, Ahmad N (1998) *Step by Step Guide to Epidemiological Health Needs Assessment for Minority Ethnic Groups.* Newcastle upon Tyne: University of Newcastle.

† Madhok R, Bhopal RS, Ramaiah RS (1992) Quality of hospital service: an 'Asian' perspective. *J Pub Health Med* 14: 271–9.

† Madhok R, Hameed A, Bhopal RS (1998) Satisfaction with health services among the Pakistani population in. Middlesbrough, England. *J Pub Health Med* 20: 295–301.

† Marmot MG, Adelstein AM, Bulusu L (1984) *Immigrant Mortality in England and Wales 1970–72. Studies of medical and population subjects, no. 47.* London: HMSO.

‡ Murphy J, Clawson N, Allard M, Harrison D, and Gocke, P (1981) *Health care provision for the Asian Community Working paper No. 45.* Manchester, Department of Social Administration, University of Manchester.

‡ NAHA (1988) *Action not Words.* Birmingham: NAHA.

† Nazroo JY (1997) *The Health of Britain's Ethnic Minorities.* London: Policy Studies Institute.

† Pilgrim S, Fenton S, Hughes A, Hine C, Tibbs N (1993) *The Bristol Black and Ethnic Minorities Health Survey Report.* Bristol: Departments of Sociology and Epidemiology, University of Bristol.

‡ Raleigh VS (1994) Public health and the 1991 census: non random underenumeration complicates interpretation. *BMJ* 309: 287–8.

† Rawaf S and Bahl V (eds) (1998) *Health Needs Assessment in Ethnic Minority Groups.* London: Royal College of Physicians.

‡ Rawaf S & Marshall F (1999) Drug Misuse: The Ten Steps for Needs Assessment. *Public Health Medicine* 1: 21–6.

† Senior P and Bhopal RS (1994) Ethnicity as a variable in epidemiological research. *BMJ* 309: 327–9.

‡ Stevens A and Raftery J (1994) *Health Care Needs Assessment: the epidemiologically based needs assessment reviews.* Oxford: Radcliffe Medical.

Tuomilheto J, Li N, Dowse G, Gareeboo H, Chitson P, Fareed D *et al.* (1993) The prevalence of coronary heart disease in the multi-ethnic and high diabetes prevalence population of Mauritius. *Journal of Internal Medicine* 233: 187–94.

Chapter 6

Am Heart J 1984; 108: 688–94.

Abbotts J (1999) Association of medical, physiological, behavioural and socio-economic factors with elevated mortality in men of Irish heritage in West Scotland. *Journal of Public Health Medicine* 21: 46–54.

† Acheson D (1998) *Independent Report into Inequalities in Health.* 1998. London: HMSO.

Anonymous (1981) X-rays, age, and immigration. *The Lancet* 1301.

Anonymous (1989) Contemporary lessons from Nazi Germany. *Institute of Medical Ethics Bulletin*, February: 13–20.

Armstead C, Lawler K, Gorden G, Cross J, Gibbons J (1989) Relationship of racial stressors to blood pressure responses and anger expression in Black college students. *Health Psychology* 8: 541–6.

† Ayanian JZ, Udvarhelyi S, Gatsonis CA, Pashos CL, Epstein A (1993) Racial differences in the use of revascularisation procedures after coronary angiography. *JAMA* 269: 2642–6.

† Balarajan R & Bulusu L (1990) *Mortality among immigrants in England and Wales, 1979–83.* In Britton, M. (ed.), Mortality and Geography: A review in the mid 1980's: 103–121. London: HMSO.

* Bhopal RS and Donaldson LJ (1988) Health education for ethnic minorities: current provision and future directions. *Health Ed J* 47: 137–40.

* Bhopal R (1997) Is research into ethnicity and health racist, unsound, or important science? *BMJ* 314: 1751–6.

3 * Bhopal RS (1998) The spectre of racism in health and health care: lessons from history and the USA. *BMJ* 316: 1970–3.

* Bhopal R (2001) Racism in medicine. *BMJ* 322: 1503–4.

* Bhopal RS (2002) *Concepts of Epidemiology.* Oxford: Oxford University Press.

* Bhopal R, Hayes L, White M, Unwin N, Harland J, Ayis S *et al.* (2002) Ethnic and socio-economic inequalities in coronary heart disease, diabetes and risk factors in Europeans and South Asians. *Journal of Public Health Medicine* 24: 95–105.

* Bhopal RS (2005) Hitler on race and health in Mein Kampf: a stimulus to anti-racism in the health professions. *Diversity in Health and Social Care* 2: 119–25.

‡ Biddiss MD (1979) *Images of Race.* Leicester: Leicester University Press.

Black E (2003) *War Against the Weak: eugenics and America's campaign to create a master race.* London: Turnaround.

‡ Bos V, Kunst AE, Garseen J, Mackenbach JP (2005) Socioeconomic inequalities in mortality within ethinic groups in the Netherlands, 1995–2000. *J Epidemiol Community Health* 59: 329–35.

† Bos V, Kunst AE, Deerenberg IMK, Garseen J, Mackenbach JP (2004) Ethnic inequalities in age- and cause-specific mortality in the Netherlands. International Epidemiological Association 33: 1112–1119.

† Bos V, Kunst AE, Keij-Deerenberg IM, Mackenbach JM (2002) Mortality amongst immigrants in the Netherlands. European Journal of Public Health 12: S41.

† Bos V (2005) Ethnic Inequalities in Mortality in the Netherlands. And the Role of Socioeconomic Status. University Medical Center Rotterdam.

Bramley D, Hebert P, Tuzzio L, Chassin M (2005) Disparities in indigenous health: a cross-country comparison between New Zealand and the United States. *American Journal of Public Health* 95: 844–50.

‡ Brandt AM (1978) *Racism and Research: the case of the Tuskegee Syphilis Study. Hastings Centre Report.* The Hastings Centre.

Carlisle DM (1998) The entry of underrepresented minority students into US medical schools: an evaluation of recent trends. *American Journal of Public Health* 88: 1314–18.

† Carlisle DM, Leake BD, Shapiro MF (1995) Racial and ethnic differences in the use of invasive cardiac procedures among cardiac patients in Los Angeles County, 1986 through 1988. *Am J Public Health* 85: 352–6.

† Chadwick J and Mann WN (1950) *The Medical Works of Hippocrates.* London: Blackwell Scientific Publications, Ltd.

Chandola T (2001) Ethnic and class differences in health in relation to British South Asians: using the new National Statistics socio-economic classification. *Soc Sci Med* 52: 1285–96.

Chavkin W and Elman D (1997) Mortality from cardiovascular causes among blacks and whites in New York City. *New England Journal of Medicine* 336: 1321.

† CMO (1992) *On the State of the Public Health. 1992.* London: Department of Health.

† Coker NE (2001) *Racism in Britain. An agenda for change.* London: King's Fund.

Cooper LA, Hill MN, Powe NR (2002) Designing and evaluating interventions to eliminate racial and ethnic disparities in health care. *J Gen Intern Med* 17: 477–86.

† Council on ethical and judicial affairs (1990) Black–white disparities in health care. *JAMA* 263: 2344–6.

‡ Davey Smith D, Chaturvedi N, Harding S, Nazaroo J & Williams R (2000) Ethnic inequalities in health: a review of UK epidemiological evidence. *Critical Public Health* 10: 375–408.

DeVille K (1999) Defending diversity: affirmative action and medical education. *American Journal of Public Health* 89: 1256–61.

Dominguez-McNeilly M (1996) Perceived Racism Scale. *Ethnicity & Disease,* 6: 154–66.

Dressler WW (1991) Social class, skin colour, and arterial blood pressure in two societies. *Ethnicity and Disease* (Winter): 60–77.

† Escarce JJ, Epstein KR, Colby DC, Schwartz JS (1993) Racial differences in the elderly's use of medical procedures and diagnostic tests. *Am J Public Health* 83: 948–54.

† Gamble VN (1993) A legacy of distrust: African Americans and medical research. *American Journal of Preventive Medicine* 9: 35–8.

‡ Geiger HJ (1996) Race and Health care—an American dilemma? *New England Journal of Medicine* 335: 815–16.

* Gill PS, Kai J, Bhopal RS, Wild S (2006) Health care needs assessment: black and minority ethnic groups. In Raftery J (ed.) *Health Care Needs Assessment. The epidemiologically based needs assessment reviews,* 3rd series, pp. 000–000. Abingdon: Radcliffe Medical Press Ltd. (book version in press, expected 2006). At http://www.hcna.radcliffe-oxford.com/bemgframe.htm

† Goldberg KC, Hartz AJ, Jacobsen SJ, Krakauer H, Rimm AA (1992) Racial and community factors influencing coronary artery bypass graft surgery rates for all 1986 Medicare patients. *JAMA* 18: 1473–7.

† Gornick ME, Eggers P, Reilly TEA (1986) Effects of race and income on mortality and use of services among Medicare beneficiaries. *New England Journal of Medicine* 335: 791–9.

† Gould SJ (1984) *The Mismeasure of Man.* London: Pelican.

‡ Guinan ME (1993) Black communities' belief in 'AIDS as genocide'. A barrier to overcome for HIV prevention. *Ann.Epidemiol,* 3: 193–95.

† Hannan EL, Kilburn H, O'Donnell JF, Lukacic G, Shields EP (1991) Interracial access to selected cardiac procedures for patients hospitalised with coronary artery disease in New York State. *Medical Care* 29: 430–41.

† Harding S, Maxwell, R. Differences in mortality of migrants. In: Drever F, Whitehead, M., editor. Health Inequalities. London: Office for National Statistics. p. 108–121.

Hernstein R and Murray C (1994) *The Bell Curve.* New York: Free Press.

‡ Hitler A (1992) *Mein Kampf,* trans. R. Manheim. London: Pimlico.

Hjern A, Haglund B, Persson G, Rosen M (2001) Is there equity in access to health services for ethnic minorities in Sweden? *Eur.J Public Health* 11: 147–52.

Jeffreys M, Stevanovic V, Tobias M, Lewis C, Ellison-Loschmann L, Pearce N *et al.* (2005) Ethnic inequalities in cancer survival in New Zealand: Linkage study. *Research and Practice* 95: 834–7.

† Jones JH (1993) *Bad Blood. The Tuskegee Syphilis Experiment*, 2nd edn. New York: Free Press.

Karlsen S and Nazroo JY (2004) Fear of racism and health. *J Epidemiol Community Health* 58: 1017–18.

† Karmi G and McKeigue P (1993) *The Ethnic Health Bibliography*. London: NE and NW Thames RHA.

† Kiple KF and King VH (1981) *Another Dimension to the Black Diaspora*. London: Cambridge University Press.

Krieger N and Sidney S (1996) Racial discrimination and blood pressure: the CARDIA study of young black and white adults. *Am J Public Health* 86: 1370–8.

† Krieger ND, Rowley DL, Herman A (1993) Racism, sexism and social class: implications for studies of health, disease, and wellbeing. *Am J Med* 9(6) (Suppl.): 82–122.

Kushnick L (1988) Racism, the National Health Service and the health of black people. *Int J Health Services* 18: 457–70.

La Veist T, Wallace J, Howard D (1995) The color line and the health of African Americans. *Humboldt Journal of Social Relations* 21: 119–37.

Lawrence D (2002) Which diseases contribute to life-expectancy differences between races? *The Lancet* 360: 1571.

‡ Lawrence E (1982) Just plain commonsense: the 'ropes' of racism. In Centre for Contemporary Cultural Studies. *The Empire Strikes Back: Race and Racism in 70s Britain*. London: Hutchinson and Co (Publishers) Ltd.

Lowry S and Macpherson G (1988) A blot on the profession. *BMJ* 296: 657–8.

‡ Macpherson WH (1999) *Report on the Stephen Lawrence Inquiry*, Cm 4262–1. London: HMSO.

† Madhok R, Bhopal R, Ramaiah S (1992) Quality of hospital service: a study comparing 'Asian' and 'non-Asian' patients in Middlesborough. *J Public Health Med* 14: 217–79.

† Madhok R, Hameed A, Bhopal R (1998) Satisfaction with health services among Pakistani population in Middlesborough, England. *J Pub Health Med* 20: 295–301.

† Marmot MG, Adelstein AM, Bulusu L (1984) *Immigrant mortality in England and Wales 1970–78*. London, HMSO.

Marmot MG, Adelstein AM, Bulusu L (1984) Lessons from the study of immigrant mortality. *The Lancet* i: 1455–8.

‡ McIntosh. Daily effects of white privilege in a racist society. *Grassroots Leadership*: 2.

* Mackintosh J, Bhopal RS, Unwin N, Ahmad N (1998) *Step-by-step Guide to Epidemiological Health Needs Assessment for Ethnic Minority Groups*. Newcastle upon Tyne: Department of Epidemiology and Public Health, University of Newcastle upon Tyne.

† McKeigue PM, Miller GJ, Marmot MG (1989) Coronary heart disease in south Asians overseas: a review. *Journal of Clinical Epidemiology* 42: 597–609.

† McKeigue PM, Richards JDM, Richards P (1990) Effects of discrimination by sex and race on the early careers of British Medical graduates during 1981–87. *BMJ* 301: 961–4.

McKenzie K ( ) Racial discrimination in medicine. *BMJ* 310: 478–9.

McKenzie K (2003) Racism and health. *BMJ* 326: 65–6.

McManus IC, Richards P, Winder W, Sproston KA, Styles V (1995) Medical school applicants from ethnic minority groups: identifying if and when they are disadvantaged. *BMJ* 310: 496–500.

McNeilly M, Robinson E, Anderson N *et al.* (1995) Effects of racist provocation and social support on cardiovascular reactivity in African American women. *Int J Behavioral Med* 2: 321–38.

† Modood T, Berthoud R, Lakey J, Nazroo J, Smith P, Virdee S, Beishon S (1997) *Ethnic Minorities in Britain: diversity and disadvantage*. London: PSI Publications.

‡ Montagu A (1998) *Man's most dangerous myth—the fallacy of race*. London: AltaMira Press, USA.

Moss KL (1995) Race and poverty data as a tool in the struggle for environmental justice. *Journal of Poverty and Race Research Action Council* 5: 1–6.

Muntaner C (1999) Invited commentary: Social mechanisms, race and social epidemiology. *American Journal of Epidemiology* 150: 121–6.

Muntaner C, Nieto J, O'Campo P (1996) The Bell curve: On race, social class, and epidemiologic research. *Am J Epidemiol* 144: 531–6.

† Nazroo JY (1997) *The Health of Britain's Ethnic Minorities: findings from a national survey*. London: Policy Studies Institute.

† Nazroo JY (2001) South Asian people and heart disease: an assessment of the importance of socioeconomic position. *Ethnicity and Disease* 11: 401–11.

Nerenz DR, Bonham VL, Green-Weir R, Joseph C, Gunter M (2002) Eliminating racial/ethnic disparities in health care: can health plans generate reports? *Health Affairs* 21: 259–63.

Oberman A and Cutter G (1984) Issues in the natural history and treatment of coronary heart disease in African American populations: surgical treatment. *American Heart Journal* 108: 688–94.

† Osborne NG and Feit MD (1992) The use of race in medical research. *JAMA* 267: 275–9.

Parker H (1997) Beyond ethnic categories: why racism should be a variable in ethnicity and health research. *J Health Service Research and Policy* 2: 256–9.

† Peterson ED, Wright SM, Daley J, Thibault GE (1994) Racial variation in cardiac procedure use and survival following acute myocardial infarction in the Department of Veterans Affairs. *JAMA* 271: 1175–80.

Polednak AP (1989) *Racial and Ethnic Differences in Disease*. New York: School of Medicine, State University of New York.

Ren XS (1996) Race and self-assessed health status: the role of socioeconomic factors in the USA. *Journal of Epidemiology and Community Health* 50: 269–73.

† Rothschild H (ed.) (1981) *Biocultural Aspects of Disease*. London: Academic Press.

† Sheth T, Nair C, Nargundkar M, Anand S, Yusuf S. Cardiovascular and cancer mortality among Canadians of European, south Asian and Chinese origin from 1979 to 1993: an analysis of 1.2 million deaths. *Canadian Medical Association Journal* 1999 Jul 27; 161(2): 132–8.

† Silver JR (2003) The decline of German medicine, 1933–45. *Journal of the Royal College of Physicians (Edin)* 33: 54–66.

‡ Smith R (1987) Prejudice against doctors and students from ethnic minorities. *BMJ* 294: 328–9.

Stronks K, Ravelli ACJ, Reijneveld SA (2001) Immigrants in the Netherlands: equal access for equal needs? *Journal of Epidemiology and Community Health* 55: 701–7.

Varma J (1996) Eugenics and immigration restriction: lessons for tomorrow. *JAMA* 275: 734.

Wailoo K (2006) Stigma, race, and disease in 20th century America. *The Lancet* 367: 531–3.

† Warren R (1993) The morbidity/mortality gap: what is the problem? *Ann Epidemiology* 3: 127–9.

† Wenneker M and Epstein A (1989) Racial inequalities in the use of procedures for patients with ischemic heart disease in Massachusetts. *JAMA* 261: 253–7.

‡ Whitridge Williams J (1926) *A text-book for the use of students and practitioners*. New York: D Appleton & Co.

‡ Whittle J, Conigliaro J, Good CB, Lofgren RP (1993) Racial differences in the use of invasive cardiovascular procedures in the Department of Veterans Affairs medical system. *New England Journal of Medicine* 329: 621–.

† Wild S and McKeigue P (1997) Cross-sectional analysis of mortality by country of birth in England and Wales, 1970–1992. *BMJ* 314: 705–10.

‡ Williams R and Hunt K (1997) Psychological distress among British South Asians: the contribution of stressful situations and subcultural differences in the West of Scotland Twenty-07 Study. *Psychol Med* 27: 1173–81.

† Williams R, Wright W, Hunt K (1998) Social class and health: the puzzling counter-example of British South Asians. *Social Science and Medicine* 47: 1277–88.

Chapter 7

‡ Amaro H & Zambrana RE (2000) Criollo, mestizo, mulato, LatiNegro, indigena, white, or black? The US Hispanic/Latino population and multiple responses in the 2000 census. *American Journal of Public Health* 90: 1724–7.

† Balarajan R & Bulusu L (1990) *Mortality among immigrants in England and Wales, 1979–83*. In Britton, M. (Ed.), Mortality and Geography: A review in the mid 1980's: 103–121. London: HMSO.

† Balarajan R, Bulusu L, Adelstein AM, Shukla V (1984) Patterns of mortality among migrants to England and Wales from the Indian subcontinent. *BMJ* 289: 1185–7.

* Bhopal R and Donaldson L (1988) Health promotion for ethnic minorities: current provision and future directions. *Health Education Journal* 47: 137–40.

* Bhopal RS and Rankin J (1996) Cancer in minority ethnic populations: priorities from epidemiological data. *Br J Cancer* 74: S22–S32.

* Bhopal RS (1998) Setting priorities for health care. Chapter 4 (pp. 57–63) in Rawaf S, Bahl V (eds) *Assessing Health Needs of Ethnic Minority Groups*. London: Department of Health.

* Bhopal RS (2006) The public health agenda and minority ethnic health: a reflection on priorities. *J R Soc Med* 99: 58–61.

‡ Bottomley V (1993) *Priority setting in the NHS*. Rationing in Action: 25–32. London: BMJ Publishing Group.

‡ Bradby H (1999) *Genetics and racism*. In Marteau, T. & Richards, M. (Eds), The troubled helix: social and psychological implications of the new human genetics: 295–316. Cambridge: Cambridge University Press.

Brandt AM (1985) *Racism and Research: The case of the Tuskegee syphilis study*. In Judith Walzer Leavitt & Ronald L Numbers (Eds.), Sickness and Health in America: Readings in the History of Medicine and Public Health: 331–343. Madison: University of Wisconsin Press. Notes: Originally published in the Hastings Center Report, December 1978, v.8(6), pp. 21–29.

Cameron WI, Moffitt PS, Williams DRR (1986) Diabetes mellitus in the Australian Aborigines of Bourke, New South Wales. *Diabetes Research and Clinical Practice* 2: 307–14.

† Donaldson LJ and Clayton DG (1984) Occurrence of cancer in Asians and Non-Asians. *J Epidemiol Community Health* 38: 203–7.

† Dunnigan MG, McIntosh WB, Sutherland GR, Gordee R *et al.* (1981) Policy for prevention of Asian Rickets in Britain: a preliminary assessment of the Glasgow Rickets Campaign. *BMJ* 288: 357–60.

† Grimley Evans J (1993) *This patient or that patient? Rationing in Action*: 118–124. London: BMJ Publishing Group.

Farooq S and Coleman MP (2005) Breast cancer survival in South Asian women in England and Wales. *J Epidemiol Community Health* 59: 402–6.

† Grulich AE, Swerdlow AJ, Head J, Marmot MG (1992) Cancer mortality in African and Caribbean migrants to England and Wales. *Br J Cancer* 66: 905–11.

Health Education Authority (1998) *Effectiveness of Interventions to Promote Healthy Eating in People from Minority Ethnic Groups: a review*. London: Health Education Authority.

† Hopkins A and Bahl V (eds) *Access to Health Care for People from Black and Ethnic Minorities*. London: Royal College of Physicians of London.

Johnson MRD, Clark M, Owen D, and Szczepura A (1988). *The Unavoidable Costs of Ethnicity: A Review for the NHSE, CRER and CHESS*. Warwick, University of Warwick.

‡ Karmi G and McKeigue P (1993) *The Ethnic Health Bibliography*. London: North West Thames Regional Health Authority.

† Klein R (1993) Dimensions of rationing: who should do what. *Rationing in Action*: 96–104. London: BMJ Publishing Group.

Lin SS & Kelsey JL (2000) Use of race and ethnicity in epidemiologic research: Concepts, methodological issues, and suggestions for research. *Epidemiologic Reviews* 22: 187–202.

* Marmot MG, Adelstein AM, Bulusu L (1984) *Immigrant Mortality in England and Wales 1970–78.* London: HMSO.

† Muir KR, Parkes SE, Mann JR, Stevens MCG, Cameron AH (1992) Childhood cancer in the West Midlands: incidence and survival 1980–1984 in a multi-ethnic population. *Clinical Oncology* 4: 177–82.

† Powell JE, Parkes SE, Cameron AH, Mann JR (1994) Is the risk of cancer increased in Asians living in the UK? *Arch Dis Childhood* 71: 398–403.

† Rankin J and Bhopal R (2001) Understanding of heart disease and diabetes in a South Asian community: cross-sectional study testing the 'snowball' sample method. *Pub Health* 115: 253–60.

Rankin J, Carlin L, White M (1998) *Interventions to Reduce Mortality from Breast and Cervical Cancer in Minority Ethnic Groups.* Newcastle upon Tyne: University of Newcastle upon Tyne, Department of Epidemiology and Public Health.

† Rawaf S and Bahl V (1998) *Assessing Health Needs of People from Minority Ethnic Groups.* London: Royal College of Physicians.

Salmon Jon and Law Alastair (1993). *The Ethnic Timebomb.* Sunday Express, 1. 13-8-1993. London.

* Senior P and Bhopal RS (1994) Ethnicity as a variable in epidemiological research. *BMJ* 309: 327–9.

† Smaje C (1995) *Race, Ethnicity and Health.* London: King's Fund Institute.

† Stiller CA and McKinney PA (1991) Childhood cancer and ethnic group in Britain: a United Kingdom children's cancer study group (UKCCSG) study. *Br J Cancer* 64: 543–8.

† Tunstall Pedoe H, Clayton D, Morris JN, Bridge W, McDonald L (1975) Coronary heart-attack in East London. *The Lancet* ii: 833–8.

Whitridge Williams J (1926) *A text-book for the use of students and practitioners.* New York: D Appleton & Co.

Chapter 8

Many of the materials relating to this chapter are in the list of web sites.

† Acheson D (1998) *Independent Report into Inequalities in Health.* 1998. London: HMSO.

Adelstein AM (1963) Some aspects of cardiovascular mortality in South Africa. *Brit J Prev Soc Med* 17: 29–40.

Agyemang C, Bindraban N, Gideon M, Gert van M, Koopmans R, Stronks K (2005) Prevalance, awareness, treatment, and control of hypertension among Black Surinamese, South Asian Surinamese and White Dutch in Amsterdam, The Netherlands: the SUNSET study. *Journal of Hypertension* 23: 1971–7.

Anand SS, Yusuf S, Jacobs R, Davis AD, Yi Q, Gerstein H (2001) Risk factors, atherosclerosis, and cardiovascular disease among Aboriginal people in Canada: the study of health assessment and risk evaluation in Aboriginal people (SHARE-AP). *The Lancet* 358: 1147–52.

Anand S, Yusuf S, Vuksan V *et al.* (2000) Differences in risk factors, atherosclerosis, and cardiovascular disease between ethnic groups in Canada: the Study of Health Assessment and Risk in Ethnic Groups. *The Lancet* 356: 279–84.

Anonymous (2001) American Indian health: insights and reservations. *The Lancet* 357: 1810.

Balarajan R and Raleigh VS (1993) *Ethnicity and Health. A guide for the NHS.* London: Department of Health.

† Bartlett C, Davey P, Dieppe P, Doyal L, Ebrahim S *et al.* (2003) Women, older persons, and ethnic minorities: factors associated with their inclusion in randomised trials of statins 1990 to 2001. *Heart* 89: 327–8.

Baxter C and Ginnety P (2003) A comprehensive strategy for travellers health. *Public Health Medicine* 4: 88–92.

* Bhopal RS and Parsons L (1993) A draft policy for adoption by Health Authorities, purchasers and providers of health care. In Hopkins A, Bahl V (eds) *Access to Health Care for People from Black and Ethnic Minorities*. London: Royal College of Physicians of London.

† Bhopal R, Unwin N, White M, Yallop J, Walker L, Alberti KG, Harland J, Patel S, Ahmad N, Turner C, Watson B, Kaur D, Kulkarni A, Laker M, & Tavridou A (1999). Heterogeneity of coronary heart disease risk factors in Indian, Pakistani, Bangladeshi, and European origin populations: cross sectional study. *BMJ* 319: 215–20.

Bhopal R, Fischbacher C, Vartiainen E, Unwin N, White M, Alberti G (2005) Predicted and observed cardiovascular disease in South Asians: application of FINRISK, Framingham and SCORE models to Newcastle Heart Project data. *Journal of Public Health* 27: 93–100.

‡ British Heart Foundation (2004) *Heart Disease and South Asians*. London: Department of Health.

† Chandra J (1996) *Facing up to Difference: A toolkit for creating culturally competent health services for black and minority ethnic communities*. London: King's Fund.

Clark M, Owen D, Szczepura A, Johnson MRD (1998) *Assessment of the costs to the NHS arising from the need for interpreter and translation services*. CRER and CHESS: University of Warwick.

‡ Clyne MB (1964) Indian patients. *Practitioner* 793: 195–9.

Denktas S and Bruijnzeels M (2002) Equal access for equal needs: role of cultural differences and language proficiency. *European Journal of Public Health* 12: S50.

Department of Health (2000) *National Service Frameworks for Coronary Heart Disease: Modern Standards and Service Models*. Department of Health.

* Elliott B for the Newcastle Strategy Group (1997) *Taking Heart. Reducing diabetes and cardiovascular disease among Newcastle's South Asian and Chinese communities*. Newcastle upon Tyne: University of Newcastle upon Tyne.

Fall CHD and Barker DJP (1997) The fetal origins of coronary heart disease and non-insulin dependent diabetes in India. *Indian Pediatrics* 34: 5–8.

† Fuller J (1987) Contraceptive services for ethnic minorities. *BMJ (Clin Res Ed)* 295: 1365.

‡ Gunaratnam G (1993) *Checklist: Health and Race: a starting point for managers on improving services for black populations*. London: King's Fund Centre.

‡ Grudzinskas JG (1987) Tower Hamlets' health. *British Medical Journal* 295: 503–4.

Henley A (1991) *Caring for Everyone: Ensuring Standards of Care for Black and Ethnic Minority Patients*. National Extension College, Cambridge.

‡ Home Office (2001) Race Relations (Amendment) Act 2000. New laws for a successful multi-racial Britain. London: Home Office.

* Ineson A and Bhopal R (2000) *Meeting the Health Needs of Minority Ethnic Groups in Lothian*. Report of the Director of Public Health. Edinburgh: Lothian Health Board.

Johnson MRD, Clark M, Owen D, Szczepura A (1998) *The Unavoidable Costs of Ethnicity: A Review for the NHSE*. CRER and CHESS: University of Warwick.

Krasnik A, Joost MJ, Sonne NA, Norredam M (2002) Communication, attitudes and knowledge among Danish hospital staff in relation to immigrants. *European Journal of Public Health* 12: S69–S70.

Leeds Health Promotion Service (1992) *Chinese Health Care in Britain*. University of Leeds: Leeds Health Promotion Service.

‡ Lothian Health Board (2002) Strategic Action Plan on Minority Ethnic Health: Being Fair For All in the NHS in Lothian (Draft for Consultation), May 2002. Edinburgh, Lothian Health Board.

* Lothian NHS Minority Health Group (2003) *Strategic Action Plan on Minority Ethnic Health: being fair for all in the NHS in Lothian*. Edinburgh: NHS Lothian.

‡ McNaught A (1985) Black and ethnic minority women and the National Health Service. *Radical Comm Med* Spring: 29–34.

† McNaught A (2004) Health policy and race equality: an illusion of progress? *J R Soc Med* 97: 579–81.

‡ MacPherson W (1999) *The Stephen Lawrence Inquiry Report.* London: The Stationery Office.

† Madhok R, Bhopal RS, Ramaiah RS (1992) Quality of hospital service: an 'Asian' perspective. *J Pub Health Med* 14: 271–9.

† Madhok R, Hameed A, Bhopal RS (1998) Satisfaction with health services among the Pakistani population in Middlesbrough, England. *J Pub Health Med* 20: 295–301.

† National Institutes of Health (2000) *Strategic Research Plan to Reduce and Ultimately Eliminate Health Disparities.* Bethesda, National Institutes of Health.

† Nazroo JY (1997) *The Health of Britain's Ethnic Minorities: findings from a national survey.* London: Policy Studies Institute.

* Patel KC, Bhopal RS (eds) (2004) *The Epidemic of Coronary Heart Disease in South Asian Populations: causes and consequences* Brimingham: South Asian Health Foundation.

† Race Equality Advisory Forum (2001) *Making it Real A Race Equality Strategy for Scotland.* Edinburgh: Scottish Executive.

† Ranganathan M and Bhopal R (2006) Exclusion and inclusion of nonwhite ethnic minority groups in 72 North American and European cardiovascular cohort studies. *PLoS Medicine* 3: 1–8.

‡ Rehman H, Edwards C, Lincoln P (1999) *Meeting the Needs of Black and Minority Ethnic Groups: a policy paper for the Health Education Authority.* Report No. R10/99. London, Health Education Authority (Unpublished).

Robinson M (2002) *Communication and Health in a Multi-ethnic Society.* Bristol: The Policy Press.

† Rocheron Y and Dickinson R (1990) The Asian mother and baby campaign: a way forward in health promotion for Asian women? *Health Educ J* 49: 128–33.

‡ *Rooting Out Racism: A Joint Declaration of Intent and Action Against Racism in the Lothian and Borders Area,* 2001.

‡ Scottish Executive (1999) White Paper, Towards a Healthier Scotland, Cm 4269. Edinburgh: The Stationery Office.

Scottish Executive (2000). Researching Ethnic Minorities in Scotland. 1–65. Edinburgh, Scottish Executive Central Research Unit.

Scottish Executive (2002) *Translating, Interpreting and Communication Support Services Across the Public Sector in Scotland: a literature review,* 2227. Edinburgh: Scottish Executive.

‡ Scottish Executive Health Department (2002) *Fair For All: working together towards culturally competent services,* HDL 51. Edinburgh, Scottish Executive.

Shaper AG & Jones KW (1959) Serum-Cholesterol, diet and coronary heart-disease in Africans and Asians in Uganda. *Lancet,* 11: 534–7.

† Shaw J (1994) *Collection of Ethnic Group data for Admitted Patients* (EL(94)77). Leeds: NHS Executive.

‡ Steinbrook R (2004) Disparities in health care—from politics to policy. *New England Journal of Medicine* 350: 1486–8.

‡ Taylor AL, Ziesche S, Yancy C, Carson P, D'Agostino R Jr, Ferdinand K *et al.* (2004) Combination of isosorbide dinitrate and hydralazine in blacks with heart failure. *New England Journal of Medicine* 351: 2049–57.

Tunstall Pedoe H, Clayton D, Morris JN, Bridge W, McDonald L (1975) Coronary heart-attack in East London. *The Lancet* 2: 833–8.

US Department of Health and Human Services (1985) *Report of the Secretary's Task Force on Black and Minority Health.* Washington, DC: US Government Printing Office.

US Department of Health and Human Services (1999) *Pocket Guide to Minority Health Resources.* Washington, DC: US Government Printing Office.

Van Oort M, Deville W, De Bakker DH (2002) Health care for asylum seekers in the Netherlands. *European Journal of Public Health* 12: 106.

‡ Woolhandler S, Himmelstein DU, Silber R, Bader M, Harnly M, & Jones AA (1985) Medical care and mortality: racial differences in preventable deaths. *Int. J Health Serv.* 15: 1–22.

Chapter 9

Agyemang C, Bindraban N, Gideon M, Gert van M, Koopmans R, Stronks K (2005) Prevalance, awareness, treatment, and control of hypertension among Black Surinamese, South Asian Surinamese and White Dutch in Amsterdam, The Netherlands: the SUNSET study. *Journal of Hypertension* 23: 1971–7.

Allmark P (2004) Should research samples reflect the diversity of the population? *J Med Ethics* 30: 185–9.

† American College of Epidemiology (1995) Statement of principles: epidemiology and minority populations. *Ann Epidemiol* 5: 505–8.

† Balarajan R and Bulusu L (1990) Mortality among immigrants in England and Wales, 1979–1983. In Britton M (ed.) *Mortality and Geography* London: HMSO.

Balarajan R, Bulusu L, Adelstein AM, Shukla V (1984) Patterns of mortality among migrants to England and Wales from the Indian subcontinent. *BMJ* 289: 1185–7.

Barkan E (1992) *The Retreat of Scientific Racism.* London: Cambridge University Press.

‡ Barker J (1984) *Black and Asian Old People in Britain.* Research perspectives on ageing. 1–53 Surrey. Age Concern Research Unit.

† Barker RM and Baker MR (1990) Incidence of cancer in Bradford Asians. *J Epidemiol Community Health* 44: 125–9.

Bartlett C, Davey P, Dieppe P, Doyal L, Ebrahim S *et al.* (2003) Women, older persons, and ethnic minorities: factors associated with their inclusion in randomized trials of statins 1990 to 2001. *Heart* 89: 327–8.

Bennett T (1997) 'Racial' and ethnic classification: two steps forward and one step back? *Public Health Reports* 112: 477–80.

Bhopal RS (1986a). The interrelationship of folk, traditional and western medicine within an Asian community in Britain. *Soc Sci Med* 22: 99–105.

Bhopal RS (1986b). Bhye Bhaddi: a food and health concept of Punjabi Asians. *Soc. Sci. Med* 23: 687–88.

* Bhopal RS (1990) Future research on the health of ethnic minorities: back to basics. A personal view. *Ethnic Minorities Health. A current awareness bulletin.* 1(3): 1–3.

* Bhopal RS (1997) Is research into ethnicity and health racist, unsound, or important science? *BMJ* 314: 1751–6.

* Bhopal RS (2000) Race and ethnicity as epidemiological variables. Centrality of purpose and context. Chapter 2 in Macbeth H (ed.) *Ethnicity and Health,* pp. 21–40. London: Taylor and Francis.

* Bhopal RS (2002) *Concepts of Epidemiology.* Oxford: Oxford University Press.

* Bhopal R (2004) Glossary of terms relating to ethnicity and race: for reflection and debate. *Journal of Epidemiology and Community Health* 58: 441–5.

† Bhopal RS and Donaldson LJ (1988) Health education for ethnic minorities—current provision and future directions. *H Educ J* 47: 137–40.

† Bhopal RS and Donaldson LJ (1998) White, European, Western, Caucasian or what? Inappropriate labelling in research on race ethnicity and health. *Am J Pub Health* 88: 1303–7.

† Bhopal R., Vettini A, Hunt S, Wiebe S, Hanna L, Amos A (2004) Review of prevalence data in, and evaluation of methods for cross cultural adaptation of, UK surveys on tobacco and alcohol in ethnic minority groups. *BMJ* 328: 76–80.

Biddiss MD (ed.) (1970) *Gobineau Selected Political Writings.* London: Jonathan Cape.

Biddiss MD (1979) *Images of Race.* Leicester, Leicester University Press.

‡ Black N (1987) Migration and health. *BMJ* 295: 566.

† *BMJ* (1996) Ethnicity, race and culture: guidelines for research, audit and publication. *BMJ* 312: 1094.

Bowes A and Fox-Rushby A (2003) A systematic and critical review of the process of translation and adaptation of generic health-related quality of life measures in Africa, Asia, Eastern Europe, the Middle East, South America. *Social Science and Medicine* 57: 1289–306.

† Bowling A (2002) *Research Methods in Health*. Buckingham: Open University Press.

† Bowling A and Ebrahim S (2006) *Handbook of Health Research Methods: investigation, measurement and analysis*. Maidenhead: Open University Press.

Burchard EG, Ziv E, Coyle N, Gomez SL, Tang H, Karter AJ *et al.* (2003) The importance of race and ethnic background in biomedical research and clinical practice. *New England Journal of Medicine* 348: 1170–5.

‡ Cartwright Dr (1851). *Africans in America—Diseases and Peculiarities of the Negro Race*. DeBow's Review, v11: New Orleans. http://www.pbs.org/wgbh/aia/part4/4h3106t.html

‡ Comstock RD, Castillo EM, Lindsay SP (2004) Four-year review of the use of race and ethnicity in epidemiologic and public health research. *Am. J Epidemiol* 159: 611–19.

† Cooper R, Rotimi C, Ataman S, McGee D, Osotimehin B, Kadiri S *et al.* (1997) The prevalence of hypertension in seven populations of West African origin. *Am J Public Health* 87: 160–8.

‡ Corbie-Smith G, Miller WC, Ransohoff DF (2004) Interpretations of 'appropriate' minority inclusion in clinical research. *Am J Med* 116: 249–52.

Corbie-Smith G, St George DMM, Moody-Ayers S, Ransohoff DF (2003) Adequacy of reporting race/ethnicity in clinical trials in areas of health disparities. *Journal of Clinical Epidemiology* 56: 416–20.

‡ Donaldson LJ and Clayton DG (1984) Occurrence of cancer in Asians and Non-Asians. *J Epidemiol Community Health* 38: 203–7.

Donaldson LJ and Taylor JB (1983) Patterns of Asian and non-Asian morbidity in hospitals. *BMJ* 286: 949–51.

‡ Donovan JH (1984) Ethnicity and health: a research review. *Soc Sc. Med* 19: 663–70.

‡ Down JLH (1867) *Observations on an Ethnic Classification of Idiots*. Reprinted in: Mental Retardation, 1995, 54–57.

Ebling FJ (ed.) (1974) *Racial Variation in Man*. London: Institute of Biology.

Ecob R and Williams R (1991) Sampling Asian minorities to assess health and welfare. *J Epidemiol Community Health* 45: 93–101.

* Elliott B for the Newcastle Strategy Group (1997) *Taking Heart. Reducing diabetes and cardiovascular disease among Newcastle's South Asian and Chinese communities*. Newcastle upon Tyne: University of Newcastle upon Tyne.

† Ellison GTH and De Wet T (1997) *Re-examining the content of the South African Medical Journal during the formalisation of 'racial' discrimination under apartheid. Health and Human Rights Project*. In: The Final Submission of the HHRP to the Truth and Reconciliation Commission.: 112–131. Cape Town: Health and Human Rights Project.

Fischbacher CM, Bhopal R, Unwin N, White M, Alberti KG (2001) The performance of the Rose angina questionnaire in South Asian and European origin populations: a comparative study in Newcastle. *Int J Epidemiol* 54: 786.

Foster MW and Sharp RR (2004) Beyond race: towards a whole-genome perspective on human populations and genetic variation. *Nat Rev Genet* 5: 790–6.

Fullilove MT (1998) Comment: abandoning 'race' as a variable in public health research—an idea whose time has come. *Am J Public Health* 88: 1297–8.

† Gamble V (1993) A legacy of distrust: African Americans and medical research. *Am J Preventive Medicine* 9(6) (Suppl.): 35–7.

† Gould SJ (1984) *The Mismeasure of Man*. London: Pelican.

Gould SJ (1990) *Hen's Teeth and Horse's Toes*. London: Penguin.

Gunaratnam Y (2003) *Researching Race and Ethnicity: methods, knowledge and power*. London: Sage Publications.

† Hahn RA and Stroup DF (1994) Race and ethnicity in public health surveillance: criteria for the scientific use of social categories. *Public Health Reports* 109: 4–12.

† Hanna L, Hunt S, Bhopal R (in press) Cross-cultural adaptation of a tobacco questionnaire for Punjabi, Cantonese, Urdu and Sylheti speakers: qualitative research for better clinical practice, cessation services and research. *Journal of Epidemiology and Community Health*.

† Health Education Authority (1994) *Health and Lifestyles: black and minority ethnic groups in England*. London: HEA.

† Hernstein R and Murray C (1994) *The Bell Curve*. New York: Free Press.

Hoare T, Thomas C, Biggs A, Booth M, Bradley S, Friedman E (1994) Can the uptake of breast screening by Asian women be increased? A randomised controlled trial of a linkworker intervention. *J Public Health Medicine* 16: 179–85.

Howard CA (1983) Survey research in New Mexico Hispanics: some methodological issues. *American Journal of Epidemiology* 117: 27–34.

Hughes AO (1995) Strategies for sampling black and ethnic minority populations. *Journal of Public Health Medicine* 17: 187–92.

Hussain-Gambles M (2003) Ethnic minority under-representation in clinical trials: Whose responsibility is it anyway? *J Health Organ Manag* 17: 138–43.

Hussain-Gambles M, Atkin K, Leese B (2004) Why ethnic minority groups are under-represented in clinical trials: a review of the literature. *Health Soc Care Community* 12: 382–8.

Huxley JS, Haddon AC, Carr-Sunders AM (1936) We Europeans: a survey of 'Racial' problems. New York: Harper.

Ineichen B (1994) Methods for epidemiological surveys of ethnic minorities. *Journal of Epidemiology and Community Health* 48: 526.

† Jones JH (1993) *Bad Blood. The Tuskegee Syphilis Experiment*, 2nd edn. New York: Free Press.

‡ Kaplan JB and Bennett T (2003) Use of race and ethnicity in biomedical publication. *JAMA* 289: 2709–16.

Kaufman J and Cooper R (1995) In search of the hypothesis. *Public Health Reports* 110: 662–6.

† Kaufman JS, Cooper RS, McGee DL (1997) Socioeconomic status and health in blacks and whites: the problem of residual confounding and the resiliency of race. *Epidemiology* 8: 621–8.

Kaufman JS and Hall SA (2003) The slavery hypertension hypothesis: dissemination and appeal of a modern race theory. *Epidemiology* 14: 111–26.

Kelleher D and Hillier S (1996) *Researching Cultural Differences in Health*. London: Routledge.

† Kiple KF and King VH (1981) *Another Dimension to the Black Diaspora*. London: Cambridge University Press.

† Krieger ND, Rowley DL, Herman A (1993) Racism, sexism and social class: implications for studies of health, disease, and wellbeing. *Am J Prev Med* 9 (6) (Suppl.): 82–122.

Krieger N and Sidney S (1996) Racial discrimination and blood pressure: the CARDIA study of young black and white adults. *Am J Public Health* 86: 1370–8.

† Krieger N (2002) *Shades of Difference Theoretical Underpinnings of the Medical Controversy on Black-White Differences in the United States, 1830–70*. In La Veist, T. A. (ed.), Race, Ethnicity and Health: 11–33. San Francisco: Jossey-Bass.

‡ Kuper L (ed.) (1975) *Race, Science and Society*. London: Allen and Unwin.

‡ Leaning J (2001) Ethics of research in refugee populations. *The Lancet* 357: 1432–3.

Lee MM, Wu-Williams A, Whittemore AS, Zheng S, Gallagher R, Teh CZ *et al.* (1994) Comparison of dietary habits, physical activity and body size among Chinese in North America and China. *Int J Epidemiol* 23: 984–90.

Leslie C (1990) Scientific racism: reflections on peer review, science and ideology. *Soc Sci Med* 31: 891–912.

Li L, Wang HM, Shen Y (2003) Chinese SF-36 Health Survey: translation, cultural adaptation, validation, and normalisation. *Journal of Epidemiol Community Health* 57: 259–63.

† Lillie-Blanton M, Anthony JC, Schuster CR (1993) Probing the meaning of racial/ethnic group comparisons in crack cocaine smoking. *JAMA* 269: 993–7.

Lin SS and Kelsey JL (2001) Use of race and ethnicity in epidemiologic research: concepts, methodological issues, and suggestions for research. *Epidemiologic Reviews* 187–202.

‡ London Chinese Health Resource in partnership with Kensington, Chelsea and Westminster Health Authority, London 1995. *Needs Assessment: A study of the family planning and sexual health needs of the Chinese Community in Kensington, Chelsea and Westminster*. London, London Chinese Health Resource Centre.

† Lynn R, Rushton P, Jenson A, Murray C, Brand C, Nyborg H *et al*. (2006) Racial IQ research. *Sunday Times* April 2.

Makridakis NM, Ross RR, Pike MC, Crocitto LE, Kolonel LN, Pearce CL *et al*. (1999) Association of mis-sense substitution in SRD5A2 gene prostate cancer in African-American and Hispanic men in Los Angeles, USA. *The Lancet* 354: 975–8.

‡ Marmot MG, Adelstein AM, Bulusu L (1984) *Immigrant Mortality in England and Wales 1970–78*. Studies on medical and populations subjects, No 47. London: HMSO.

Marquez MA, Muhs JM, Tosomeen A, Riggs BL, Melton III LJ (2003) Costs and strategies in minority recruitment for osteoporosis research. *Journal of Bone and Mineral Research* 18: 3–8.

† Mason S, Hussain-Gambles M, Leese B, Atkin K, Brown J (2003) Representation of South Asian people in randomised clinical trials: analysis of trials' data. *BMJ* 326: 1244–5.

† Mather HM and Keen H (1985) The Southall Diabetes Survey: prevalence of known diabetes in Asians and Europeans. *BMJ* 291: 1081–4.

† Matheson LM, Dunnigan MG, Hole D, Gillis CR *et al*. (1985) Incidence of colo-rectal, breast and lung cancer in a Scottish Asian population. *Health Bulletin (Edin)*. 43: 245–9.

McKeigue PM (1989) Diet and fecal steroid profile in a South Asian population with a low colon-cancer rate. *American Journal of Clinical Nutrition* 50: 151–4.

‡ McKeigue PM (1997) Mapping genes underlying ethnic differences in disease risk by linkage disequilibrium in recently admixed populations. *American Journal of Human Genetics* 60: 188–96.

† McKeigue PM, Marmot, MG, Syndercombe-Court YD, Cottier DE, Rahman S, Riemersma RA (1991) Relation of central obesity and insulin resistance with high diabetes prevalence and cardiovascular risk in South Asians. *The Lancet* 337: 382–6.

‡ McKenzie K and Crowcroft NS (1996) Describing race, ethnicity and culture in medical research. *BMJ* 312: 1054.

Melia RJW, Chinn S, Rona RJ (1988) Respiratory illness and home environment of ethnic groups. *BMJ* 296: 1438–40.

† Modood T, Berthoud R, Lakey J, Nazroo J, Smith P, Virdee S, Beishon S (1997) *Ethnic Minorities in Britain: diversity and disadvantage*. London: PSI Publications.

‡ Muntaner C, Nieto J, O'Campo P (1996) The bell curve: On race, social class, and epidemiologic research. *Am J Epidemiol* 144: 531–6.

† Nazroo JY (1997) *The Health of Britain's Ethnic Minorities: findings from a national survey*. London: Policy Studies Institute.

Nazroo JY (1998) Genetic, cultural or socio-economic vulnerability? Explaining ethnic inequalities in health. *Sociology of Health & Illness*, 20: 710–730.

Netto G, Arshad R, De Lima P, Diniz FA, MacEwen M, Patel V *et al*. (2001) *Audit of Research on Minority Ethnic Issues in Scotland from a 'Race' Perspective*.

† Office of Management and Budget (1977) *Race and Ethnic Standards for Federal Statistics and Administrative Reporting*. Directive No. 15. Washington, Office of Management and Budget.

† Osborne NG and Feit MD (1992) The use of race in medical research. *JAMA* 267: 275–9.

Ossorio P and Duster T (2005) Race and genetics: controversies in biomedical, behavioral, and forensic sciences. *Am Psychol* 60: 115–28.

‡ Parker H (1997) Beyond ethnic categories: why racism should be a variable in ethnicity and health research. *J Health Service Research and Policy* 2: 256–9.

† Patel S, Unwin N, Bhopal R, White M, Harland J, Ayis SA, Watson W, Albert KGMM (1999) A comparison of proxy measures of abdominal obesity in Chinese, European and South Asian adults. *Diabetic Medicine* 16: 853–60.

‡ Pilgrim S, Fenton S, Hughes A, Hine C, Tibbs N (1993) *The Bristol Black and Ethnic Minorities Health Survey Report*. Bristol: Departments of Sociology and Epidemiology, University of Bristol.

† Polednak AP (1989) *Racial and Ethnic Differences in Disease*. New York: Oxford University Press.

President's Cancer Panel, Report of the Chairman (1997) *The Meaning of Race in Science—recommendations from the Interagency Committee for the review of federal measurements of race and ethnicity*. Report to the Office of Management and Budget. A1-A39. Bethesda, National Institues of Health, National Cancer Institute.

† Rahemtulla T and Bhopal R (2005) Pharmacogenetics and ethnically targeted therapies. *BMJ* 330: 1036–7.

† Ranganathan M and Bhopal R (2006) Exclusion and inclusion of nonwhite ethnic minority groups in 72 North American and European cardiovascular cohort studies. *PLoS Medicine* 3: 1–8.

Rathore SS and Krumholz HM (2003) Race, ethnic group, and clinical research. *BMJ* 327: 763–4.

‡ Rothschild H (ed.) (1981) *Biocultural Aspects of Disease*. London: Academic Press.

Rotimi CN (2004) Are medical and nonmedical uses of large-scale genomic markers conflating genetics and 'race'? *Nat Genet* 36: S43–S47.

† Rudat K (1994) *Black and Minority Ethnic Groups in England: Health and Lifestyles, 1994*. London: Health Education Authority.

‡ Salmon J and Law A (1995) The ethnic time-bomb. *Sunday Express*.

Salomon JA, Tandon A, Murray CJL (2004) Comparability of self-rated health: cross sectional multi-country survey using anchoring vignettes. *BMJ* 328: 258–62.

† Savitz DA (1994) In defense of black box epidemiology. *Epidemiology* 5: 550–52.

Schwartz MD (2001) Racial profiling in medical research. *New England Journal of Medicine* 18: 1392–3.

† Sheikh A (2006) Why are ethnic minorities under-represented in US research studies? *PLoS Med* 3: e49.

Sheikh A, Netuveli G, Kai J, Panesar SS (2004) Comparison of reporting of ethnicity in US and European randomised controlled trials. *BMJ* 329: 87–8.

Sheikh A, Panesar SS, Lasserson T, Netuveli G (2004) Recruitment of ethnic minorities to asthma studies. *Thorax* 59: 634.

Sheldon TA and Parker H (1992) Race and ethnicity in health research. *J Public Health Med* 14: 104–10.

† Skrabanek P (1994) The emptiness of the black box. *Epidemiology* 5: 553–5.

Smith KW, McGraw SA, Crawford SL, McKinlay JB (1998) Do blacks and whites differ in reporting Rose questionnaire angina? Results of the Boston health care project. *Ethnicity and Disease* 3: 278–89.

Stepan N (1982) *The Idea of Race in Science*. London: Macmillan.

Svensson CK (1989) Representation of American Blacks in clinical trials of new drugs. *JAMA* 261: 263–5.

‡ Taylor AL, Ziesche S, Yancy C, Carson P, D'Agostino R Jr, Ferdinand K *et al.* (2004) Combination of isosorbide dinitrate and hydralazine in blacks with heart failure. *New England Journal of Medicine* 351: 2049–57.

† Terry PB, Condie RG, Mathew PM, Bissenden JG (1983) Ethnic differences in the distribution of congenital malformations. *Postgraduate Medical Journal* 59: 657–8.

Unwin N, Alberti KGMM, Bhopal R, Harland J, Watson W, White M (1998) Comparison of the current WHO and new ADA criteria for the diagnosis of diabetes mellitus in three ethnic groups in the UK. *Diabetic Medicine* 15: 554–7.

Unwin N, Harland J, White M, Bhopal R, Winocour P, Stephenson P, Watson W, Turner C, Alberti KGMM (1997) Body mass index, waist circumference, waist–hip ratio, and glucose intolerance in Chinese and Europid adults in Newcastle, UK. *J Epidemiol Comm Health* 51: 160–6.

Vernon SW, Roberts RE, Lees ES (1984) Ethnic participation in longitudinal health studies. *Am J Epidemiol* 119: 99–113.

Warnecke RB, Johnson TP, Chavez N, Sudman S, O'Rourke DP, Lacey L *et al.* (1997) Improving question wording in surveys of culturally diverse populations. *Ann Epidemiol* 7: 334–42.

‡ Warren RC, Hahn RA, Bristow L, Yu ESH (1994) The use of race and ethnicity in public health surveillance. *Public Health Reports* 109: 4–6.

Watt IS, Howel D, Lo L (1993) The health care experience and health behaviour of the Chinese: a survey based in Hull. *J Pub Hlth Med* 15: 129–36.

‡ Wendler D, Kington R, Madans J, Van Wye G, Christ-Schmidt H, Pratt LA *et al.* (2006) Are racial and ethnic minorities less willing to participate in health research? *PLoS Med* 3: e19.

‡ Whitridge Williams J (1926) *A Text-book for the use of Students and Practitioners.* D Appleton and Co.

† Wild SH, Fischbacher CM, Brock A, Griffiths C, Bhopal R (2006) Mortality from all cancers and lung, colorectal, breast and prostate cancer by country of birth in England and Wales, 2001–2003. *Br. J Cancer* 94: 1079–85.

Williams DR, Lavizzo-Mourey R, Warren RC (1994) *The concept of race and health status in America. Public Health Reports* 109: 26–41.

Williams DRR, Moffitt PS, Fisher JS, Bashir HV (1987) Diabetes and glucose tolerance in New South Wales coastal Aborigines: possible effects of non-Aboriginal genetic admixture. *Diabetologia* 30: 72–7.

‡ Williams JW, (1926). *Obstetrics—A text book for the use of students and practitioners.* New York: D Appleton & Co.

‡ Williams R, Bhopal R, Hunt K (1993) Health of a Punjabi ethnic minority in Glasgow: a comparison with the general population. *J Epi Comm Health* 47: 96.

Witzig R (1996) The medicalization of race: scientific legitimization of flawed social construction. *Annals of Internal Medicine* 125: 675–9.

† Woywodt A, Haubitz, Haller, Matteson EL (2006) Wegener's granulomatosis. *The Lancet* 367: 1362–6.

Chapter 10

‡ Ahmad WIU (ed.) (1993) *'Race' and Health in Contemporary Britain.* London: Open University Press.

Ahmad WIU (1989) Policies, pills and political will: a critique of policies to improve the health status of ethnic minorities. *The Lancet* i: 148–9.

Balarajan R and Yuen P (1986) British smoking and drinking habits: regional variations. *Comm Med* 8: 131–7.

‡ Banton M (1987) *Racial Theories.* Cambridge: Cambridge University Press.

‡ Barnett A (1950) *The Human Species.* Bungay, Suffolk: The Chaucer Press Ltd.

Bhopal RS (1986*a*) The interrelationship of folk, traditional and western medicine within an Asian community in Britain. *Soc Sci Med* 22: 99–105.

* Bhopal RS (1997) Ethnicity. In Boyd KM *et al.* (eds) *The New Dictionary of Medical Ethics* pp 89–90. London: BMJ Books.

Bhopal R (2006) Race and Ethnicity: Responsible Use from Epidemiological and Public Health Perspectives. *Journal of Law, Medicine and Ethics* 32: 500–7.

Bhopal RS, Phillimore P, Kohli HS (1991) Inappropriate use of the term 'Asian': an obstacle to ethnicity and health research. *J Pub Health Med* 13: 244–6.

Bloche MG (2004) Race-based therapeutics. *New England Journal of Medicine* 351: 2035–7.

Bolt C (1970) *Victorian Attitudes to Race.* London: Routledge and Kegan Paul.

Brown MJ (2006) Hypertension and ethnic group. *BMJ* 332: 833–6.

‡ Caldwell SH and Popenhoe R (1995) Perception and misperceptions of skin colour. *Annals of Internal Medicine* 122: 614–17.

† Chief Medical Offices (1992) *On the State of Public Health 1991.* London: HMSO.

‡ Coon CS (1963) Growth and development of social groups. In Wolstenholm G (ed.) *Man and his Future,* pp. 120–31. London: J and A Churchill Ltd.

Cooper RS and Kaufman JS (1999) Is there an absence of theory in social epidemiology? The authors respond to Muntaner. *American Journal of Epidemiology* 150: 127–8.

Cruikshank JK and Beevers DG (1989) *Ethnic Factors in Health and Disease*. Oxford: Butterworth-Heinemann.

Dogra N, Connin S, Gill P, Spencer J, Turner M (2005) Teaching of cultural diversity in medical schools in the United Kingdom and Republic of Ireland. *BMJ* 330: 403–4.

Duster T (2005) Medicine. Race and reification in science. *Science* 307: 1050–1.

‡ Elliot C and Brodwin P (2002) Identity and genetic ancestry tracing. *BMJ* 325: 1469–71.

† Golby AJ, Gabrieli JDE, Chiao JY, Eberhardt JL (2001) Differential responses in the fusiform region to same-race and other-race faces. *Nature Neuroscience* 4: 845–50.

Hernstein R and Murray C (1994) *The Bell Curve*. New York: Free Press.

Hopkinson ND, Doherty M, Powell RJ (1994). Clinical features and race-specific incidence/prevalence rates of systemic lupus erythematosus in a geographically complete cohort of patients. *Annals of the Rheumatic Diseases* 53: 675–80.

Huth EJ (1995) Identifying ethnicity in medical papers. *Ann Intern Med* 122: 619–21.

Johnson M (1984) Ethnic minorities and health. *J Roy Coll Physicians, London* 18: 228–23.

Jones D, Gill P, Harrison R, Meakin R, Wallace P (2003) An exploratory study of language interpretation services provided by videoconferencing. *Journal of Telemedicine and Telecare* 9: 51–56.

Kai J (1999) Valuing ethnic diversity in primary care. *British Journal of General Practice* 49: 171–3.

‡ Kai J, Spencer J, Wilkes M, Gill PS (1999) Learning to value ethnic diversity—what, why and how? *Medical Education* 33: 616–23.

Kohn M (1996) *The Race Gallery: the return of racial science*. London, Cape.

† Kuhn TS (1996) *The Structure of Scientific Revolutions*, 3rd edn. Chicago, Il.: The University of Chicago Press.

‡ Kuper L (ed.) (1975) *Race, Science and Society*. London: Allen and Unwin.

§ La Veist TA (1994) Beyond dummy variables and sample selection: what health services researchers ought to know about race as a variable. *Health Services Research*, 29: 1–16.

† Lynn R, Rushton P, Jenson A, Murray C, Brand C, Nyborg H et al. (2006) Racial IQ research. *Sunday Times* 2 April (letters).

Matheson LM, Henderson JB, Hole D, Dunnigan MG (1988) Changes in the incidence of acute appendicitis in Glasgow Asian and white children between 1971 and 1985. *J Epidemiol Community Health* 42: 290–3.

† Modood T, Berthoud R, Lakey J, Nazroo J, Smith P, Virdee S, Beishon S (1997) *Ethnic Minorities in Britain: diversity and disadvantage*. London: PSI Publications.

‡ Muntaner C, Nieto J, O'Campo P (1996) The bell curve: on race, social class, and epidemiologic research. *Am J Epidemiol* 144: 531–6.

‡ Nazroo JY (1998) Genetic, cultural or socio-economic vulnerability? Explaining ethnic inequalities in health. *Sociology of Health & Illness*, 20: 710–730.

O'Donnell M (1991) *Race and Ethnicity*. New York: Longman.

‡ Oppenheimer GM (2001) Paradigm lost: race, ethnicity, and the search for a new population taxonomy. *Am J Public Health* 91: 1049–55.

Osborne, RT, Noble CE, Weyl N (1978) *Human Variation: the biopsychology of age, race and sex*. New York, Academic press.

Pearson M (1990) *Sociology of race and health*. In Cruikshank, JK & Beevers DG (eds.), Ethnic factors in health and disease.: 71–3. London.: Wright.

‡ Pfeffer N. Theories of race, ethnicity and culture. *BMJ* 1998; 317: 1381–1384.

Ramaiya KL, Swai ABM, McLarty DG, Bhopal RS, Alberti KGMM (1991) Prevalence of diabetes and cardiovascular risk factors in Hindu Indian sub-communities in Tanzania. *BMJ* 303: 271–6.

Rothschild H (ed.) (1981) *Biocultural Aspects of Disease*. London: Academic Press.

† Schoenbach VJ, Reynolds GH, Kumanyika SK (1994) Racial and ethnic distribution of faculty, students, and fellows in US epidemiology degree programs, 1992. Committee on Minority Affairs of the American College of Epidemiology. *Ann.Epidemiol* 4: 259–265.

§ Stronks K, Uniken Venema P, Dahhan N, Gunning-Schepers LJ (1999) Allochtoon, dus ongezond? Een conceptueel model ter verklaring van de samenhang tussen etnische herkomst en gezondheid. [Being an immigrant implies being unhealthy? A conceptual model integrating the mechanisms lying behind the association between ethnicity and health]. *T Soc Gezondheidsz* 77: 33–40.

Takwani NH (1996) The importance of mentioning ethnicity in the clinical presentation. *Journal of the American Medical Association* 275: 733.

Taylor AL, Ziesche S, Yancy C, Carson P, D'Agostino R Jr, Ferdinand K *et al.* (2004) Combination of isosorbide dinitrate and hydralazine in blacks with heart failure. *New England Journal of Medicine* 351: 2049–57.

Weissman JS, Betancourt J, Campbell EG, Park ER, Kim M, Clarridge B *et al.* (2005) Resident physicians' preparedness to provide cross-cultural care. *JAMA* 294: 1058–67.

§ Williams DR, Lavizzo-Mourey R, Warren RC (1994) The concept of race and health status in America. *Public Health Reports* 109: 26–41.

§ Williams DR (1997). Race and health: basic questions, emerging directions. *Ann. Epidemiol*, 7: 322–333.

† Woywodt A, Haubitz M, Haller H, Matteson EL (2006) Wegener's granulomatosis. *The Lancet*; 367: 1362–6.

Ethnicity and health web sites: a selection

All web site addresses were checked for access in April or May 2006.
With special thanks to by Mark Johnson of the UK-CEEHD at De Montfort University and University of Warwick Medical School, and the National Resource Centre for Ethnic Minority Health for sharing information.
Web site material that has been reworked, invariably in part, for the purposes of this book are marked with the symbol*
Web sites that have been cited in the text are marked with the symbol[†]
Web sites that are sources of quotations are marked with the symbol[#]

Organizations' web sites

[†]American College of Epidemiology
http://www.acepidemiology2.org/policystmts/SoPrinEndorse.asp

[†]ASH Scotland—Action on Smoking and Health
http://www.ashscotland.org.uk/ash/ash_display_home.jsp?p_applic=CCC&p_service=Content.show&pContentID=3752&

Center for Healthy Families and Cultural Diversity
http://www2.umdnj.edu/fmedweb/chfcd/INDEX.HTM

Centre for Asian and Migrant Health Research, New Zealand
http://www.aut-camhr.ac.nz

Centre for Asian Migrant Health Research (New Zealand)
http://www.aut.ac.nz/research/research_institutes/niphmhr/centre_for_asian_and_migrant_health_research/

Centre for Caribbean Health
http://www.kcl.ac.uk/depsta/ccm/index.html

Centre for Evidence in Ethnicity Health and Diversity
http://www.dmu.ac.uk/msrc

Centre for Evidence in Ethnicity, Health and Diversity—England
http://www2.warwick.ac.uk/fac/med/clinsci/research/ethnicityhealth/

Centre for Minority Health—USA
http://www.cmh.pitt.edu/home1.html

†Commission for Racial Equality-UK
http://www.cre.gov.uk/

†Daily Effects of White Privilege in a Racist Society by Peggy McIntosh
http://members.aol.com/tillery/effects.html

†Department of Health, England—Minority Ethnic Communities and Health,
   Publications
http://www.minorityhealth.gov.uk/publications.htm

DiversityRx (USA)
http://www.diversityRx.org

Equality Commission for Northern Ireland—Guide to Equality Impact Assessment based
   on legislation in Northern Ireland
http://www.equalityni.org

European Centre for the Study of Migration & Social Care (MASC)
http://www.kent.ac.uk

European Migration Centre
http://www.emz-berlin.de/start/animation.htm

Excellence Centres to Eliminate Ethnic/Racial Disparities (EXCEED)—USA
http://www.ahrq.gov/research/exceed.htm

Health Institute Clearinghouse Australia
http://www.dhi.gov.au/clearinghouse.

*Institute of Medicine-USA
http://www.iom.edu/CMS/18007.aspx

The International Epidemiological Association
http://www.dundee.ac.uk/iea/

*Lothian NHS Board Scotland—Publications
http://www.nhslothian.scot.nhs.uk/publications/ethnic_health/background_material.
html

Minority Health Project to eliminate health disparities—UNC-CH-USA
http://www.minority.unc.edu/reports/

National Centre for Languages Information
http://www.cilt.org.uk/

National Race and Health programme
http://www.raceforhealth.org

*National Resource Centre for Ethnic Minority Health
http://www.nrcemh.nhsscotland.com/

†Office of Minority Health (USA)
http://www.omhrc.gov

PAHO (Pan American Health Organization) Equity List:
http://www.paho.org/English/AD/GE/Ethnicity.htm

Research Centre for Transcultural Studies in Health
http://www.mdx.ac.uk/www/rctsh/homepage.htm

*Scottish Association of Black Researchers
http://www.sabreuk.org/

South Asian Health Foundation (U.K.)
http://www.sahf.org.uk/

South Asian Health Research Institute (SAHRI)
http://www.sahri.org

South Asian Public Health Association
http://www.sapha.net/

United States Department of Health and Human Services—Office of Civil Rights
http://www.hhs.gov/ocr/

WHO (World Health Organization)
http://www.who.int/en/

†WHO-HPH Taskforce on Migrant Friendly Hospitals
http://www.hph-hc.cc/projects.php#mfh

Journals specializing in ethnicity and health

Diversity in Health and Social Care
http://www.radcliffe-oxford.com/journals/J18_Diversity_in_Health_and_Social_
Care/

Ethnicity and Disease Journal
http://www.ishib.org/ED_index.asp

Ethnicity and Health
http://www.tandf.co.uk/journals/carfax/13557858.html

Journal of Immigrant and Minority Health
http://www.springer.com/uk/home/generic/search/results?SGWID=3-40109-70-
35544009-0

Journal of Transcultural Nursing
http://www.tcn.sagepub.com/

Transcultural Psychiatry
http://www.tps.sagepub.com/

Reports and general information on specific topics

American Anthropological Association, Response to OMB Directive 15: Race and Ethnic Standards for Federal Statistics and Administrative Reporting. Available at http://www.aaanet.org/gvt/ombdraft.htm

Adolf Hitler—from Wikipedia, the free encyclopedia
http://www.en.wikipedia.org/wiki/Adolf_Hitler

*Aryan Nations—Membership Application
http://www.aryan-nations.org/application.htm

Australian Government Department of Health and Ageing Publications—Aborigenes
http://www.health.gov.au/internet/wcms/publishing.nsf/Content/health-oatsih-pubs-index.htm

*Commission for Racial Equality—The Race Equality Duty
http://www.cre.gov.uk/duty/reia/how.html

Council on Ethical and Judicial Affairs: Reports on Managed Care
http://www.search.ama-assn.org/Search/query.html?qp=&TR=amasection%3A%22
Ethics%22&TD=Ethics&qc=public+amnews+pubs&qt=Race

CSDI—The International Workshop on comparative Survey Design and Implementation
http://www.gesis.org/en/research/eccs/csdi/

CultureMed—Health Materials in Languages other than English
http://www.culturedmed.sunyit.edu/foreign/index.html

Deadly Medicine. Creating the Master Race
http://www.ushmm.org/museum/exhibit/online/deadlymedicine/overview/index.php?
content=overview_300k

*‡Department of Health, Ten Point Plan of the Chief Executive, Nigel Crisp
http://www.dh.gov.uk/PublicationsAndStatistics/Bulletins/BulletinArticle/fs/en?
CONTENT_ID=4072494&chk=1e/oI7&qid=Leadership+and+Race+Equality+&coll=10
&Z=1

Emergency Multilingual Phrasebook—Department of Health, England.
http://www.dh.gov.uk/PublicationsAndStatistics/Publications/PublicationsPolicyAnd
Guidance/PublicationsPolicyAndGuidanceArticle/fs/en?CONTENT_ID=4073230&chk=
8XboAN

†Ethnic Monitoring in the NHS and Social Care. London, Department of Health.
http://www.dh.gov.uk/PublicationsAndStatistics/Publications/PublicationsPolicyAnd
Guidance/PublicationsPolicyAndGuidanceArticle/fs/en? CONTENT_ID=4116839& chk
=xfG3pr

#Ethnic Monitoring Toolkit. ISD Scotland, 2005
http://www.isdscotland.org/isd/collect2.jsp?pContentID=3393&p_applic=CCC&p_
service=Content.show

FDA Issues Guidance on Race and Ethnicity Data
http://www.fda.gov/fdac/features/2003/303_race.html

Forty Years of Law Against Racial Discrimination: An online exhibition from the CRE
http://www.cre.gov.uk/40years

*Heathcare Needs Assessment—Black And Minority Ethnic Groups
http://www.hcna.radcliffe-oxford.com/bemgframe.htm

†Health Survey for England—The Health of Minority Ethnic Groups '99
http://www.archive.official-documents.co.uk/document/doh/survey99/hse99-00.htm

*Mein Kampf by Adolf Hitler
http://www.hitler.org/writings/Mein_Kampf/index.html

My Pil Resources in multilingual format
http://www.mypil.com/level2/contents.htm

National Healthcare Disparities Report, 2005
http://www.ahrq.gov/qual/nhdr05/nhdr05.htm

#Neurodiversity.com History of Scientific Racism
http://www.neurodiversity.com/racism.html

New Zealand—Ruth DeSouza's home page
http://www.wairua.com/ruth/

†NIII Program of Action—USA
http://www./ncmhd.nih.gov/

Office of Management and Budget—Data on Race and Ethnicity
http://www.whitehouse.gov/omb/inforeg/backgrd_docs2.html

†Race/Ethnicity and Medicine: An Online Resource on BiDil—Archive
http://www.nottingham.ac.uk/igbis/reg/bidil.htm

Race, Racism and the Law
http://www.academic.udayton.edu/race/

†Race Relations legislation—UK
http://www.communities.homeoffice.gov.uk/raceandfaith/

Racial Privacy Initiative—USA
http://www.adversity.net/RPI/rpi_mainframe.htm

Report of World Conference against Racism
http://www.un.org/WCAR

*Right to Equal Treatment
http://www.phrusa.org/research/domestic/race/race_report/bibliography.html

*Royal College of Nursing (Online Course For Cultural Competence)—UK
http://www.rcn.org.uk:8080/query.html?qt=on-Line+course+for+cultural+competence
&x=2&y=8

*Scottish Executive Health Department, Fair for All: Working Together Towards Cultur-
ally Competent Services, NHS HDL (2002) 51, Edinburgh, Scottish Executive.
http://www.phis.org.uk/pdf.pl?file=pdf/FAIR%20FOR%20ALL%20-
%20SEHD%20DOCUMENT%20(June%202002)1.pdf

†Scottish Executive's response to the Race Equality Advisory Forum's Recommendations
http://www.scotland.gov.uk/library5/equality/reaf-21.asp

†Stephen Lawrence Inquiry
http://www.archive.official-documents.co.uk/document/cm42/4262/sli-47.htm

†Transcultural Health Care Practice: An educational resource for nurses and health care
practitioners
http://www.rcn.org.uk/resources/transcultural/index.php

Tuskegee Timeline
http://www.cdc.gov/nchstp/od/tuskegee/time.htm

Networks

British Sociological Association race and ethnicity group
http://www.britsoc.co.uk/specialisms/RaceandEthnicitySG

Minority Health e-network
http://www.minority-ethnic-health@jiscmail.ac.uk

Muslim Health Network
http://www.muslimhealthnetwork.org/

Statistics and census (these and other websites were used in chapter 2)

*Australian Bureau of Statistics ABS Census Dictionary
http://www.abs.gov.au/ausstats/abs@.nsf/web+pages/statistics?opendocument

*Brazil's Statistical Agency, IBGE, Demographic Census
http://www1.ibge.gov.br/english/

General Register Office for Scotland
http://www.gro-scotland.gov.uk/

National Centre for Health Statistics
http://www.cdc.gov/nchs/fastats/Default.htm

*National Statistics Online—Census 2001—Ethnicity and Religion in England and Wales
http://www.statistics.gov.uk/census2001/profiles/commentaries/ethnicity.asp

*Singapore Department of Statistics, Definitions
http://www.singstat.gov.sg/

*South Africa Statistics, Census in Brief, 1996
http://www.statssa.gov.za/

*Statistics Canada
http://www12.statcan.ca/english/census01/home/index.cfm

Statistical Resources on the Web—Health
http://www.lib.umich.edu/govdocs/sthealth.html

United Nations Statistics Division, Population and housing census dates
http://www.un.org/depts/unsd/demog/cendate/index.html

*US Census Bureau, Racial and Ethnic Classifications Used in Census 2000 and Beyond
http://www.census.gov/population/www/socdemo/race/racefactcb.html

Index

Note: page numbers in bold denote diagrams, tables and boxes